DrExam Clinical Examination & OSCE Revision Guide

Clinical Examination,
Communication Skills
& History Taking

Editors:

Prof. B.H. Miranda
M.K. Sood
Prof. J. Kinnear
Prof. V. Ramakrishnan

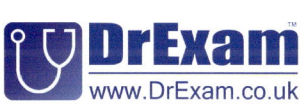
www.DrExam.co.uk

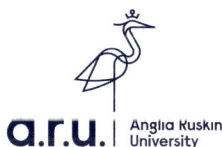
a.r.u. | Anglia Ruskin University

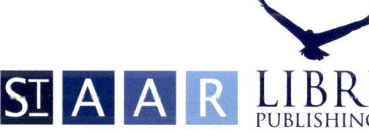
STAAR LIBRI PUBLISHING

First published in 2024 by Libri Publishing

ISBN 978-1-911450-88-7

A CIP catalogue record for this book is available from The British Library

Design by Carnegie Book Production

Printed in the UK by Halstan

Libri Publishing
Brunel House
Volunteer Way
Faringdon
Oxfordshire
SN7 7YR

Tel: +44 (0)845 873 3837

www.libripublishing.co.uk

CONTENTS

BH Miranda, MJ Portou, MC Winslet

SECTION C: HISTORY TAKING 413

Chapter 16:   **STRUCTURED HISTORY** 415

AD Ebinesan, BH Miranda

VIDEO MATERIAL

https://drexam-clinical.libripublishing.co.uk

ABOUT THE EDITORS

Professor Ben H Miranda

ALCM, BSc, MBBS (Lond), MRCS (Eng), FRCS (Plast), EBHS (FESSH), DipHandSurg (BSSH), PhD

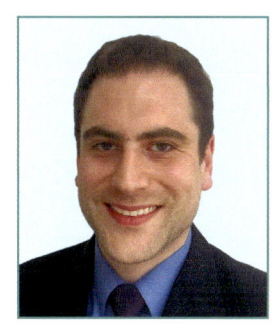

Professor Ben Miranda is a Consultant Plastic & Hand Surgeon at the internationally renowned St Andrew's Centre for Plastic Surgery & Burns (Chelmsford, UK), a Visiting Professor at Anglia Ruskin University and the head of the St Andrew's Anglia Ruskin (StAAR) Research Group; he is also a Tutor for the University of Manchester-British Society for Surgery of the Hand (BSSH) Diploma and an Honorary Senior Clinical Lecturer at the Anglia Ruskin University School of Medicine. He completed his Specialty Training in the London Deanery Plastic Surgery & Burns Training Rotation in 2018 and was previously a Research Registrar at the Plastic Surgery & Burns Research Unit, University of Bradford. His research interest in hair follicle biology and growth control led him to complete a PhD within three years.

Having graduated from the Royal Free & University College Hospital School of Medicine (London) in 2004, he has won over 20 academic prizes and awards, primarily at postgraduate level. He has over 130 published journal papers, features, books and international / national presentations, including a front cover publication in the British Journal of Dermatology on part of his PhD research. Professor Miranda has gained training exposure to a wide variety of medical and surgical sub-specialities, including A&E, Burns, Cardiovascular, ENT, Gastrointestinal, Nephrology, Neurosurgery, Plastic Surgery, Respiratory, Urology and Vascular Surgery.

Professor Miranda's passion for education developed since 1998, when he began teaching Mathematics to GCSE and A-Level students. He continued this throughout medical school, and in 2006 was drafted to teach Royal Free & University College Hospital School of Medicine MBBS finalists. In 2007 he helped to establish DrExam as a leading educational provider, in association with and in support of the Plastic Surgery & Burns Research Unit. His dedication to medical and surgical education, and the future progress of surgery, has been proven by his many extracurricular activities; these include integral participation in the well-publicised £200,000 fundraising appeal for the Research Unit's 25th anniversary in 2010.

Mr Manu K Sood

MS, MCh (Plast), FRCS (Plast)

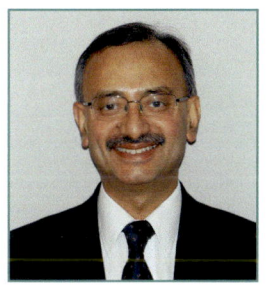

Mr Manu Sood is a Consultant Plastic & Hand Surgeon at St Andrews Centre for Plastic Surgery and Burns (Chelmsford, UK). He is currently the Medical Director for Plastic Surgery and Dermatology for the Mid and South Essex NHS Foundation Trust, is a member of the British Association for Plastic, Reconstructive and Aesthetic Surgeons (BAPRAS) and the British Society for Surgery of the Hand (BSSH); he has also previously been a member of the BSSH Council.

Mr Sood's primary interest is Hand Surgery; in particular, his subspecialty interests include small joint arthroplasty in the hand, management of nerve palsy, management of the spastic upper limb and management of children's hand conditions. He has published on Hand Surgery in peer reviewed journals. He has been an Examiner for the BSSH Diploma in Hand Surgery for ten years and was on the Committee of Examination for the BSSH Diploma in Hand surgery for five years.

Mr Sood has been actively involved in teaching and training Hand Surgery to all levels ranging from undergraduate students to experienced Consultant surgeons. He has taught regularly on international and national courses such as the BSSH Hand Course, Manchester and the Advanced Course of Hand Surgery at the Royal College of Surgeons of England.

Professor John Kinnear

MBBCh MSc(MedEd) MBA DCH(SA) DObst(SA) DA(SA) DA(UK) FRCA FFICM FAcadMEd FHEA

Professor John Kinnear is the founding Head of the Anglia Ruskin School of Medicine, as well as an Honorary Consultant in Critical Care Medicine at Mid & South Essex NHS Foundation Trust. He graduated from the University of Witwatersrand in Johannesburg in 1985 and trained in Paediatrics, Obstetrics & Gynaecology before completing training as a Specialist Anaesthetist at the Barts & London School of Anaesthetics.

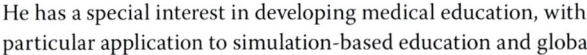

He has a special interest in developing medical education, with particular application to simulation-based education and global healthcare improvement. He co-designed and was the founding director of the high-fidelity simulation centre for the Postgraduate Medical Institute at Anglia Ruskin University and founded the Zambia MMed Anaesthesia programme based in Lusaka, which he designed specifically to address the high surgical mortality associated with anaesthesia in resource-challenged environments. He also founded the Global Anaesthesia Development Partnerships charity to support projects in low-income countries.

Professor Kinnear's research interests include global healthcare education, simulation-based education and the impact of human factors on clinical decision-making in acute medicine.

Professor Venkat Ramakrishnan

MS, FRCS, FRACS (Plastic Surgery)

Professor Venkat Ramakrishnan is a Consultant Plastic Surgeon at St Andrew's Centre for Plastic Surgery and Burns (Chelmsford, UK). His main area of work is microsurgical reconstruction of the breast and aesthetic surgery of the breast. His secondary interests are microsurgical reconstruction of the chest wall, abdomen, and lower limb.

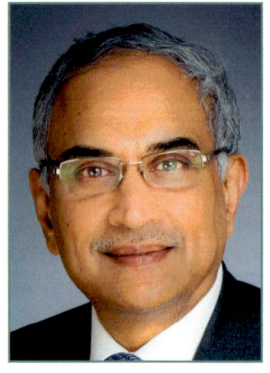

He has a major role as a trainer in microsurgery and was the inaugural Tutor in plastic surgery at the Royal College of Surgeons of England, London. He was the Director of the St Andrew's Centre and has held roles in the British Association of Plastic Reconstructive & Aesthetic Surgeons (BAPRAS) Council and the project board of the National Mastectomy & Reconstruction audit. He is a member of the Editorial Board of the Journal of Plastic, Reconstructive and Aesthetic Surgery (JPRAS) and Archives of Plastic Surgery (APS), and is Chairman of the Microsurgery Sub-Committee of the British Association of Plastic, Reconstructive and Aesthetic Surgeons (BAPRAS). He is a fellow of the Royal College of Surgeons of England and the Royal Australasian College of Surgeons.

Professor Ramakrishnan has over 100 publications in peer reviewed journals. He has given numerous presentations and keynote addresses at international meetings, including the *Susruta* Oration at the Association of Plastic Surgeons of India and the *Gillies* oration at the British Association of Plastic Surgeons. His main areas of research and audit work are in microsurgical techniques, service delivery and microcirculation in free flaps. He is a visiting Professor at the Anglia Ruskin University.

AUTHORS & CONTRIBUTORS

Mr Sharif Kaf Al-Ghazal MS, MD, FRCS
Consultant Plastic Surgeon
Bradford Teaching Hospitals
Honorary Senior Lecturer
School of Medicine, University of Leeds

Dr John Annaradnam MB BS, MRCGP
General Practitioner
The Southgate Surgery, London

Mr Kamil Asaad BSc MBChB MPhil FRCS (Plast)
Consultant Plastic Surgeon
Oxford University Hospitals NHS Foundation Trust

Mr Omer Baldo MBBS, MRCS, FRCS, FRCS (Urol)
Consultant Urologist
Airedale NHS Foundation Trust

Dr Heike I Bauer
Consultant Dermatologist
Bradford Teaching Hospitals NHS Foundation Trust

Carly Betton MA, BA (Hons), MIMI, RMIP
Senior Clinical Photographer
University Hospitals Birmingham NHS Foundation
Trust

Mr Waseem Bhat MuDr, MA, MRCS
Consultant Plastic Surgeon
Leeds Teaching Hospitals NHS Trust

Wendy Birch BSc (Hons), MSc, MBIE, LIAS
Anatomist & Dissection Room Manager
Research Department of Cell and Developmental
Biology
University College London Medical School

Mr Quamar MK Bismil MB ChB (Hons), MRCS, Dip
SEM, MFSEM, FRCS (Tr & Orth)
Consultant Orthopaedic Surgeon
London

Professor Peter EM Butler MD, FRCSI, FRCS, FRCS
(Plast)
Professor of Plastic Surgery & Honorary Senior
Lecturer
Royal Free & University College Hospitals London

Laurence Clarke MBIE, LIAS, FAAPT
Senior Anatomy Technician
Research Department of Cell and Developmental
Biology
University College London Medical School

Paul Creasey BSc MIMI, RMIP
Senior Clinical Photographer
Bradford Teaching Hospitals NHS Trust

Ms Prita Daliya
MBChB, MRCS, PGDip Hons (MedEd), PhD
Specialty Registrar in General Surgery
East Midlands Deanery
King's Mill Hospital, Sherwood Forest Hospitals NHS
Foundation Trust

Antony Dook BSc, MIMI, RMIP
Chief Clinical Photographer
Bradford Teaching Hospitals NHS Trust

Dr Nicola Downer
MBChB, FRCP, MMedSci (MedEd)
Consultant in Respiratory Medicine
King's Mill Hospital, Sherwood Forest Hospitals NHS
Foundation Trust

Mr AD Ebinesan MB ChB, MRCS (Eng), FRCS (Tr
& Orth)
Consultant in Trauma & Orthopaedics
Manchester University Hospitals NHS Foundation
Trust

Dr Marc Epstein BSc, MBBS, MRCGP, MRCP
General Practitioner
The Humbleyard Practice, Norwich

Ms Edwina Ewart BSc (Hons), MBChB, MRCS (Ed)
MD Research Registrar
Northern Lincolnshire & Goole Hospitals NHS Trust

Carol Fleming BSc, FIMI, RMIP
Principal Clinical Photographer & Medical
Illustration Manager
Bradford Teaching Hospitals NHS Foundation Trust

Mr Ivan Foo FRCS Eng (Plast), FRCS Ed
Consultant Plastic & Reconstructive Surgeon
Bradford Teaching Hospitals NHS Foundation Trust

Miss Sheila Fraser MB ChB, MRCS, FRCS
Consultant Endocrine Surgeon
Leeds Teaching Hospitals NHS Trust

Dr Brian Geffin MB BCh, MRCGP
General Practitioner
The Southgate Surgery, London

Dr Brijanand Sharma Ghoorun MD, FRCA
Consultant ITU & Trauma Anaesthetist
Huddersfield Royal Infirmary

Katherine Grice BA, MIMI, RMIP
Senior Clinical Photographer
Bradford Teaching Hospitals NHS Trust

Dr Ayshea Hameeduddin MBBS, BA (Hons) Med
Journalism, FRCR
Consultant Radiologist
Barts Health NHS Trust, London

Dr Brian Holloway MRCS, FRCR
Consultant Radiologist
Royal Free Hospital, London

Mr Jonathan A Joseph BSc (Hons), MBBS, DOHNS,
FRCS (ORL-HNS)
Consultant ENT Surgeon
Royal National Throat, Nose & Ear Hospital, London

Mr Vishal Kakar BSc, MBBS (Lond), MRCS (Eng)
Specialty Registrar Neurosurgery
Northern Ireland Deanery

Mr Senthil Kamalasekaran MB ChB, MS (Orth),
MRCS
Consultant in Trauma & Orthopaedics
Apollo Hospital, Chennai, India

Professor Simon P Kay FRCS, FRCS (Plast), FRCS
Ed (Hon)
Professor of Plastic & Reconstructive Surgery &
Surgery of the Hand
Leeds Teaching Hospitals NHS Trust

Mr Malcolm Keene MBBS, FRCS
Consultant ENT Surgeon
Barts and the London NHS Trust

Professor John Kinnear MBBCh, MSc (MedEd),
MBA, DCH (SA), DObst (SA), DA (SA), DA (UK),
FRCA, FFICM, FAcadMEd, FHEA
Founding Head of School, School of Medicine,

Anglia Ruskin University, Chelmsford, UK.
Honorary Consultant in Critical Care Medicine, Mid
& South Essex NHS Foundation Trust, Southend
University Hospital, UK

Mr R Linforth MD, FRCS Ed, FRCS (Gen Surg)
Consultant Breast & Oncoplastic Surgeon
Bradford Teaching Hospitals NHS Foundation Trust

Dr KM London
Consultant Dermatologist
Bradford Teaching Hospitals NHS Foundation Trust

Ms Joanna Lorains BSc, MB ChB, MRCS
Specialty Registrar General Surgery
North Western Deanery

Dr Anmol Malhotra BSc (Hons), MRCP, FRCR
Consultant Radiologist
Royal Free Hospital, London

Dr Katherine Lindsay
BMedSci, BMBS, MRCP, MRCGP
Specialty Registrar in Haematology
Mersey Deanery

Dr Christopher Lutterodt
MBBS, BSc (Hons), MRCS
Specialty Registrar in General Practice
Surrey

Mr JC May MB, BCh, FRCS Ed (Gen)
Consultant General Surgeon
Bradford Teaching Hospitals NHS Foundation Trust

Laura McMurray BSc, PGCMCH, PGCCBT,
PGDipCBT
Psychological Therapist
Camden & Isllington NHS Foundation Trust, London

Dr Emily McDonald
BMedSci, BMBS, FRCP, MMedSci (MedEd), MRCP
Consultant in Acute Medicine
Royal Derby Hospital, Derby Teaching Hospitals
NHS Foundation Trust

Adela Miranda
Hand Trauma Coordinator & Registered Nurse
Chelsea & Westminster Hospital, London

Professor Benjamin H Miranda ALCM, BSc,
MBBS, (Lond), MRCS (Eng), FRCS (Plast), EBHS
(FESSH), DipHandSurg, (BSSH), PhD.
Consultant Plastic & Hand Surgeon, St Andrew's
Centre for Plastic Surgery & Burns, Mid & South
Essex NHS Foundation Trust, Broomfield Hospital,
Chelmsford, UK.

Visiting Professor, Anglia Ruskin University, UK.
St Andrew's Anglia Ruskin (StAAR) Research Group Lead.
Honorary Visiting Senior Clinical Lecturer, School of Medicine, Anglia Ruskin University, UK.

Mr Jabir Nagaria MBBS, FRCS (Surgical Neurology)
Consultant Neurosurgeon
Royal Victoria Hospital
Belfast

Mr Marios Nicolaou BMedSci, BMBS, MRCS, FRCS (Plast), EBOPRAS, PhD
Consultant Plastic Surgeon
Salisbury NHS Foundation Trust

Dr Selva Nithiyananthan MB BS, MRCP, DipMedRehab, MRCGP
General Practitioner
The Southgate Surgery, London

Dr Stephen Oakey MBBS, FRCA
Consultant in Anaesthesia & Burns Critical Care
St Andrew's Centre for Plastic Surgery & Burns
Broomfield Hospital, Chelmsford

Mr Kanak K Patel FDS, RCPS, FRCS (OMFS)
Consultant Oral & Maxillofacial Surgeon
Bradford Teaching Hospitals NHS Foundation Trust

Mr Mark James Portou MB ChB (Hons), MRCS
Consultant General Surgeon
Royal Free London NHS Foundation Trust, London

Mr N Rhodes FFDRCS, FRCS (Plast)
Consultant Plastic & Reconstructive Surgeon
Bradford Teaching Hospitals NHS Foundation Trust

Professor Venkat Ramakrishnan MS, FRCS, FRACS (Plastic Surgery)
Consultant Plastic & Reconstructive Surgeon
St Andrew's Centre for Plastic Surgery & Burns, Mid & South Essex NHS Foundation Trust, Broomfield Hospital, Chelmsford, UK

Mr J Saksena BMSc (Hons), MB ChB, MRCS, FRCS (Tr&Orth)
Consultant Orthopaedic & Trauma Surgeon
The Whittington Hospital London

Professor DJA Scott MD, MB ChB, FRCS, FEBVS
Professor of Vascular Surgery
Division of Cardiovascular and Diabetes Research
Leeds Institute of Genetics, Health and Therapeutics

Professor David T Sharpe OBE, MA, Bchir, FRCS
Professor of Plastic & Reconstructive Surgery
Plastic Surgery & Burns Research Unit Director
University of Bradford

Mr Masha Singh MBBS, BSc, MRCS
Consultant Plastic & Reconstructive Surgeon
St George's University Hospitals NHS Foundation Trust

Mr Niroshan Sivathasan BSc, MBBS, MRCS, DU, AFACP, FCPCA, FFMACCS, FACCS, FASCBS
Consultant Plastic & Cosmetic Surgeon
Ignite Medispa, Australia

Sarah Slade BA (Hons), MIMI, RMIP
Clinical Photographer
Bradford Teaching Hospitals NHS Trust

Mr Mark S Soldin MB ChB, FCS (SA), FRCS (Plast)
Consultant Plastic & Reconstructive Surgeon
St George's Healthcare NHS Trust London

Mr Manu K Sood MS, MCh (Plast), FRCS (Plast)
Consultant Plastic & Hand Surgeon
St Andrew's Centre for Plastic Surgery & Burns, Mid & South Essex NHS Foundation Trust, Broomfield Hospital, Chelmsford, UK

Mr M A Steward FRCS (Ed)
Consultant Colorectal & General Surgeon
Bradford Teaching Hospitals NHS Foundation Trust

Mr D N Sutton BDS, FRCDS (Ed), FRCS (Ed), FRCS (Eng)
Consultant Oral & Maxillofacial Surgeon
Bradford Teaching Hospitals NHS Foundation Trust

Mr Michael J Timmons MA, MChir, FRCS
Consultant Plastic & Reconstructive Surgeon
Bradford Teaching Hospitals NHS Foundation Trust

Professor Desmond J Tobin PhD, FRCPath, FIBiol
Professor of Cell Biology
Director of the Charles Institute for Investigative Dermatology, University College Dublin
Honorary Visiting Professor, University of Bradford

Mr David A L Watt MB ChB, FRCS (Plast)
Consultant Plastic & Reconstructive Surgeon
Bradford Teaching Hospitals NHS Foundation Trust

Professor Marc C Winslet MS, FRCS (Ed), FRCS
(Eng), MEWI
Professor of Surgery, Head of Department
Chairman of Division of Surgery & Interventional
Science
School of Medicine
Faculty of Biomedical Science
University College London

Dr A L Wright BMedSci (Hons), LRCP, MRCS, MB
ChB, FRCP
Consultant Dermatologist & Lead Clinician
Bradford Teaching Hospitals NHS Foundation Trust

'The Anatomy Dissection Team'
**Rachel Eyre, Rebecca Gayner, Emma
Williams, James Davis, Lucy Collison, David
Reynolds, Alexander Morton, Gopigia Thana-
Balasundaram, Timothy Chan, Oliver White,
Zoya Georgieva, James Lewis, Brett Packham,
Kevin Cao, Radoslaw Rippel, Donald Leith**

ACKNOWLEDGEMENTS

'Putting this Clinical Examination & OSCE revision guide
together has been one of the most challenging & rewarding
experiences to date.

It could not have been achieved without the help of teachers past & present,
co-contributors – Professors, Consultants, other professional colleagues
& the DrExam students...

... BUT...

In particular I would like to thank the following people in no particular order:
Gladys, David, Adela, Zac & Amelie Miranda.

I thank you & will never forget your unconditional love & support.'

Ben

PREFACE

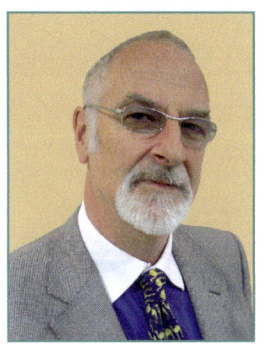

The DrExam Clinical Examination & OSCE revision guide adopts an innovative approach which addresses the needs of candidates for their upcoming exams; the authors have tackled subjects that are common, complicated or important. This was only achievable through the collaborative efforts of over 80 Professors, Consultants & Specialists from across the United Kingdom & worldwide.

DrExam has several decades of experience in teaching candidates on revision courses that have evolved & adapted to the changes in their exams. The highly successful courses (www.DrExam. co.uk) have become internationally attended & this book series has developed following glowing reviews by the Royal College of Surgeons & British Journal of Surgery regarding the contained material, high candidate success rates & positive feedback about the teaching quality, knowledge imparted & detailed academic content provided.

What differentiates this book from others is that it is targeted specifically to all Medical Professionals, Undergraduate Students & Allied Healthcare Professionals who want to learn how to perform & are being assessed on their Clinical Examination Skills & OSCEs. The material in this book is presented in structured question-answer format throughout & covers the most common & complicated clinical OSCE topics encountered by examination candidates. The material is illustrated by fantastic high-resolution colour images that were contributed by anatomists, radiologists, clinical photographers & medical illustrators. Each chapter, or sections within a chapter, has been written or verified by specialists within the field.

Topics covered in detail within this book include: Clinical Examination Protocols, Lumps 'n' Bumps, Head & Neck, Cardiology, Respiratory, Breast, Abdomen, Herniae & Scrotum, Stoma, GALS & Rheumatology, Orthopaedics, Hands, Vascular, Neurosciences, Upper Limb Nerves, Communication Skills, Ethics & History Taking. In addition, clinical examination is taught not only with written words & pictures, but also with video material available containing all major examination routines. This allows the candidate to pick up 'nuances' of clinical examination that are not readily communicated through still images alone.

The Bradford Burns & Plastic Surgery Research Unit evolved following the Bradford City Football Club stadium fire disaster in 1985. DrExam continues to be an active supporter of the skin sciences research undertaken by this unit & the future patient care that it will improve. Ben Miranda was a Research Registrar at the Unit, was involved in the 25th Anniversary fund raising appeal where over £200,000 was raised in support of it, & it is rewarding to see his continuing contribution to Plastic Surgery & Hand Surgery.

The DrExam series is the most colourful, complete & structured Clinical Examination OSCE revision guide to be released on the market to date & I thank all those who were involved in making this project a success. It will not only be of great value to any OSCE candidate, but also to training Doctors, Surgeons, General Practitioners, Physiotherapists, Occupational Therapists, Nurses, Medical Practitioners & Students who are required to revise these vital core subjects.

Professor David T Sharpe OBE

This book is dedicated to the memory of the 56 who died, 270 who were injured & thousands more who were affected by the Bradford City Football Club stadium fire disaster on 11th May 1985.

INTRODUCTION
(IMPORTANT – READ ME!)

B H Miranda
M K Sood
J Kinnear
V Ramakrishnan

CONTENTS

How to Use this Book

What to wear!

Approaching the Clinical Examination Stations, Start & Finish!

- Start
- Clinical Examination
- Finish

Please read the following sections carefully, they provide the candidate with vital tips regarding the use of this book, accompanying video material, how to approach the OSCE & maintain good clinical practice in the future.

HOW TO USE THIS BOOK

- The primary objective of this book is to present **structured clinical examination routines that are reproducible in both the OSCE & in everyday clinical practice**. These routines represent a thorough framework, reviewed by Professors, Consultants & Specialists in their respective fields, which may be modified to accommodate normal variations in clinical practice. *These appear at the beginning of each chapter.*
- The **accompanying clinical examination tutorial video material** also covers these examination routines & should be used in conjunction with the routines in this book.
- An additional objective is to provide the candidate with **questions & structured / categorised answers relating to clinical topics that are commonly asked during this OSCE & in everyday clinical practice**. *These appear at the end of each chapter.*
- Candidates are advised to **learn & consistently practice these routines**, so that they may be reproduced almost involuntarily, in order to become competent clinicians! This may be achieved via use of books, attendance at courses & on the wards / in clinic.

WHAT TO WEAR!

Modern infection control practices have precipitated a review of dress code for the OSCE as follows:

- Arms bare below the elbow
- No jewellery on hands or wrists except wedding rings / bands
- No ties or dangling clothing.

Female candidates may wish to present themselves as follows:

- Smart haircut with tied-back hair (if long)
- Smart blouse, sleeves rolled up to above the elbows
- Smart skirt / trousers
- Smart & comfortable shoes (not open)
- Minimal jewellery & makeup.

Male candidates may wish to present themselves as follows:

- Smart haircut
- Smart shirt, sleeves rolled up to above the elbows.
- No tie
- Smart trousers
- Smart & comfortable shoes
- No jewellery other than a wedding ring / band.

APPROACHING THE CLINICAL EXAMINATION STATIONS, START & FINISH!

It is important to conduct yourself throughout the OSCE stations, in a manner that is appropriate to real clinical settings. It is therefore important to establish a good rapport with your 'patient' & examiner by using effective communication strategies *(see communication skills chapter)*. Remember to be calm, clear & calculative when talking to both the examiner & patient. Never 'bleat' out an answer that hasn't been thought through systematically. It doesn't hurt to smile & be friendly either!

Passing the clinical examination stations requires a systematic approach that appears almost involuntary. Examiners are unlikely to interrupt or prompt the candidate, so it is vital to display an award-winning performance. The best way for the candidate to ensure that they perform successfully during clinical examination stations, is to practise, practise & practise beforehand! This will ensure that the candidate develops a structured & systematic approach that is easily identifiable to the examiner.

A structured & systematic clinical examination performance may be thought of in 3 stages:

1. **START**

2. **CLINICAL EXAMINATION**

3. **FINISH**

Memory:	**START:**	**FINISH:**
	I Want PC PEG	*To Happily Wave at Safe Drivers*
	Introduction	**Th**ank Patient
	Wash Hands	**H**elp Patient Dress
	Permission	**W**ash Hands
	Chaperone	**S**ummary
	Position	**D**ifferential Diagnosis
	Exposure	
	General Inspection	

It is also useful to have a standard introduction strategy for the start & finish of the clinical examination stations.

START

Introduction, Wash Hands & Permission:

It is important to have a standard introduction strategy that is easily recallable under the influence of OSCE nerves! This should also include obtaining consent for the examination & hand washing. It is important to remember to wash your hands before & after each case. Here is an example opening statement:

> *'Hello, my name is Dr X. I am one of the candidates for today's examination. Is it alright for me to examine your head / neck / chest / back / hip / legs etc?'*

You may be required to communicate your findings to the examiner as you go along. If so you can add:

> *'... & talk to the examiner as I go along?'*

You may have to adjust your introduction according to the scenario as follows:

> **Scenario: You are the doctor on call & have been asked to see Mrs Deyton who has a blocked catheter. You are informed that she is in pain & you arrive at her bedside. Begin the consultation.**
>
> *'Hello Mrs Deyton, my name is Dr X. I am the doctor on call & I understand that you have a blocked catheter. Are you in any pain at all? ...'*

Chaperone:

All sensitive examination areas require a chaperone e.g. breast & scrotum. It is also important to maintain patient dignity via the use of a bed sheet. You should communicate to the examiner that you are considering these points, by interacting with the patient:

> *'I will need a chaperone in order to examine your breasts. Is this alright?'*
>
> *'Yes doctor!'*
>
> *'Thank you, we will get some sheets to keep you covered up.'*

Position & Exposure:

Remember that each clinical examination routine requires careful consideration of the relevant position & exposure of the patient. These will be discussed at the relevant START sections of the structured routines throughout this book.

General Inspection:

General inspection precedes every clinical examination routine. Stand a step away from the foot of the bed, in line with the patient's midline. If the patient is sitting in a chair & it is appropriate, stand opposite the patient. In this position, with your **hands behind your back**, comment on:

1. **The general health of the patient:**

   'Standing at the end of the bed, the patient looks comfortable at rest...'

2. **Peripheral markers of disease:**

   '... & there are no peripheral markers of disease.'

Comment on peripheral markers of disease by looking purposefully around the patient & bedside. Peripheral markers of disease may be classified as follows:

Classification	Examples
General Surgical	Cannula, Catheter, Drain & Fluid Line
Breast	Prosthesis & Support Bra
Cardiovascular	Cardiac Monitor, Cigarettes & ECG Leads
Gastrointestinal	Commode, Kidney Dish & Stoma Bag
Neurological	Hearing Aid & Walking Stick
Orthopaedic	Crutches, Plaster Cast, Prosthesis & Walking Stick
Respiratory	Cigarettes, Inhaler, Peak Flow Meter & Pulse Oximeter Probe
Vascular	Cigarettes, Compression Bandage & Prosthesis

CLINICAL EXAMINATION

Move to the relevant examination position that is specific to each examination routine. These will be discussed in the relevant START sections of the structured routines throughout this book. **Remember to conduct all examinations, which require the patient to be on an examination couch, standing to the right side of the patient.**

FINISH

Thank Patient & Wash Hands:

Thank the patient for their time & wash your hands. **It is important to remember to wash your hands before & after each case.**

Summary & Differential Diagnosis:

Summarise the relevant positive & negative findings from your clinical examination of the patient. Your findings should be reported in a similar order & format to your clinical examination routine i.e. inspection, palpation, percussion & auscultation. Offer a differential diagnosis that is classified, in a similar manner to those that are presented throughout this book.

SECTION A:
CLINICAL EXAMINATION STRUCTURED ROUTINES & OSCE QUESTIONS

SECTION A1:
LUMPS 'N' BUMPS, HEAD & NECK

CHAPTER 1
LUMPS 'N' BUMPS

BH Miranda
MS Soldin

CHAPTER CONTENTS

THE CRUCIAL LUMP EXAMINATION

The examination of a lump may be important in all surgical specialities:

Speciality	Examples
ENT	Head & Neck Cancer
General Surgery	Organomegaly
Orthopaedics	Bone Tumours
Plastic Surgery	Benign Lumps & Skin Cancer
Urology	Bladder & Penile Cancer
Vascular Surgery	Aneurysms & Varicose Veins

For this reason in the OSCE, it is vital for the candidate to demonstrate an examination protocol that covers all the important clinical features of the lump. The protocol presented in this chapter is universal, so it is important to remember that some parts may not be relevant to all lumps e.g. do not auscultate a lump in the neck for bowel sounds!

LUMPS 'N' BUMPS EXAMINATION

START: Ensure adequate exposure of the lump & surrounding region:

          Memory: The 6 x S's of inspection.

INSPECTION	Interpretation
Site	Anatomical location e.g. dorsum of the right hand or anterior triangle of the neck.
Size	Approximate size of base e.g. 3cm x 2cm.
Shape	Approximate shape of base & indicate dimensions e.g. hemispherical & protuberant.
Symmetry	Remember that lumps may be asymmetrical e.g. melanoma, symmetrical about the midline e.g. goitre or symmetrical about their own axis e.g. cyst.
Skin	Comment on the overlying & surrounding skin e.g. erythematous, punctum visible or ulcerated.
Scars	Comment on the presence of scars that may be indicative of previous surgery.

Ask about pain.

Feel for temperature changes with the back of your hand.

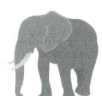   Memory: 'SEC FFP TR' or Sister Entered Clinic, Frowning at Frightened
                              Peter's Terrible Result

PALPATION	Interpretation
Surface	Rough or smooth.
Edge	Irregular, infiltrative or well defined.
Consistency	Comment if the consistency is: • **Hard** (feels like the nasal bridge). • **Firm** (feels like the nasal tip). • **Soft** (feels like the nares).
Fixed	Comment if the lump is: • **Fixed to skin** (the skin will not move freely over the lump). • **Fixed to underlying tissue** (the lump will not move freely over underlying tissue). • **Fixed to the muscle surface** (the lump becomes more prominent with contraction of underlying muscle). • **Within muscle** (the lump will become less prominent with muscle contraction).
Fluctuant	**Paget's Sign:** Use the index & middle finger of 1 hand to stabilise the base of the lump. Press the middle of the lump with the index finger of the other hand. A lump is fluctuant if the edges press / spill over the tops of the stabilising fingers e.g. cyst. This should be done in 2 planes.
Pulsatile / Expansile	Use the index fingers of both hands, in parallel, to demonstrate. Place a finger on each edge of the lump. Pulsatile lumps will move your fingers up & down in a vertical plan e.g. lump overlying an artery or a well-vascularised tumour. Expansile lumps will move your fingers outward & inward in a radial plane e.g. aneurysm.
Transilluminable	Shine a torch into one side of the lump & look at the contralateral side. Fluid-filled lumps will glow brightly on the contralateral side e.g. cyst.
Reducible	Always ask a patient to reduce their lump first, then ask if you may reduce it e.g. hernia.

It may not be appropriate to percuss some lumps e.g. scrotal hernias.

PERCUSSION	Interpretation
Sternum	Fluid-filled lumps may have a fluid thrill or be stony dull to percussion.

It may not be appropriate to auscultate for bowel sounds or bruits in all lumps e.g. neck lumps where you would listen for bruits, not bowel sounds. Remember to auscultate for bowel sounds in all scrotal lumps that may be hernias containing bowel loops.

AUSCULTATION	Interpretation
Lump	Auscultate for bowel sounds or bruits.

COMPLETION	Interpretation
Lymphadenopathy	Check draining regional lymph nodes. Compare with contralateral side where possible. Watch for normal structures that may be mistaken for lymphadenopathy e.g. the greater horn of the hyoid bone, a prominent transverse arch of the atlas & the submandibular gland.
Neurovascular Status	Ensure no encroachment on nerves or vessels by performing a distal neurological & vascular examination.
General Examination	Lumps may be a cause or consequence of metastasis so it is important to perform an appropriate general examination e.g. breast lumps should prompt an abdominal, respiratory & spinal examination.
Cosmetic & Quality of Life	Establish if the patient is affected by the appearance of the lump & whether it affects their quality of life in any way.

FINISH:

ULCER EXAMINATION

Ulcers are clinically examined like all lumps, however it is important that the following features are also addressed when inspecting ulcers:

 Memory: Ulcers have BEDS

Ulcer Inspection	Interpretation	
Base	Granulation Tissue, Slough	
Edge	**Sloping:**	Traumatic & Venous Ulcers
	Punched:	Arterial Ulcers
	Undermined:	TB
	Rolled:	BCC
	Everted:	SCC & Marjolin's Ulcer
Discharge	Serous, Sanguinous, Serosanguinous, Purulent	
Structures Visible	Muscles, Vessels, Bone	

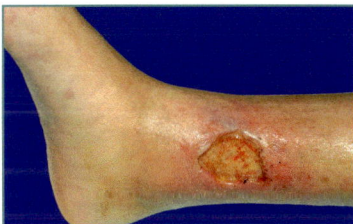

Fig 1.1: Venous ulceration of the gaiter area & medial malleolus of the right lower limb.

There is healthy granulation tissue at the ulcer base, with some slough. There is associated haemosiderin deposition & lipodermatosclerosis.

OSCE QUESTIONS

Q: What are the differential diagnoses for a lump?

The differentials for any lump are classified by location as follows:

Location	Examples		
Cutaneous	Benign:	Actinic Keratosis, Campbell de Morgan Spots, Dermatofibroma, Keratoacanthoma, Naevus, Seborrhoeic Keratosis	
	Malignant:	Epidermal:	BCC, SCC, Melanoma
		Dermal:	DFSP, Malignant Fibrous Histiocytoma
Subcutaneous	Cyst		
Fat	Lipoma		
Artery	Aneurysm		
Vein	Varicosity		
Nerve	Neuroma		
Lymph Node	Lymphadenopathy		
Muscle	Tumour		
Bone	Tumour, Malunited Fracture, Osteoma		
Anatomical Region	Ganglion (dorsum of hand), Liver (right hypochondrium), Hernias (groin) etc.		

Q: What is actinic keratosis?

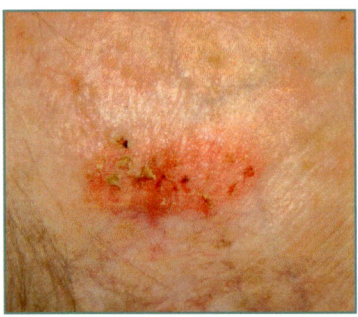

Fig 1.2: Actinic keratosis.

This is the most common pre-malignant lesion of the skin, caused by chronic sun damage. Actinic keratoses are common on the face & present as rough white patches stuck onto an erythematous base. Histology reveals thickening of the keratin (hyperkeratosis) & prickle cell (acanthosis) layers of the skin, increased cell mitoses & dysplasia; 10% may progress to SCC over 2 years.

Q: What treatment options are available for actinic keratosis?

Like all treatment options, they may be classified as conservative, medical & surgical:

Conservative	Medical	Surgical
Sun Protection	Diclofenac Sodium Gel (Solarase™)	Cautery
(prevention is the best treatment)	5- Fluorouracil Cream	Cryosurgery
	Cryotherapy	Laser
		Surgical Excision

Q: What are Campbell de Morgan spots?

These are cherry haemangiomas formed by a proliferation of dilated venules. They are more common with increasing age & are seen as small, bright red papules on the skin. Treatment is conservative, however cryotherapy, curettage & shave excision are also options.

Q: What is a dermatofibroma?

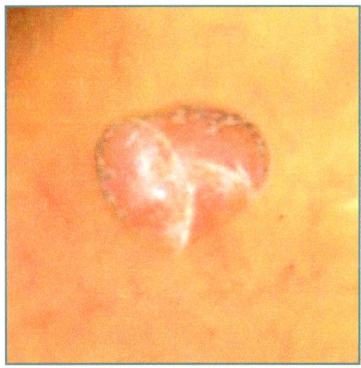

Fig 1.3: Dermatofibroma.

A benign neoplasm of dermal fibroblasts or 'histiocytoma'. A history of trauma is usually present e.g. insect bite. The lesion is a firm papule, usually 5–8 mm in size & roughly circular within the dermis. As rapid growth & pigmentation is possible, so is confusion with melanoma. The 'dimple sign' is characteristic for dermatofibromas, where lateral compression results in central dimpling inwards. Treatment is conservative, but if in doubt of the diagnosis, excision biopsy is preferable.

Q: What is a furuncle & carbuncle?

Furuncles & carbuncles may affect any hair-bearing skin e.g. face, axilla & groin. They may be tender to palpation but have distinct differences as follows:

Terminology	Explanation
Furuncle	Perifollicular bacterial infection by *Staphylococcus aureus*. This results in a small, pus-containing swelling or 'boil'. As pus accumulates there is enlargement & punctum development. When the punctum bursts, the furuncle discharges spontaneously.
Carbuncle	A carbuncle is a cluster of furuncles that merge to form a larger lesion. They are often located at the back of the neck & are more common in diabetic patients. If present, investigation of blood glucose should be undertaken. Treatment may initially be conservative, however antibiotics may help. Good diabetic control will help to prevent further lesions in these patients. Large resistant lesions should be treated by surgical incision & drainage.

Q: What is a keratoacanthoma?

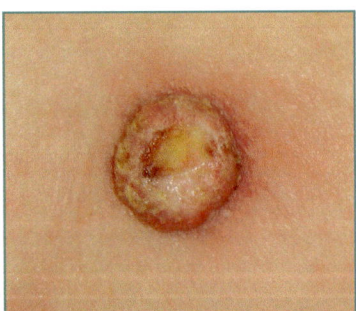

Fig 1.4: **Keratoacanthoma.**

A benign overgrowth of hair follicles, with a central keratin plug. Some consider this a type of self-limiting SCC. Keratoacanthomas may resemble some forms of BCC, SCC & melanoma, however spontaneously regress, leaving a depressed scar. Small biopsies will not be of diagnostic assistance, so an accurate history is important. They enlarge in weeks, remain static for 2–3 months & then resolve. The total cycle is 4–6 months.

Q: What are the treatment options for a keratoacanthoma?

Treatment	Examples
Conservative	**Monitoring** needs to be frequent due to the possibility of malignancy. This is very intense on outpatient clinics.
Surgical	**Treatment is usually by excision biopsy** as it is difficult to differentiate between a keratoacanthoma & SCC. This provides enough tissue for an accurate histological diagnosis.

Q: What is a naevus?

A benign proliferation of the normal constituent cells of the skin. Naevi may be classified as follows:

Classification	Example	Explanation
MELANOCYTIC	**Congenital**	Present at birth, often protuberant, hairy & pigmented (light brown-black). Often >1cm in diameter. There is a small risk of developing malignant melanoma (<5%).
	Junctional	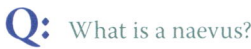 Fig 1.5: Junctional naevus. Flat, round / oval pigmented macules that are often multiple. Lesions vary in size (typically 2–10mm) & colour (light–dark brown).
	Intradermal	Dome-shaped, flesh-coloured papules. Often seen on the face / neck.
	Compound	Pigmented nodules that appear warty / hairy & have variable pigmentation. They are usually <1cm in diameter.
	Blue	Usually solitary & named due to blue colour.
	Becker's	Pigmented, hairy naevus, commonly on the back / shoulder.
	Dysplastic	Irregular shape & pigmentation, with a high risk of malignant change.
VASCULAR	**Port Wine Stain**	Irregular red / purple macule, often affecting 1 side of the face.
	Salmon Patch	The most common vascular naevus, affecting almost 50% of neonates. Patches on the face often disappear, however posterior neck patches (stork marks) often persist.
	Strawberry Naevus	Also known as a capillary haemangioma, this usually develops during the 1st few weeks of life, reaching maximum size by 1 year. It is recognisable as a fleshy, red naevus that may affect the skin anywhere. Most regress spontaneously by the age of 8 years, leaving an area of atrophy.
EPIDERMAL	**Warty Naevus**	These may be present at birth or may develop during childhood. They are linear, pigmented, warty lesions that may grow to several centimetres in length. Recurrence is common after surgical excision.
CONNECTIVE TISSUE	**Shagreen Patches**	Rare soft, yellow, connective tissue naevus, associated with tuberose sclerosis, often found in the lumbar / sacral region.

Q: What is seborrhoeic keratosis?

A benign overgrowth of the basal cell layer of the epidermis. The following 3 features apply:

1. **Hyperkeratosis:** Thickening of the keratin layer.
2. **Acanthosis:** Thickening of the prickle cell layer.
3. **Hyperplasia:** Increased division of variably pigmented basaloid cells.

Q: What are the clinical features of seborrhoeic keratosis & how would you treat it?

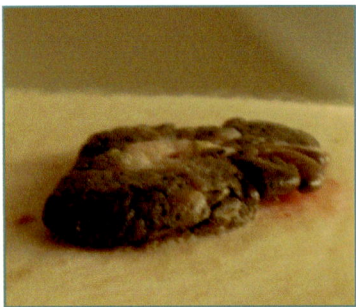

Fig 1.6: Seborrheoic keratosis.

Often seen on the face & trunk as variably pigmented lesions with a 'stuck on skin' warty appearance. They may be numerous & may scratch off easily & bleed. It is this & the pigmentation that causes concern, but they are benign. Patients may present with discomfort & irritation if they catch on clothing. Treatment is usually conservative & surgical treatment options include curettage, cryotherapy & cautery.

Q: What is a neurofibroma?

A benign hamartoma of peripheral nerve schwann cells. They may been seen as soft & fleshy pedunculated lesions of the skin. Altered sensation, pain & compressive symptoms may be present e.g. intra-abdominal neurofibromas may result in bowel obstruction & impingement on the spinal column may cause scoliosis or bone cysts. Treatment is usually conservative & surgical excision is possible.

Q: What is neurofibromatosis?

Neurofibromatosis represents 2 similar conditions, both inherited as autosomal dominant, classified into types I & II as follows:

Neurofibromatosis	Condition	Features
TYPE I	**Von Recklinghausen's Disease**	• ≥6 café-au-lait spots ≥0.5cm in diameter. • Multiple cutaneous neurofibromas that may be very large & can undergo sarcomatous change. • Increased risk of meningioma, acoustic neuroma & optic nerve glioma. • Kyphosis & tibial bowing may also occur.
TYPE II	**Bilateral Acoustic Neurofibromatosis**	These are more central than type I. Neurofibromas & café-au-lait spots are therefore not hallmark features, although may be present. Features include: • Bilateral acoustic neurofibromas. • Intracranial meningiomas. • Cranial nerve schwannomas.

Q: What is a papilloma?

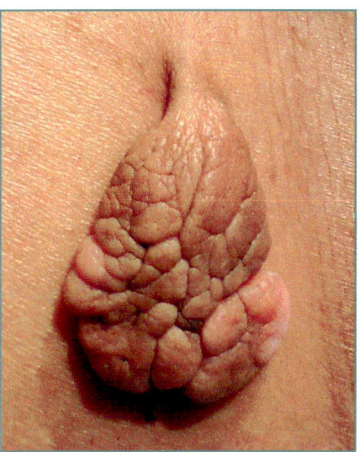

Fig 1.7:   Large pedunculated papilloma.

A benign overgrowth of all skin layers, with a central vascularised core. Papillomas are fleshy, may vary in size & are also known as 'skin tags'. They may occur anywhere but are often seen on the face & neck. Treatment is by surgical excision.

Q: What is a pyogenic granuloma?

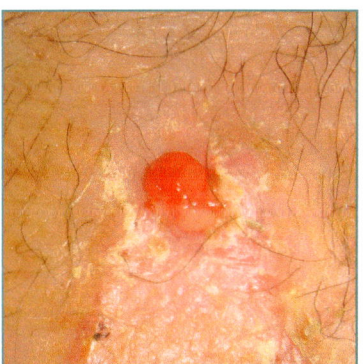

Fig 1.8: Pyogenic granuloma.

Unlike the name suggests, this is an acquired capillary haemangioma. Pyogenic granulomas are associated with a history of trauma. They present as soft raised lesions with a colour range from light red to deep purple. They may be painful & can bleed either spontaneously or with little trauma. They are best excised as this fixes the problem of bleeding & ensures tissue for histological diagnosis. **Note: Do not miss the amelanotic melanoma that looks like a pyogenic granuloma, especially if subungal.**

Q: What is a sebaceous (epidermoid) cyst?

An abnormal membrane-lined sac, composed of epithelial cells, containing a caseous substance with a 'cheesy odour'. This substance is comprised of:

- Fibrous tissue
- Fluid
- Keratin

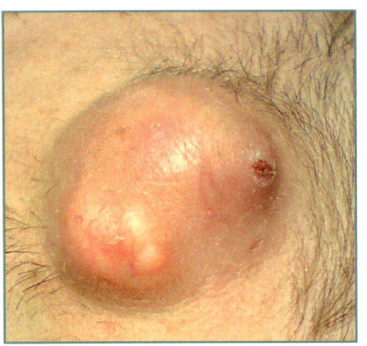

Fig 1.9: Sebaceous cyst.

Sebaceous cysts originate in the subcutaneous tissues so often seem fixed to skin. They may be of variable size with a central punctum. Discharge, ulceration & infection (abscess) may occur. Treatment is conservative unless symptomatic when surgical excision is indicated.

Q: What is a lipoma?

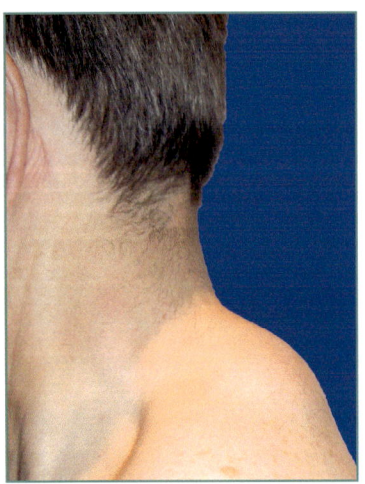

Fig 1.10: Large lipoma of the posterior neck / upper back.

A benign tumour of mature fat cells. Commonly seen on the neck & trunk & may become quite large. They originate in the fat layer, so are neither fixed to skin nor to underlying structures. They are freely mobile & it may be possible to demonstrate the 'slip sign' as the lump 'slips away' on palpation. Treatment is either conservative or surgical e.g. liposuction & excision biopsy. Liposuction leaves less scarring, but is associated with a higher recurrence.

Ulcers

Q: What is an ulcer?

A breakdown in all layers of an epithelial surface.

Q: What are the causes & 'edge features' of ulcers?

Classification	Notes	Edge
Traumatic	Ill fitting shoes / pressure sores.	Sloping
Venous (Fig 1.1)	Due to deep venous insufficiency & venous hypertension. Commonly seen over the malleoli.	Sloping
Infective	May be primary or secondary to infection of colonised chronic ulcers by e.g. Staphylococcus / Streptococcus.	Sloping
Arterial	Painful. Often associated with peripheral arterial disease, particularly at pressure points e.g. between toes, plantar surface of foot, heel, metatarsal heads. May also be related to embolism or vasculitis.	Punched-Out
Neuropathic	Painless. Causes of neuropathy include diabetes, chronic alcohol abuse, leprosy or syphilis.	Punched-Out
Neoplastic	May be primary / secondary.	• Everted e.g. SCC / Marjolin's Ulcer • Rolled e.g. BCC

Q: What are the treatment options for ulcers?

- Treatment is of the underlying cause & complications.
- General strategies include:

Conservative	Medical	Surgical
Dressings	Antibiotics (if infective)	Ligation & Stripping (varicose veins)
Foot Elevation	Diabetic Control	Surgical Excision (neoplastic)
Orthopaedic Foot Wear		Skin Graft
Compression Stockings	**Note: 4 x layer compression bandaging of venous ulcers may be contraindicated in concurrent peripheral arterial disease e.g. ankle-brachial pressure index <0.8.**	

SKIN CANCER

Basal Cell Carcinoma (BCC)

Q: What is a BCC?

A basal cell carcinoma (or rodent ulcer) is a malignant, locally infiltrative, neoplasm of the basal cells of the epidermis. It is the most prevalent form of skin cancer. Metastasis is very rare, but aggressive when present.

Q: How are BCCs classified?

Histologically there are many different sub-types. BCCs may be classified as:

Classification	Examples
Localised	• Nodular (most common)
	• Nodulocystic
	• Pigmented
Superficial	• Superficial Spreading
	• Multifocal
Infiltrative	• Morphoeic
	• Morpheaform

Q: How are BCC risk factors classified?

Congenital	Acquired
Fitzpatrick Skin Type I	UV Exposure
Gorlin's Syndrome	Increased Age

Q: What are the clinical features of BCCs?

- More common on sun-exposed sites e.g. head & neck.
- Appearance may be variable.
- Nodular is the most common sub-type.

Sub-type	Description
Nodular	• Raised Lesion
(Fig 1.11)	• 'Rolled Edges' with 'Pearly Sheen'
	• Central Depression / Ulceration
	• Superficial Telangiectasia
Superficial	• Erythematous Patches
Infiltrative	• Flat Pale Areas

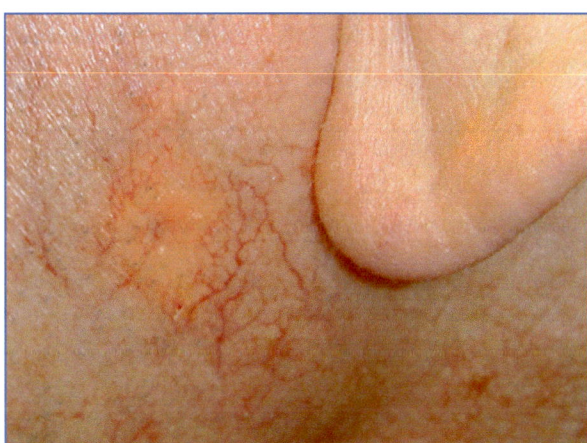

Fig 1.11: Nodular basal cell carcinoma. The lesion is raised with central depression & telangiectasia. The edges are 'rolled' with a 'pearly sheen'.

Q: What are the treatment options for BCCs?

This depends on the BCC sub-type, location, patient co-morbidities, patient wishes & should be discussed within an MDT environment. In addition to excision, reconstruction may be required.

Medical	Surgical
Chemotherapy e.g. 5-FU Cream	Curettage & Cautery
Cryotherapy	Excision
Phototherapy	Moh's Micrographic Surgery
Radiotherapy	

Q: What excision margins are suitable for excision of a BCC?

BCC	Excision Margins		
Primary	Small (<2cm):	3mm	= 85% Clearance (e.g. Face)
		4–5mm	= 95% Clearance
	Large (>2cm) / Morphoeic:	5mm	= 85% Clearance
		13–15mm	= 95% Clearance
Recurrent	Gold standard is Moh's Micrographic Surgery		
	Previous guidelines suggest 5-10mm otherwise		
Incomplete Excision	Re-excision		
	Consider alternative treatment depending on patient / site e.g. radiotherapy		
	Consider surveillance		

Q: What is Moh's Micrographic Surgery?

- Sequential horizontal tumour excision with immediate frozen section examination.
- Histological analysis is performed intra-operatively by the surgeon.
- If the margins are not adequately clear, more is removed from the patient & re-examined.
- This is repeated until clear margins are achieved.

Squamous Cell Carcinoma (SCC)

Q: What is a cutaneous SCC?

A cutaneous squamous cell carcinoma is a malignant skin cancer arising from keratinising cells of the epidermis. It is the 2nd most prevalent form of skin cancer & has metastatic potential.

Q: How are SCC risk factors classified?

Congenital	Exposure Related	Acquired
Fitzpatrick Skin Type I	UV Exposure	Immunosuppression e.g. HIV, Iatrogenic
Xeroderma Pigmentosum	Chemicals e.g. Arsenic, Organic Hydrocarbons	Chronic Wounds e.g. Marjolin's Ulcer
	HPV Infection	Increased Age

Q: Do you know of any pre-malignant lesions of SCC?

Lesion	Description
Actinic Keratosis	• Rough White Patches 'Stuck Onto' Erythematous Base
	• 10–15% Progress to SCC
Bowen's Disease	• Red, Scaly Patch
	• Considered as SCC *in situ*
	• 5% progress to SCC
Leukoplakia	• White Patch on Oral / Other Mucosal Surface
	• 15% Progress to SCC

Q: What is the clinical appearance of SCC?

This is variable, but the classic appearance is an ulcerated lesion, with hard raised edges (Fig 1.12).

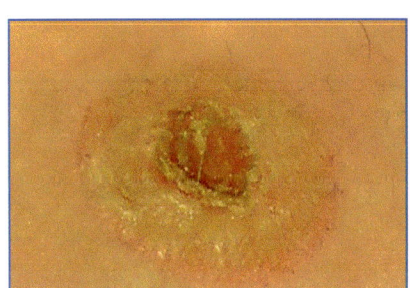

Fig 1.12: Squamous cell carcinoma. The lesion has central ulceration & raised edges.

Q: How is cutaneous SCC staged?

Cutaneous SCC is staged according to the AJCC TNM classification system.

Primary Tumour Extent (T)		Regional Lymph Nodes (N)	
Tx	Primary tumour cannot be evaluated.	Nx	Regional nodal status cannot be evaluated.
T0	No evidence of primary tumour.	N0	No regional lymph node involvement.
Tis	Carcinoma *in situ*.	N1	Single node metastasis longest axis ≤3cm.
T1	Primary tumour longest axis ≤2cm.	N2	Single ipsilateral node metastasis longest axis >3cm & ≤6cm / multiple ipsilateral node metastases.
T2	Primary tumour longest axis >2cm & ≤4cm	N3	Single node metastasis longest axis >6cm.
T3	Primary tumour longest axis >4cm or deeper subcutaneous soft tissue structures invasion / minor cortical bone invasion.	Metastasis & Distant Lymph Nodes (M)	
		Mx	Distant metastasis & lymph nodes cannot be evaluated.
T4	Primary tumour gross cortical bone or marrow invasion / skull base or axial skeleton or foraminal involvement.	M0	No distant metastasis.
		M1	Distant metastasis or contralateral lymph node involvement.

Q: What are the treatment options for cutaneous SCC?

These should be considered within an MDT environment & include:

Medical	Surgical
Cryotherapy	Excision ± Reconstruction
Radiotherapy	Moh's Micrographic Surgery

Q: What excision margins are suitable for excision of a SCC?

Excision margins should be according to British Association of Dermatologists guidelines, in order to achieve complete excision rates of ≥95%; further excision is usually required after incomplete excision, unless alternative treatment options are deemed more appropriate after MDT discussion.

SCC	Excision Margins
≤2cm Diameter / Low Risk	4mm
>2cm Diameter / High Risk	6mm
>4cm Diameter / Very High Risk	10mm

Note: Moh's micrographic surgery may also be considered for SCC excision.

Malignant Melanoma

Q: What is a malignant melanoma?

A malignant neoplasm of melanocytes, predominantly in the skin, but also occurring in the leptomeninges, eyes, gastrointestinal tract, oral & genital mucous membranes. It has the greatest mortality of all skin cancers.

Q: What are the risk factors for malignant melanoma?

Congenital	Exposure Related	Acquired
Family History	UV Exposure	Immunosuppression
Fitzpatrick Skin Type I		
Xeroderma Pigmentosum		
Dysplastic Naevus Syndrome		

Q: What clinical features make you suspicious of malignant melanoma?

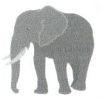

Memory: **ABCDE**   for suspicious features of malignant melanoma

Asymmetry
Border Irregularity
Colour Variegation
Diameter >6mm
Evolving e.g. Size, Shape, Symptoms

Q: What sub-types of malignant melanoma do you know?

Sub-Type	Notes
Superficial Spreading (Fig 1.13)	• 50% of all sub-types. • Presents as a flat / slightly raised brown lesion with heterogeneous (irregular) pigmentation & irregular borders. • Usually affects the trunk (males) or legs (females).
Nodular	• 15–30% of all sub-types. • Presents as a blue-black nodule, with smooth borders, that may ulcerate / bleed. • 5% are amelanotic.
Lentigo Maligna Melanoma	• 10–15% of sub-types. • Presents on sun-damaged skin of elderly patients. • The precursor lesion is known as Hutchinson's Freckle / lentigo maligna.
Acral Lentiginous	• 30–70% of sub-types in dark skinned & 5% in fair skinned races. • Lesions present on the palms & soles or subungual (below the nail plate). • Hutchinson's Sign describes extension of an acral lentiginous melanoma to the nail folds.
Amelanocytic	• <5% of sub-types. This refers to an unpigmented melanoma. • Commonly affects nodular melanomas / metastases (due to incapability of poorly differentiated cells to synthesise melanin).

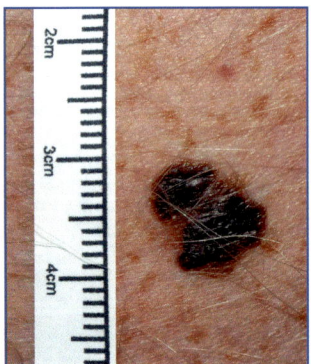

Fig 1.13: Superficial spreading malignant melanoma.

Q: What is the surgical management of suspected malignant melanoma?

+ Excision biopsy (2mm margin) to confirm diagnosis & Breslow thickness.
+ Once diagnosis is confirmed, this is **discussed in an MDT**; treatment is then guided by the outcome of this discussion & according to national melanoma treatment guidelines e.g. BAD, NICE.
+ Wider local excision is performed for positive biopsies, with margins based on Breslow thickness.
+ SLNB may also be considered at the time of wider local excision.

Q: What is Breslow thickness & why is it important?

The depth of penetration (mm) of the melanoma, from the stratum granulosum. It is important as it guides excision margins & prognosis as follows:

Breslow Thickness (mm) (malignant melanoma)	Excision Margins (cm) (malignant melanoma)	5 Year Survival (%)
In situ	0.5	95
<1	1	95
1–2	1–2	80
2.1–4	2–3	65
>4	2–3	50

Q: What do you understand by Clark's Levels?

This is an anatomical measure of tumour depth.

Level	Notes
I	Confined to epidermis.
II	Extends to papillary dermis.
III	Extends to junction between papillary & reticular dermis.
IV	Extends into reticular dermis.
V	Extends into subcutaneous fat.

Q: How would you stage malignant melanoma?

Melanoma is staged according to the AJCC TNM classification system.

Primary Tumour Extent (T)		Regional Lymph Nodes (N)	
Tx	Primary tumour cannot be evaluated.	Nx	Regional nodal status cannot be evaluated.
T0	No evidence of primary tumour.	N0	No regional lymph node involvement.
Tis	Carcinoma *in situ*.	N1	**N1a:** 1 enlarged regional lymph node & micro-metastases present.
T1	**T1a:** ≤1mm depth, without ulceration. **T1b:** ≤1mm depth, with ulceration.		**N1b:** 1 enlarged regional lymph node & macro-metastases present.
T2	**T2a:** 1.01–2mm depth, without ulceration. **T2a:** 1.01–2mm depth, with ulceration.	N2	**N2a:** 2–3 enlarged regional lymph nodes with micro-metastases present.
T3	**T3a:** 2.01–4mm depth, without ulceration. **T3b:** 2.01–4mm depth, with ulceration.		**N2b:** 2–3 enlarged regional lymph nodes with macro-metastases present.
T4	**T4a:** >4mm depth, without ulceration. **T4b:** >4mm depth, with ulceration.	N3	≥4 enlarged regional lymph nodes / matted nodes / in-transit metastases / satellite lesions.

Metastasis & Distant Lymph Nodes (M)			
Mx	Distant metastasis & lymph nodes cannot be evaluated.	M1a	Distant skin metastases present.
		M1b	Distant lung metastases present.
M0	No distant metastasis / lymphadenopathy.	M1c	Other visceral / distant metastases present. Any melanoma with elevated LDH.

Q: When would you perform a sentinel lymph node biopsy for malignant melanoma?

- This is decided according to national guidelines & following MDT discussion.
- At the time of wider local excision.
- Patients with thick melanomas.
- Presence of >1 malignant melanoma.
- Consider in melanomas with adverse features e.g. ulceration, lymphovascular invasion, mitotic rate ≥1mm^2.
- Role in melanomas <1mm thick remains controversial.

Q: Who makes up the malignant melanoma multidisciplinary treatment team?

This will vary according to each unit, but should comprise of:

- Dermatologist
- Plastic Surgeon
- Clinical Oncologist
- Pathologist
- Clinical Nurse Specialist
- Psychologist

CHAPTER 2
HEAD & NECK

JA Joseph
BH Miranda
M Keene

CHAPTER CONTENTS

Thyroid Examination

Thyroid Status Examination

Neck Lump Examination

Parotid Gland Examination

Submandibular Gland Examination

OSCE Questions

- Thyroid Embryology
- Goitre & Thyroid Cancer
- Head & Neck Lumps
- Head & Neck Lymph Nodes
- Neck Dissection
- Salivary Glands & Cancer
- Facial Nerve Palsy
- Tonsillitis
- Epistaxis

THYROID EXAMINATION

START: Patient sitting on chair, with shirt unbuttoned / off.

Ask the patient to point out the lump if it is not clearly visible.

Inspect from FRONT, BACK, SIDES & ABOVE as follows:

INSPECTION	Interpretation
Lump	Goitre (Fig 2.1) & thyroglossal duct cysts are in the anterior triangle usually within 2cm of the midline.
6 x S's	Describe lump site, size, shape, symmetry, overlying skin & associated scars. **Note: The goitre may be butterfly shaped & symmetrical about the midline.**
Distended Veins	Distended neck veins imply SVC obstruction.
Swallow Water	Ask the patient to look up & swallow water. Goitres will move up.
Protrude Tongue	Ask the patient to look up & protrude tongue. Thyroglossal duct cysts will move up.

Ask about pain.

To prevent causing distress, explain to the patient that you will be feeling from behind.

Examine each side, accentuating the lobe by gently pressing the contralateral lobe towards the midline.

Examine the good side first.

Feel for temperature changes with the back of your hand.

PALPATION	Interpretation
SEC FFP TR	Palpate lump surface, edge, consistency, fixity to skin & underlying structures, fluctuance, pulsatility & expansility, transilluminability & reducibility. **Note: The goitre surface may be smooth or nodular.**
Feel Below Lump	Inability to get below the lump suggests retrosternal extension.
Swallow Water	Ask the patient to look up & swallow water. Goitres will move up.
Protrude Tongue	Ask the patient to look up & protrude tongue. Thyroglossal duct cysts will move up.
Trachea	Check for deviation.
Lymphadenopathy	Submental, submandibular, pre-auricular, post-auricular, occipital, posterior cervical, anterior cervical, pre-tracheal & supraclavicular.

PERCUSSION	Interpretation
Sternum	Percuss down sternum, checking for a dull-resonant interface. This suggests retrosternal goitre extension.

AUSCULTATION	Interpretation
Lump	Thyroid bruit in Graves' Disease.

COMPLETION	Interpretation
Thyroid Status	*See later.*
Vocal Fold Check	Refer to ENT specialist for FNE.

FINISH:

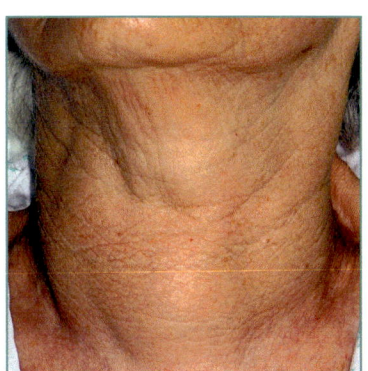

Fig 2.1: Goitre.

This is a large bilateral thyroid goitre. The right lobe is clearly visible & more enlarged than the left.

THYROID STATUS EXAMINATION

START: Patient sitting on chair, with shirt unbuttoned / off.

Inspect from FRONT, BACK & SIDES as follows:

General Appearance	Hyperthyroid	Hypothyroid
Demeanour	Restless	Docile
Hair	Normal	Brittle, Dry & Thin
Face	Wasting	Myxoedema Facies
Neck	Thyroid Swelling & Scars	Thyroid Swelling & Scars
Trunk	Weight Loss	Weight Gain

Hands	Hyperthyroid	Hypothyroid
Fingertips	Acropachy (Fig 2.2)	Normal
Palpation	Warm & Sweaty	Cold, Dry, Rough & Inelastic Skin
Paraesthesia	Usually Not Present	Carpal Tunnel Syndrome
Tremor	Present	Absent
Radial Pulse	Tachycardic / Irregular	Bradycardic

Eyes	Hyperthyroid	Hypothyroid
Lid Retraction	Present in Graves' Disease	Absent
Exophthalmos	Present in Graves' Disease	Absent
Lid Lag	Present in Graves' Disease	Absent
Sunken Eyes	Absent	Present
Periorbital Puffiness	Absent	Present
Loss of Outer Third of Eyebrow	Absent	Present

Shins	Hyperthyroid	Hypothyroid
Pretibial Myxoedema	Present in Graves' Disease	Absent

To test ankle reflexes position the patient with one knee on a chair & foot hanging over the edge.

Reflexes	Hyperthyroid	Hypothyroid
Ankle Reflex	Normal / Brisk	Slow Relaxing

To complete, perform a thyroid lump examination & ask questions relating to thyroid status as follows:

Question	Hyperthyroid	Hypothyroid
Mood Change	Anxiety	Depression
Appetite Change	Increased	Decreased
Body Temperature	Always Hot	Always Cold
Weight Change	Decreased	Increased
Hand Sensation	Usually Unaltered	Carpal Tunnel Syndrome
Heart Beat	Tachycardia & AF	Bradycardia
Bowel Habit	Diarrhoea	Constipation
Period	Menorrhagia	Oligomenorrhoea
Medication	Carbimazole & Propanolol	Levothyroxine
Operations / Radiotherapy	Total thyroidectomy is the commonest cause of hypothyroidism.	
Voice Change	Pressure of goitre on recurrent laryngeal nerve.	
Breathing Difficulty Lying Down	Pressure of goitre on trachea. This may also cause stridor.	
Swallowing Difficulty	Pressure of goitre on oesophagus causing dysphagia.	
Anaemia / DM / Pigmentation	Associated autoimmune disease.	

FINISH:

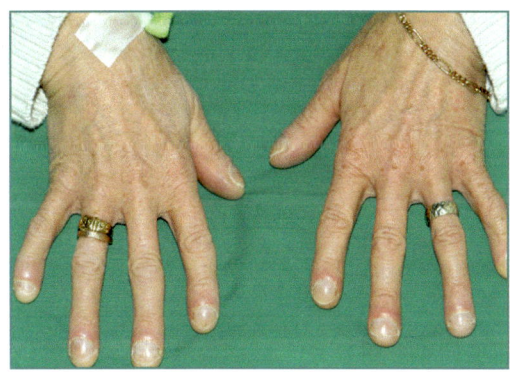

Fig 2.2: Digital Clubbing.

Digital clubbing associated with Grave's disease is known as thyroid acropachy.

NECK LUMP EXAMINATION

START: Patient sitting on chair, with shirt unbuttoned / off.

Ask the patient to point out the lump if it is not clearly visible.

Inspect from FRONT, BACK, SIDES & ABOVE as follows:

INSPECTION	Interpretation
General Appearance	*See thyroid status.*
6 x S's	Describe lump site, size, shape, symmetry, overlying skin & associated scars.
Distended Veins	Distended neck veins imply SVC obstruction.

If the lump is confined to the anterior triangle, test for thyroid swellings by asking the patient to look up & swallow water, then look up & protrude tongue. If the lump moves up on swallowing or with tongue protrusion, continue palpation as for thyroid examination.

If the lump is confined to the posterior triangle, continue neck lump palpation as follows:

Ask about pain.

To prevent causing distress, explain to the patient that you will be feeling from behind.

Examine both sides of the neck, starting with the good side.

Feel for temperature changes with the back of your hand.

PALPATION	Interpretation
SEC FFP TR	Palpate lump surface, edge, consistency, fixity to skin & underlying structures, fluctuance, pulsatility & expansility, transilluminability & reducibility.
Neck Regions	Do not forget to palpate the remaining neck regions as there may be another lump.
Lymphadenopathy	Submental, submandibular, pre-auricular, post-auricular, occipital, posterior cervical, anterior cervical, pre-tracheal & supraclavicular.

AUSCULTATION	Interpretation
Lump	Bruit e.g. carotid / subclavian artery aneurysm.

The following examinations must be undertaken for completion if a neck lump is identified:

COMPLETION	Interpretation
ENT	Full ENT examination – refer to specialist for FNE.
Scalp & Face	Metastasis.
Axilla & Groin	Lymphadenopathy.
Breast	Metastasis.
Abdomen	Metastasis.

FINISH:

PAROTID GLAND EXAMINATION

START: Patient sitting on chair, with shirt unbuttoned / off.

Ask the patient to point out the lump if it is not clearly visible.

Inspect from FRONT, BACK, SIDES & ABOVE as follows:

INSPECTION	Interpretation
6 x S's	Describe lump site, size, shape, symmetry, overlying skin & associated scars (Fig 2.3).
Parotid Fistula	Previous operation.
Other Lumps	Do not forget to look at the contralateral side for bilateral parotid lumps. Look for possible lymphadenopathy.
Facial Nerve (VII)	Look for facial asymmetry, particularly looking at the nasolabial fold. Test muscles of facial expression 'raise eyebrows, shut eyes against resistance, blow out cheeks, show teeth, tense & flare neck muscles'. Facial nerve involvement suggests malignancy.
Oral Cavity	Using a pen torch, look for inflammation, pus & stones. Inspect the opening of **Stensen's Duct** in the buccal vestibule at the level of the maxillary 2nd molar.

Ask about pain.

To prevent causing distress, explain to the patient that you will be feeling from behind.

Examine both sides, starting with the good side.

Feel for temperature changes with the back of your hand.

PALPATION	Interpretation
SEC FFP TR	Palpate lump surface, edge, consistency, fixity to skin & underlying structures, fluctuance, pulsatility & expansility, transilluminability & reducibility. **Note: Asking the patient to clench their teeth will contract masseter, hence accentuating some parotid lumps & assisting in assessing fixity.**
Lymphadenopathy	Submental, submandibular, pre-auricular, post-auricular, occipital, posterior cervical, anterior cervical, pre-tracheal & supraclavicular.
Stensen's Duct	Palpate the opening of Stensen's Duct with the patient's mouth open. Try to milk the duct of any pus that may be present.
Bimanual	Use gloves, feeling for calculi & deep lobe tumours.

COMPLETION	Interpretation
Contralateral Side	Do not forget to examine the other side.
Chorda Tympani	Ask about change in taste sensation.
ENT	Full ENT examination – consider referral to specialist.

FINISH:

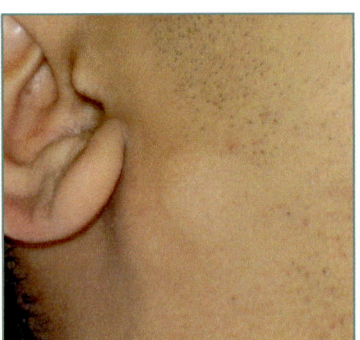

Fig 2.3: Right parotid pleomorphic adenoma.

SUBMANDIBULAR GLAND EXAMINATION

START: Patient sitting on chair, with shirt unbuttoned / off.

Ask the patient to point out the lump if it is not clearly visible.

Inspect from FRONT, BACK, SIDES & ABOVE as follows:

INSPECTION	Interpretation
6 x S's	Describe lump site, size, shape, symmetry, overlying skin & associated scars.
Other Lumps	Do not forget to look at the contralateral side for bilateral submandibular lumps. Look for possible lymphadenopathy.
Oral Cavity	Using a pen torch, look for inflammation, pus & stones. Inspect the opening of **Wharton's Duct** either side of the lingual frenulum.
Marginal Mandibular Nerve	Damage due to malignant infiltration / previous surgery results in an inability to depress the angle of the mouth. Facial asymmetry may also be seen here.
Hypoglossal Nerve (XII)	Damage due to malignant infiltration / previous surgery results in tongue deviation towards the side of the lesion with tongue protrusion.

Ask about pain.

To prevent causing distress, explain to the patient that you will be feeling from behind.

Examine both sides, starting with the good side.

Feel for temperature changes with the back of your hand.

PALPATION	Interpretation
SEC FFP TR	Palpate lump surface, edge, consistency, fixity to skin & underlying structures, fluctuance, pulsatility & expansility, transilluminability & reducibility.
Lymphadenopathy	Submental, submandibular, pre-auricular, post-auricular, occipital, posterior cervical, anterior cervical, pre-tracheal & supraclavicular.
Wharton's Duct	Palpate the opening of Wharton's Duct with the patient's mouth open. Try to milk the duct of any pus that may be present.
Bimanual	Use gloves, feeling for calculi & tumours.
Lingual Nerve	Damage due to malignant infiltration / previous surgery results in decreased touch sensation to the anterior two thirds of the tongue.

COMPLETION	Interpretation
Contralateral Side	Do not forget to examine the other side.
ENT	Full ENT examination – consider referral to specialist.

FINISH:

OSCE QUESTIONS

Thyroid Embryology

Q: What do you know about the embryology of the thyroid gland?

- 1st endocrine organ to develop.
- Development begins gestation day 24.
- Development begins between the 1st & 2nd pharyngeal pouches at the foramen caecum.
- Develops as a proliferation of endodermal cells on the pharyngeal floor, sited between the tuberculum impar & copula.
- Descent is via a pathway outlined by the thyroglossal duct (Fig 2.4).
- By gestation week 10, the thyroid gland lies with its isthmus over tracheal rings 2–4.
- The inferior parathyroid glands & thymus are derived from pharyngeal pouch 3.
- The superior parathyroid glands are derived from pharyngeal pouch 4.

Q: What are the clinical implications of disorders of thyroid gland embryology?

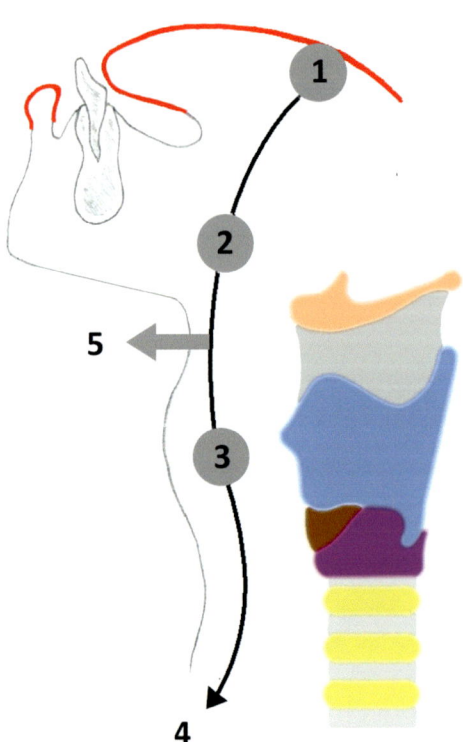

Clinical implications of thyroid gland embryology are due to the abnormalities of the normal pathway of descent & embryological development. Most of these disorders therefore lie along the pathway of the thyroglossal duct e.g. ectopic thyroid / retrostenal goitre.

Fig 2.4: Disorders of thyroid gland embryology.

1. **Lingual Thyroid:** Lump at the foramen caecum causing speech difficulty / dysphagia. Treatment is by surgical excision.
2. **Suprahyoid Thyroglossal Cyst:** *See later.*
3. **Infrahyoid Thyroglossal Cyst:** *See later.*
4. **Retrosternal Goitre:** *See above.*
5. **Thyroglossal Fistula:** Rarely congenital. Commonly due to infection / surgery. Treatment is by surgical excision.

Goitre & Thyroid Cancer

Q: How would you investigate a thyroid lump?

After taking a **full history** & performing a **thorough clinical examination**, I would consider the following tests:

Investigations	Notes
Blood Tests	FBC, U&E, LFT, CRP, TFT, Ca & Clotting.
USS & FNA	USS defines dimensions of tumour, if it is solitary / multinodular / solitary nodule / cyst. Cytology from FNA can reveal diagnosis.
Core Biopsy	Useful particularly if FNA is inconclusive.
CT / MRI	Defines complex anatomy, retrosternal extension, airway deviation or compression & oesophageal compression.
Radioisotope Scan	Identifies whether a nodule is **'hot & functioning'** (takes up isotope) or **'cold & non-functioning'** (no isotope uptake). Hot nodules are rarely malignant.

Q: How would you categorise the causes of thyroid swellings?

Goitre	Cause	Notes
NODULAR	**True Solitary Nodule**	50% have a true solitary nodule. Of these: 80% are adenomas. 10% are cysts, fibrosis or thyroiditis. 10% are cancer.
DIFFUSE	**Multinodular Goitre**	50% have a large nodule as part of a multinodular goitre.
	Physiological	Due to increased demand e.g. pregnancy.
	Dietary Iodine Deficiency	Rare but endemic to high altitude areas e.g. Alps & Himalayas.
	Dietary Goitrous Agents	Uncooked cabbage & turnips, calcium or fluoride in drinking water, various drugs.
	Graves' Disease	Patient is hyperthyroid & displays signs of Graves' Disease.
	Hashimoto's Thyroiditis	Autoimmune goitre & hypothyroid state.
	De Quervain's Thyroiditis	Self limiting & viral.
	Hereditary Errors of Thyroid Metabolism	Very rare autosomal recessive inborn errors of metabolism (8 types). They cause failure to respond to TSH or failure of T3 & T4 synthesis & release.
	Other	Lymphoma & amyloid.
	Congenital Absence or Atrophy of the Thyroid	If untreated leads to cretinism Rarely associated with Pendred's Syndrome (congenital hypothyroidism & high tone deafness).

Q: What are the treatment options for benign thyroid swelling?

Classification	Treatment	Notes
CONSERVATIVE	**Remove Goitrogens e.g. Cabbage**	Reduce Thyroid Goitre.
MEDICAL	**Carbimazole**	If Hyperthyroid.
	Propylthiouracil	If Hyperthyroid.
	β–Blocker e.g. Propanolol	Symptomatic Relief of Hyperthyroidism.
	Thyroxine	If Hypothyroid.
SURGICAL	**Lobectomy** **Total Thyroidectomy**	**Indications:** • Diagnostic • Resolution of Compressive Symptoms e.g. Dysphagia, Dyspnoea & Dysphonia • Thyrotoxicosis Refractory to Medical Treatment e.g. Graves' Disease • Cosmetic

Q: What are the common thyroid cancers?

Thyroid Cancer	%	Notes
Papillary Adenocarcinoma	70	Common in children. 90% have lymphatic metastases at presentation.
Follicular Carcinoma	20	Common around 50 years. Blood-borne spread.
Medullary Carcinoma	5	Parafollicular C cell origin. Produce calcitonin. 90% are sporadic, 10% are MEN related.
Anaplastic Carcinoma	<5%	Common in older patients.
Lymphoma	<5%	Core biopsy best for diagnosis. Treat with DXT & chemotherapy.

Q: What is the epidemiology of thyroid cancer?

• Rare.
• Accounts for approximately 0.5% of cancer related deaths.
• 2–3 times more common in females.

Q: What are the treatment options for malignant thyroid disease, diagnosed following FNAC?

Diagnosis	Treatment	Notes
Papillary Adenocarcinoma	Thyroid Hormone Suppression. Hemithyroidectomy.	Some centres advocate this when tumour <1cm (T1 stage).
	Radio-Iodine Ablation.	For tumours greater than 1cm (T2–4 stage).
	Total Thyroidectomy & Level VI Neck Dissection.	
Follicular Adenocarcinoma	Hemithyroidectomy.	Usually performed in the 1st instance as it is difficult to distinguish adenoma (benign) from adenocarcinoma (malignant) on FNAC.
	Radio-Iodine Ablation. Total Thyroidectomy.	Completion thyroidectomy & level VI neck dissection performed if histology shows malignancy, followed by radio-iodine ablation.
Medullary Thyroid Cancer	Total Thyroidectomy.	Completion thyroidectomy & level VI neck dissection, with removal of any other suspicious lymph nodes. Requires lifelong calcitonin (tumour marker) follow up.
Anaplastic Carcinoma	Surgical Debulking, DXT & Doxorubicin.	Survival is around 1 year only.

Q: Do you know any inherited syndromes causing tumours of the endocrine system?

Multiple endocrine neoplasia (MEN), is inherited in an autosomal dominant manner & may be classified by type as follows:

Type	Notes
MEN I	**Memory:** 3 x P's • **P**ancreatic Islet Cell Tumour • **P**ituitary Adenoma • **P**rimary Hyperparathyroidism
MEN IIa	**Memory:** 3 x C's • **C**atecholamines (Phaeochromocytoma) • **C**alcitonin (Thyroid Medullary Carcinoma) • **C**alcium (Primary Hyperparathyroidism)
MEN IIb	Same features as MEN IIa without parathyroid involvement. Also: • Marfanoid Habitus • Multiple Neuromas

Head & Neck Lumps

Q: Can you list some causes of neck lumps in the regions labelled 1–6?

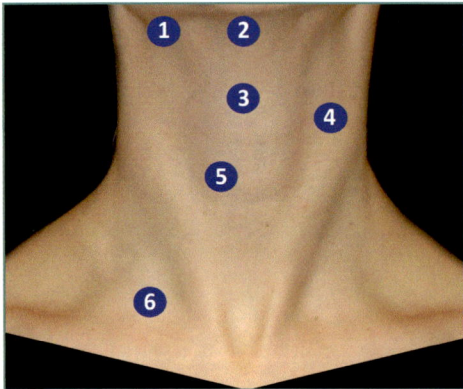

1. **Submandibular Gland Swelling**
   Chemodactoma (expansile)
2. **Submental Gland Swelling**
   Dermoid Cyst
3. **Thyroglossal Cyst**
4. **Branchial Cyst**
5. **Thyroid Nodule**
6. **Cystic Hygroma**
   Tip of Cervical Rib
   Subclavian Artery Aneurysm (expansile)

Q: What investigations would you order for a neck lump & in what order?

Investigations	Notes
Bloods	FBC, U+E, LFT, CRP & Clotting CMV, EBV, *Toxoplasma & Bartonella*.
USS & FNA	Will provide diagnosis if squamous cell carcinoma, infective or inflammatory.
CT / MRI	Helps locate primary tumour. Neck, chest, abdomen & pelvis images assist staging.
Lymph Node Biopsy	Required when FNA inconclusive e.g. Lymphoma.

Q. What are the causes of neck lumps?

These include the causes for any lump (*see lumps 'n' bumps chapter*) & those specific to the neck as follows:

Classification	Location	Cause	Notes
CONGENITAL	Anterior Triangle	**Congenital Dermoid Cyst**	Affects children & young adults. Commonly on lateral & medial aspect of eyebrow & anywhere in the midline at sites of embryological fusion.

Classification	Location	Cause	Notes
		Thyroglossal Duct Cyst	Cyst lying along the tract of the obliterated thyroglossal duct. 90% in midline. Most occur in childhood. Excised by Sistrunk's Procedure. This removes the cyst, middle third of hyoid & any thyroglossal duct remnants.
		Sternomastoid Tumour	Caused by birth trauma. Head turned away & tilted toward affected side. Painful to turn head. Treated with surgical tenotomy.
	Posterior Triangle	**Cystic Hygroma**	Type of lymphangioma. Occur in lower neck. Treat with surgical excision.
ACQUIRED	Anterior Triangle	**Implantation Dermal Cyst**	In areas subjected to repeated trauma e.g. fingers. Seen rarely in the neck. Due to forcible implantation of skin subcutaneously.
		Branchial Cyst	Thought to arise from elements of squamous epithelium in a lymph node. Usually in young adults. 60% are in males. Lie deep to anterior border of SCM at junction of upper & mid third in anterior triangle.
		Thyroid Lump	*See above*
		Parotid Tumour	*See below*
		Submandibular Swelling	*See below*
		Chemodectoma	Nearly always benign. There are many types e.g. carotid body tumour. This arises from the carotid bulb & may be pulsatile. Rare except in high altitude areas e.g. Mexico City.
		Pharyngeal Pouch	Caused by herniation of pharyngeal mucosa (pulsion diverticulum) through weak point in its muscular coat (Killian's Dehiscence) between thyopharyngeus above & cricopharyngeus below (2 muscles of inferior constrictor).
			Most commonly in elderly. Occasional cystic swelling in low anterior neck. Causes regurgitation of undigested food.
			Diagnosed with barium swallow. (Fig 2.5)
			If troublesome treated with endoscopic pouch stapling.

CHAPTER 2

HEAD & NECK OSCE QUESTIONS

41

Classification	Location	Cause	Notes
		Carotid Artery Aneurysm	Expansile mass. Caused by atheroma, infection or trauma. Resect if causing TIAs.
		Laryngocoele	Laryngeal air sac from increased intra-laryngeal pressure e.g. glassblowers.
	Posterior Triangle	**Cervical Rib**	Palpable bony swelling in supraclavicular fossa. Cause of thoracic outlet syndrome.
		Lipoma	Commonly in posterior triangle & overlying trapezius.
		Subclavian Artery Aneurysm	Sometimes palpable in supraclavicular fossa. Often due to thoracic outlet syndrome.
	All Regions	**Lymphadenopathy**	*See later* (Fig 2.6).

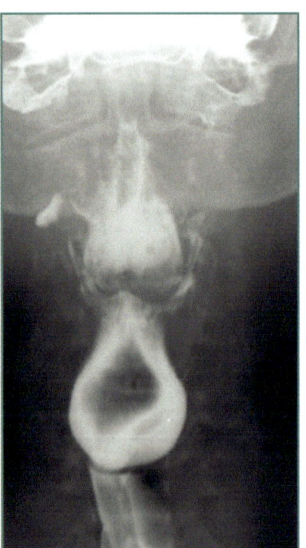

Fig 2.5: Pharyngeal pouch.

Barium swallow delineating a pharyngeal pouch.

Head & Neck Lymph Nodes

Q: What lymph nodes should be routinely examined in the head & neck?

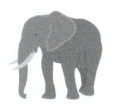

Memory: Examine for head & neck lymphadenopathy systematically, standig behind the patient. You can use the order presented (Fig 2.6). Your hands should move in a sweeping motion without going backwards & forwards. Feel & compare both sides. This looks more 'slick' to the examiner.

Nodes	Notes
Submental	Underneath chin & anterior third of mandible.
Submandibular	Underneath mandible body.
Pre-Auricular	Anterior to pinna of ear, over mandible ramus.
Post-Auricular	Behind the ear over the mastoid bone.
Anterior (Deep) Cervical Chain	Follows the course of the IJV in the neck. Can be palpated along the anterior border of sternocleidomastoid.
Posterior (Superficial) Cervical Chain	Within the posterior triangle along trapezius.
Occipital	Over the occipital bone at the back of the skull.
Supraclavicular	Within the posterior triangle along the posterior-superior border of the clavicle.
Pre-Tracheal	In midline overlying the trachea.

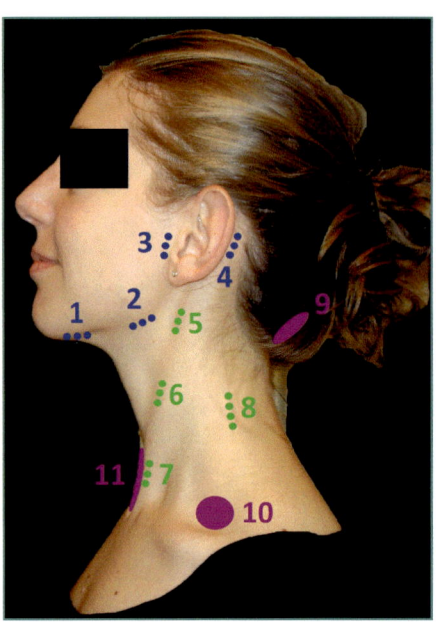

Fig 2.6: Head & neck lymphadenopathy.

Key	Nodes	Level
1	Submental	I
2	Submandibular	I
3	Pre-auricular	-
4	Post-auricular	-
5	Anterior / Deep Cervical (Upper)	II
6	Anterior / Deep Cervical (Middle)	III
7	Anterior / Deep Cervical (Lower)	IV
8	Posterior / Superficial Cervical	V
9	Occipital	-
10	Supraclavicular	VI
11	Pre-Tracheal	VI

Note: Current practice in ENT is to describe cervical lymphadenopathy in terms of levels (I–VI) as follows:

Level	Notes
I	Submental & submandibular nodes within the digastric triangle.
II	Upper anterior / deep cervical chain nodes around the upper third of the IJV, where it is crossed anteriorly by the spinal accessory nerve. This level extends from the skull base in the region of the jugular foramen to the carotid bifurcation (Fig 2.7).
III	Mid anterior / deep cervical nodes around the middle third of the IJV, from the carotid bifurcation to the cricothyroid notch.
IV	Lower anterior / deep cervical nodes around the lower third of the IJV, from the cricothyroid notch to the clavicle.
V	Posterior triangle nodes between the posterior border of SCM & anterior border of trapezius. This also includes the supraclavicular nodes.
VI	Anterior compartment of the neck adjacent to the thyroid & trachea.

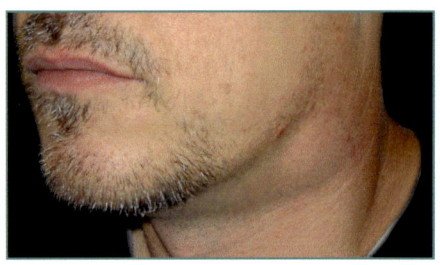

Fig 2.7: Level II lymphadenopathy.

Neck Dissection

Q: What do you understand about neck dissection?

There are several types of neck dissection described for head & neck tumours:

Dissection Type	Notes
Radical	*Removal of:* • Level I-V lymph nodes. • Accessory nerve. • Sternocleidomastoid muscle (SCM). • Internal jugular vein (IJV).
Modified Radical	*Removal of:* • Level I-V nodes... Then subclassified as: • **Type 1:** Preserve accessory nerve. • **Type 2:** Preserve accessory nerve & SCM. • **Type 3:** Preserve accessory nerve, SCM & IJV.
Extended Radical	Radical dissection with removal of paratracheal & mediastinal lymph nodes & parotid gland.
Selective	Depends on lymph node level taken.

Salivary Glands & Cancer

Q: What is the epidemiology of salivary gland neoplasms?

- 5% of all head & neck tumours.
- 80% arise in the parotid gland.
- 15% arise in the submandibular gland.
- 5% arise in the sublingual & minor salivary glands.

Q: What tests would you order to investigate a parotid lump & in what order?

Investigations	Notes
Bloods	FBC, U+E, LFT, CRP, Ca, clotting, rheumatoid factor, autoantibody screen (Sjögren's Syndrome).
USS & FNA	Will reveal stones. Delineates tumour & can provide cytological diagnosis.
Sialogram	Shows anatomy of ductal system & any stones present. Can be therapeutic intervention (crush stone or grasp & remove).
MRI	If concerned about complex anatomy or deep lobe involvement.

Q: What are the causes of diffuse parotid swelling?

Cause	Notes
Infective	Causing acute / chronic parotitis & may be:
	Viral: Coxsackie, Echovirus Mumps, & HIV.
	Bacterial: Actinomycosis, *Staphylococcus* & TB.
Inflammatory	**Sjögren's Syndrome:** An autoimmune disease often associated with rheumatoid arthritis. Symptoms include parotidomegaly, xerostomia & keratoconjunctivitis sicca.
	Mikulicz's Syndrome: Similar to Sjögren's Syndrome, characterised however by salivary & lacrimal gland enlargement. Must have an associated underlying cause e.g. TB / Sarcoid.
Drugs	Alcohol, OCP, Thiouracil, Phenylbutazone & Isoprenaline.
Metabolic	Bulimia, Cirrhosis, Cushing's Disease, Diabetes, Gout & Myxoedema.
Sialectasis	Progressive destruction of the parotid gland occurs, accompanied by duct stenosis & cyst formation. May be either congenital or acquired through epithelial debris / calculi.
Pseudo-Parotidomegaly	The following may mimic parotid swelling:
	• Cyst
	• Lipoma
	• Preauricular Lymphadenopathy
	• Facial Nerve (VII) Neuroma
	• Hypertrophic Masseter
	• Winged Mandible
	• Mandible Tumour
	• Branchial Cyst
	• Dental Cyst

Q: What are the common parotid & submandibular salivary gland neoplasms?

Gland	%	Salivary Neoplasm
Parotid	80	Pleomorphic Adenoma
	10	Mucoepidermoid Carcinoma
	5	Warthin's Tumour
Submandibular	35	Pleomorphic Adenoma
	25	Adenoid Cystic Carcinoma
	10	Mucoepidermoid Carcinoma
	5	Adenocarcinoma

Q: What are the causes of a parotid gland tumour?

Classification	Example	Notes
BENIGN	**Pleomorphic Adenoma (Fig 2.3)**	Commonest of all salivary gland neoplasms. 80% of parotid tumours. Peak incidence in 5th decade.
	Warthin's Tumour (papillary cystadenoma)	Also known as a papillary cystadenoma. Peaks around the 7th decade & is 7 times more prevalent in males.
	Monomorphic Adenoma	Group of rare tumours. Most common is basal cell adenoma. Presents in 6th decade.
	Lymphangioma	Rare congenital hamartoma. Usually present before age 2. Removed for cosmetic reasons.
	Haemangioma	Most common in children.
	Neurofibroma	Rare in parotid. Nerve sheath tumour. Originates from facial nerve (VII).
VARIABLE MALIGNANCY	**Mucoepidermoid Carcinoma**	Most prevalent salivary neoplasm in children. This can act like a benign or malignant tumour.
	Acinic Cell Carcinoma	This can act like a benign or malignant tumour.
MALIGNANT	**Adenoid Cystic Carcinoma**	The most prevalent malignant parotid tumour. Peaks around the 6th decade.
	Adenocarcinoma	Develops within secretory ducts. Local & distant metastases present in 33% of presentations.
	Undifferentiated Carcinoma	Uncommon, high-grade cancer. Tumour size is an important prognostic indicator.
	Lymphoma	Commonly affects elderly men. Biopsy is indicated as treatment includes chemotherapy / radiotherapy.

Q: What is a pleomorphic adenoma?

- Commonest of all salivary gland neoplasms.
- 80% of parotid tumours (35% of submandibular).
- Peak incidence in 5th decade of life.
- Histologically contains stromal & epithelial elements.
- Presents as a slow-growing & benign painless mass.
- Commonly in the superficial lobe of the parotid gland & treated by superficial parotidectomy.
- Small proportion may undergo malignant transformation.

Q: What are the features of Warthin's Tumour?

- Also known as a papillary cystadenoma.
- 5% of parotid tumours.
- 10% are bilateral.
- Peaks during 7th decade of life & 7 times more prevalent in males.
- Histologically is an adenolymphoma with cystic spaces surrounded by eosinophilic columnar cells.
- Presents as a slow-growing & benign painless mass of the parotid gland & treated by surgery.
- Malignant change is extremely rare.

Facial Nerve Palsy

Q: How would you classify the clinical features & causes of facial nerve palsy?

Classification	Clinical Features	Causes
UPPER MOTOR NEURON	• Hemifacial palsy. • Able to raise eybrow due to bilateral innervation of frontalis & orbicularis oculi.	**Cerebrovascular Accident:** Suspect in the elderly & those at risk of ischaemic or haemorrhagic events. **Multiple Sclerosis** **Meningitis** **Acoustic Neuroma** **Glioma**
LOWER MOTOR NEURON (Fig 2.8)	• Hemifacial palsy. • Unable to raise eyebrow.	**(55%) Bell's Palsy:** Unknown aetiology so is a diagnosis of exclusion. Theoretical viral or ischaemic cause. Treat with high dose oral steroids & acyclovir for 7 days if <72 hours. 85% fully recovered after 3 months. **(19%) Trauma:** Iatrogenic e.g. parotidectomy, Blunt or Penetrating. **(7%) Ramsay Hunt Syndrome:** Herpes zoster viral infection resulting in shingles of the facial nerve (VII). Characteristic vesicles are seen in the ear canal. **(6%) Tumour:** Either of the facial nerve (VII) e.g. schwannoma, due to invasion e.g. malignant parotid tumour or extrinsic pressure e.g. vestibular nerve schwannoma. **Infection:** Acute or chronic suppurative otitis media. Malignant otitis externa.
MIXED	Upper & lower motor neuron lesion signs.	Causes are rare e.g. sarcoid, myasthenia gravis, Guillain-Barré syndrome & drugs.

Fig 2.8: Right facial nerve lower motor neuron involvement.

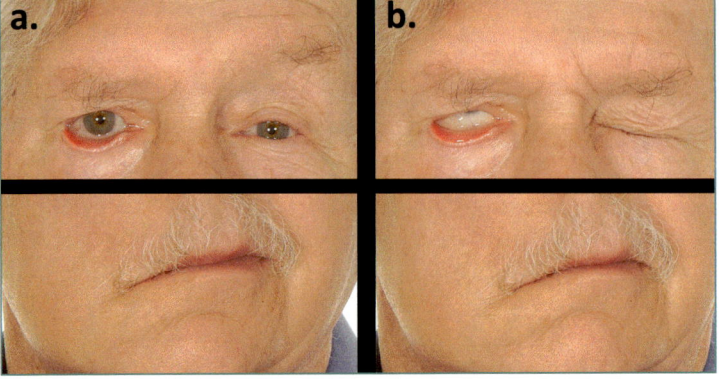

(a) This patient has a right-sided facial droop, with loss of the right forehead furrow. (b) When the patient is asked to shut his eyes, the right eye does not close & deviates superiorly (Bell's Reflex).

Q: What is Sjögren's Syndrome?

This is an autoimmune disease, 90% of which is seen in women around 50 years of age. Periductal lymphocytes in multiple organs is characteristic at histology. 50% of cases have salivary gland involvement. Lymphoma affects 1 in 6 patients. The syndrome may be classified as follows:

- **Primary:**   Keratoconjunctivitis Sicca & Xerostomia

     No Connective Tissue Disorder Association

- **Secondary:**   Connective Tissue Disorder Association:

     - Rheumatoid Arthritis

     - Systemic Lupus Erythematosus

     - Scleroderma

Q: What specific investigations would assist your diagnosis of Sjögren's Syndrome?

Investigation	Notes
Schirmer's Test	Hyposecretion: the lacrimal glands may be tested by inserting a special strip of filter paper under the lower eyelid. Hyposecretion is confirmed by wetting of the filter paper <5mm in 5 minutes (normal 15mm).
Autoantibodies	Rheumatoid factor, anti-Ro & anti-La.
Sublabial Biopsy	Salivary gland histology.

Q: What are the treatment options for a patient with Sjögren's Syndrome?

Conservative	Medical	Surgical
Meticulous Oral Hygiene	Artificial Tears	Lacrimal Punctum Diathermy
Antibacterial Mouth Wash	Steroids	
Monitoring for Lymphoma	Immunosuppressants	

Tonsillitis

Q: What are the causes of acute tonsillitis?

Viral	Bacterial
Influenza	β-Haemolytic *Streptococcus*
Parainfluenza	*Streptococcus pneumoniae*
Adenovirus	*Haemophilus influenzae*
Enterovirus	Anaerobic Organisms
Rhinovirus	
Epstein Barr Virus (EBV)	

Q: What are the clinical features of tonsillitis (Fig 2.9)?

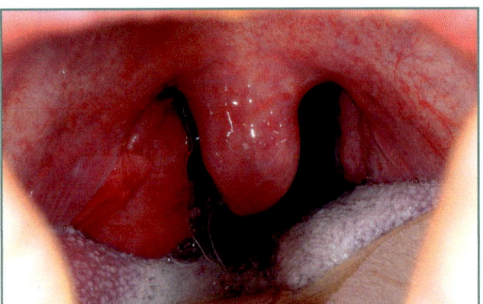

Fig 2.9: Acute right-sided tonsillitis.

The patient has an enlarged, erythematous right tonsil.

Clinical Features	Notes
Pyrexia, Malaise & Headache	Often prodromal for 24 hours.
Hyperaemic Tonsils, Pus & Debris in Crypts	Clinically diagnostic for infective tonsillitis.
Sore Throat	The predominant symptom.
Muffled Voice	Due to generalised oedema. A 'hot potato voice' may be present, so-called due to sounding like the voice of a person trying to speak with hot potatoes in their mouth! The significance is a possible **Quinsy**.
Neck Pain	There may be associated cervical lymphadenopathy.
Odynophagia	Pain on swallowing.
Trismus	Difficulty opening mouth.
Tender Jugulodigastric Lymphadenopathy	Enlarged regional nodes in upper neck (level I & II).
Quinsy	Peritonsillar abscess seen as a collection of pus around the tonsil. Requires drainage under local anaesthetic.
Respiratory Obstruction	Severe swelling causing obstruction & respiratory distress.

Q: What investigations would you consider for a patient with suspected tonsillitis?

After taking a **full history** & performing a **thorough clinical examination**, I would order the following tests:

Investigation	Example	Explanation
BLOOD TESTS	**Paul-Bunnell / Monospot Test**	Detects EBV in glandular fever (infectious mononucleosis).
	FBC	Expect raised WBC. Neutrophilia if bacterial cause. Lymphocytosis if viral cause.
	CRP	Acute phase reactant.
MICROBIOLOGY	**Throat Swab / MC+S**	Useful if empirical treatment not working.
	Blood Cultures	Detect bacteraemia.

Q: What treatment would you implement for a patient with confirmed tonsillitis?

Medical	
Analgesia & Antipyretics	Reduce pain & temperatures.
Penicillin	Aerobic cover. Erythromycin may be used if the patient is penicillin allergic. **Note: Avoid amoxicillin as it causes a generalised rash in patients with glandular fever.**
Metronidazole	Anaerobic cover.
Dexamethasone	Reduces inflammation & particularly useful in severe cases.
Hospital Admission	
IV Antibiotics	In extreme cases, when the patient is unable to tolerate fluids orally, the patient is not safe for discharge & requires hospital admission for IV treatment.
IV Fluids	
IV Analgesia	
Surgical	
Tonsillectomy	For recurrent cases (>5 episodes in each of 2 consecutive years).

Q: What are the complications of tonsillitis?

Complication	Notes
Respiratory Obstruction	Severe swelling causing obstruction & respiratory distress.
Quinsy	Peritonsillar abscess seen as a collection of pus around the tonsil. Requires drainage under local anaesthetic.
Parapharyngeal / Retropharyngeal Abscess	May require drainage under general anaesthetic.
Acute Otitis Media	Due to tracking infection along eustachian tube.
Recurrent Acute Tonsillitis	Tonsillectomy is indicated with >5 episodes in each of 2 consecutive years.

Epistaxis

Q: What is epistaxis?

Acute haemorrhage from the nostril, nasal cavity or nasopharynx. This may either be anterior (90% of cases) or posterior. Anterior bleeds mostly arise from Little's area, which is richly vascularised (Kiesselbach's plexus). Posterior bleeds mostly arise from Woodruff's plexus.

Q: What are the causes of epistaxis?

These may be classified as local / systemic as follows:

Local	Systemic
Nose Picking	Hypertension
Trauma (direct / barotrauma)	Blood Dyscrasias
Infection (upper respiratory tract)	Drugs (aspirin / warfarin / heparin)
Allergy (sinusitis / rhinitis)	Alcohol Abuse
Substance Abuse (cocaine)	Liver Failure
Tumors	Haematological Anaemias
Iatrogenic (nasal cannulae / nasogastric tube)	

Q: What are the clinical features of epistaxis?

- Overt bleeding from the nasal cavity.
- Posterior bleeding from the nasopharynx may be visualised in the oropharynx.
- Massive epistaxis may mimic haemoptysis / haematemesis.

Q: What are the treatment options for expistaxis?

This is an emergency & must be managed in the context of either the acute life support (ALS) or acute traumatic life support (ATLS) protocols, addressing ABCs (**A**irway, **B**reathing, **C**irculation). The underlying cause must also be addressed. Specific treatment options include:

Conservative	Medical	Interventional / Surgical
Direct Pressure (20 Minutes)	(IV) Fluid Resuscitation	Embolisation*
Nasal / Post-Nasal Packing	Adrenaline Spray	Ligation*
Epistaxis Balloon	Cautery	***Arteries involved include the sphenopalatine, posterior ethmoidal, maxillary.**
Stop Aspirin / Warfarin / Heparin	Antibiotics (especially after packing)	

SECTION A2: TRUNK & THORAX

CHAPTER 3
CARDIOLOGY

Ms Prita Daliya
Dr Christopher Lutterodt
Dr Emily McDonald
Dr Nicola Downer

CHAPTER CONTENTS

Cardiovascular Examination

OSCE Questions:

- Acute Coronary Syndrome (ACS), Angina & Myocardial Infarction (MI)
- Aortic Dissection
- Heart Failure
- Acute Left Ventricular Failure
- Valvular Heart Disease
- Infective Endocarditis
- Hypertension
- Atrial Fibrillation (AF)
- Heart Block
- Ventricular Tachycardia / Ventricular Fibrillation
- Bradycardia
- Cardiomyopathy
- Cardiac Tamponade
- Pericarditis
- Cardiac Pericardiocentesis

CARDIOVASCULAR EXAMINATION

START: Patient lying supine at 45°, exposed to underwear. This is to facilitate the abdominal examination for signs of right heart failure.

Use sheet appropriately, to maintain patient dignity.

Standing at the end of the bed look at the surrounding environment for any indicators of cardiovascular disease e.g. O_2, GTN spray & fluid restriction signs.

INSPECTION	Interpretation
GENERAL:	
General State	Pain, SOB & cachexia may be evident.
Pallor	Anaemia.
Xanthoma/Xanthomata	*Yellow fatty deposits.*
	Seen on tendons or joints in hypercholesterolaemia.
Signs of Clinical Syndromes	Certain associations exist:
	• **Down's:** Atrial & ventricular septal defect.
	• **Marfan's:** Mitral valve prolapse, aortic aneurysm, aortic dissection.
	• **Turner's:** Bicuspid aortic valve, aortic coarctation.
Scars	**Chest:** sternotomy, infraclavicular, thoracotomy scars (Figs 3.1-3.3).
	Limbs: previous vein harvest.
HANDS:	
Temperature	'Cold & clammy' in low cardiac output states (e.g. cardiac failure, MI).
	'Warm & sweaty' in raised cardiac output states (e.g. sepsis).
Pale Palmar Creases	Anaemia.
Peripheral Cyanosis	*Blue discolouration of the fingertips.*
	Seen in hypoxia, low cardiac output & Raynaud's phenomenon.
Tar Staining	*Yellow discolouration of the fingertips & nails.*
	Secondary to smoking.
Osler's Nodes	*Painful, raised, red lesions.*
	Due to immune complex deposition in infective endocarditis.
Janeway Lesions	*Painless, haemorrhagic lesions.*
	Due to septic emboli in infective endocarditis.
Finger Clubbing (Fig. 2.2)	*Increased nail angle curvature (also see abdomen chapter).*
	Cardiovascular causes: congenital cyanotic heart disease, atrial myxoma (rare), subacute bacterial endocarditis (rare).

Splinter Haemorrhages	*Small, linear lesions under the nails.*
	Trauma (common), infective endocarditis septic emboli (rare).
ARMS:	
Blood Pressure	If not performed earlier, offer to take a manual blood pressure reading (Table 3.1).
FACE:	
Malar Flush	*Redness of the cheeks.*
	Due to mitral stenosis.
Corneal Arcus	*Yellow-white ring around the iris.*
	Aging (arcus senilis) or hypercholesterolaemia.
Xanthelasma	*Fatty deposits seen around the eyes.*
	Seen in hypercholesterolaemia.
Conjunctival Pallor	Anaemia.
Central Cyanosis	*Bluish discolouration of the tongue & mucous membranes.*
	Hypoxia
Fundoscopy	• **Hypertensive Retinopathy:** Papilloedema (optic disc swelling), cotton-wool spots (in ischaemia), microaneurysms or flame hemorrhages.
	• **Roth's Spots:** *Haemorrhagic retinal lesions with pale centres* (in infective endocarditis)
NECK:	
Jugular Venous Pressure (JVP)	May be raised e.g. heart failure, cardiac tamponade, constrictive pericarditis (Table 3.2).
PRECORDIUM:	
Scars	Indicative of previous surgery (Figs 3.1-3.3)

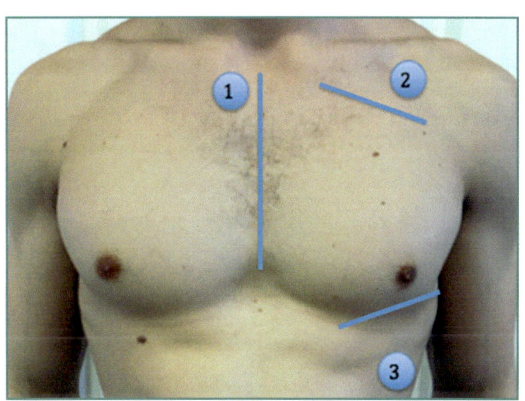

Fig 3.1: Thoracic scars.

1 **Median Sternotomy:** CABG, aortic / mitral valve replacement

2 **Infraclavicular:** Pacemaker, ICD

3 **Left Thoracotomy:** Mitral valve replacement / valvotomy

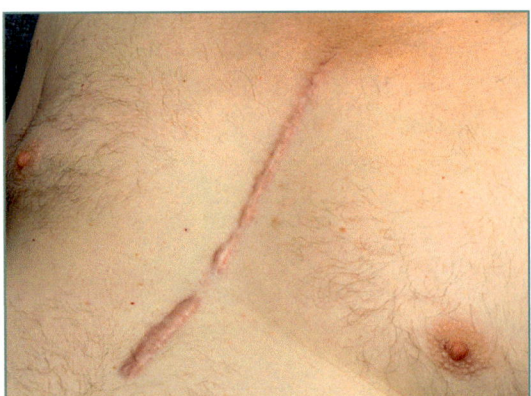

Fig 3.2: Hypertrophic median sternotomy scar.

Useful access for CABG, aortic / mitral valve replacement.

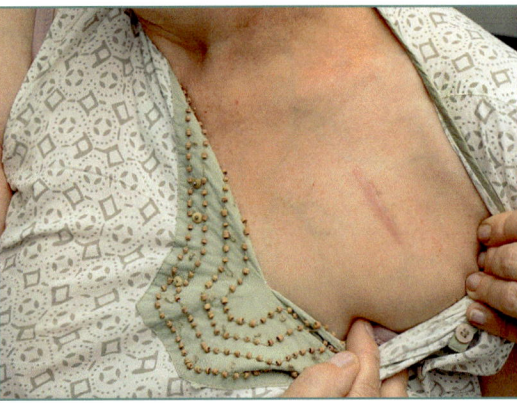

Fig 3.3: Left infraclavicular scar.

Useful access for pacemaker / ICD insertion.

Table 3.1: Blood pressure measurement.

- Position the blood pressure cuff around the upper arm, ensuring the cuff is placed over the brachial artery & is not inside out.
- Estimate the systolic pressure by inflating the cuff to a pressure where the radial pulse is no longer palpable.
- Release the pressure & repeat again to a pressure 20 mmHg higher than the estimated systolic pressure. This time place the stethoscope over the brachial artery & listen to ensure that you inflate to a pressure where the pulse becomes inaudible.
- Slowly deflate the cuff at about 2 mm/Hg per second until the pulse is audible again. This is the **systolic pressure.**
- Continue deflating the cuff until the pulse becomes inaudible again. This is the **diastolic pressure.**

Table 3.2: Jugular venous pressure (JVP) measurement.

- Ask the patient to look left whilst lying supine at 45°.
- Look for the double waveform of the JVP between the sternocleidomastoid heads.
- The height of the JVP is measured as the vertical distance from the sterno-manubrial angle (normal = 3-4cm).
- Pushing down over the liver will help to augment this if not immediately visible.
  Note: This is hepatojugular 'reflux' (not reflex).
- The JVP may be raised in congestive or right-sided heart failure, cardiac tamponade or constrictive pericarditis.

Ask about pain.

PALPATION	Interpretation
PERFUSION:	
Capillary Refill	Press the fingertips for 5 seconds, then release. Normal reperfusion (look under the nail plate) occurs over 2-3 seconds. Delayed in low cardiac output states.
PULSE:	
Rate & rhythm generally assessed via the RADIAL pulse, character & volume via the CAROTID pulse. Never palpate both carotid pulses simultaneously.	
Rate	Measure resting heart rate (HR), ideally over 1 minute: • **Bradycardia:** HR <60 beats per minute (bpm). • **Normal:** HR 60-100bpm. • **Tachycardia:** HR >100bpm.
Rhythm	Described as either: • **Regular:** Normal. • **Regularly irregular:** Heart block. • **Irregularly irregular:** AF or multiple ectopic beats.
Character	• **Collapsing (Water Hammer):** Aortic regurgitation, patent ductus arteriosus. *Note: Feel the radial pulse with 3 or 4 fingers & quickly elevate the patient's arm up above their head, supporting the elbow. When the arm is raised, a collapsing pulse will be felt trickling down your fingers with each beat.* **Remember to ask about shoulder pain first.** • **Small Volume & Slow Rising:** Aortic stenosis. • **Pulsus Alternans:** *Alternating weak-strong beats.* LVF. • **Pulsus Paradoxus:** *Abnormal drop in systolic BP & pulse amplitude on inspiration.* Cardiac tamponade & constrictive pericarditis.
Volume	'Weak/Thready' in hypovolaemia = late sign of shock. 'Strong/Bounding' in CO_2 retention & sepsis.

| Other | • **Radial-Radial Delay:** Aortic arch aneurysm & dissection, subclavian & brachial artery stenosis. |
| | • **Radial-Femoral Delay** Coarctation of the aorta. |

PRECORDIUM:

Memory: The 'Z' manoeuvre (Fig 3.4).

Apex Beat	**Note: Palpate using the radial border of the hand & index finger.**
	The most inferior-lateral position on the chest that the heartbeat can be felt (normal = 5th intercostal space, mid-clavicular line).
	Position & character may vary:
	• **Displaced:** Cardiomegaly.
	• **Tapping:** Mitral stenosis (felt with the palm of the hand).
	• **Forceful:** Mitral/aortic regurgitation, volume overload.
	• **Heaving:** Ventricular Hypertrophy e.g. aortic stenosis, hypertension, HOCM.
	• **Absent:** Obesity, emphysema, pericardial effusions, pneumothorax.
Parasternal Heave	**Note: Palpate using the palmar aspect of the hand & fingers, placed parallel & to the left of the sternum.**
	Palpable, forceful heart contraction. Right ventricular hypertrophy.
Thrill	**Note: Palpate using the palmar aspect of the hand & fingers, placed perpendicular to & across the sternum at 2nd intercostal space level.**
	Palpable cardiac murmur.

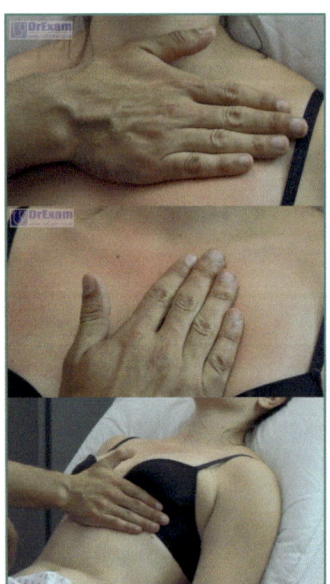

Fig 3.4: The 'Z'-manoeuvre.

Thrill: Palpable cardiac murmur.

Note: Palpate using the palmar aspect of the hand & fingers, placed perpendicular to & across the sternum at 2nd intercostal space level.

Parasternal Heave: Palpable, forceful heart contraction e.g. right ventricular hypertrophy.

Note: Palpate using the palmar aspect of the hand & fingers, placed parallel & to the left of the sternum.

Apex: The most inferior-lateral position on the chest that the heartbeat can be felt (normal = 5th intercostal space, mid-clavicular line).

Note: Palpate using the radial border of the hand & index finger.

AUSCULTATION	Interpretation
PRECORDIUM:	
Carotid Bruit	Carotid artery stenosis, radiation of aortic stenosis ejection systolic murmur.
Cardiac Areas	Listen in all 4 cardiac areas using the diaphragm of the stethoscope.
(Fig 3.5)	• **Mitral:** 5th intercostal space, mid-clavicular line (at the apex beat). • **Tricuspid:** 4th intercostal space, left sternal edge. • **Pulmonary:** 2nd intercostal space, left sternal edge. • **Aortic:** 2nd intercostal space, right sternal edge. **Note: Palpating the carotid artery during auscultation will help differentiate systolic & diastolic murmurs**
Murmurs	• **Mitral Regurgitation:** *(pan-systolic murmur)* Listen over the apex & for radiation into the axilla. • **Mitral Stenosis:** *(mid-diastolic murmur)* Low, rumbling murmur heard over the apex using the diaphragm bell with the patient rolled to the left-lateral position & in expiration. • **Aortic Regurgitation:** *(early diastolic murmur)* Heard at the lower left sternal edge (not the "aortic" area) using the diaphragm with the patient sat forward & in expiration. • **Aortic Stenosis:** *(ejection systolic murmur)* Heard over the aortic area with radiation to the carotids. Often heard throughout the precordium. **Note: An ejection systolic murmur heard at the aortic area that does not radiate to the carotid could be *aortic sclerosis* (benign).** **Memory: Left-sided heart murmurs are louder in expiration. Right-sided murmurs are louder in inspiration. This is due to changes in intra-thoracic pressure & IVC venous return.**
Crepitations	Listen to the lung bases at the back of the thorax. Crepitations may be present with pulmonary oedema.

COMPLETION	
Pitting oedema	Palpate the sacrum & ankles. Present in right ventricular failure.
Vascular Examination	Full vascular examination including assessment of all peripheral pulses.
Abdominal Examination	Look for: • **Hepatomegaly:** Right ventricular failure. If hepatomegaly is pulsatile = tricuspid valve regurgitation. • **Ascites:** Right ventricular failure.

Other Observations	• **Respiratory Rate**
	• **Oxygen Saturation**
	• **Temperature**
Urine dipstick	Microscopic haematuria may be seen in endocarditis due to renal emboli/ infarcts
Further investigations	• **ECG**
	• **CXR**
	• **Echo**
	• **Coronary Angiogram**

FINISH:

Fig 3.5: Cardiac auscultation.

<u>**M**</u>itral: 5th intercostal space, mid-clavicular line (at the apex beat).

<u>**T**</u>ricuspid: 4th intercostal space, left sternal edge.

<u>**P**</u>ulmonary: 2nd intercostal space, left sternal edge.

<u>**A**</u>ortic: 2nd intercostal space, right sternal edge.

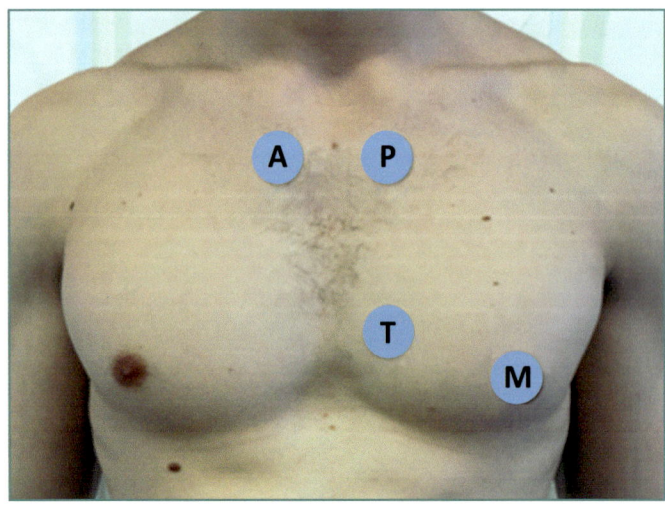

OSCE QUESTIONS

Acute Coronary Syndrome (ACS), Angina & Myocardial Infarction (MI)

Q: What is Acute Coronary Syndrome (ACS)?

- Spectrum of coronary disorders from unstable angina to Myocardial Infarction (MI):
  1. **STEMI**
  2. **Non-STEMI**
  3. **Unstable angina**
- Myocardial ischaemia or infarction occurs secondary to atherosclerotic plaque rupture & coronary thrombosis.
- Common presentation is chest pain + features of the underlying disorder.

Q: What is angina?

- Collection of symptoms associated with myocardial ischaemia due to reduced coronary blood flow in the presence of atheromatous disease.
- Commonly presents with dull/heavy central chest pain, radiating to the jaw, arms or shoulders.
- Associated symptoms include chest tightness, SOB, palpitations, sweating & nausea.

Q: What types of angina do you know of?

Angina	Notes
Stable	Symptoms are precipitated by exercise, cold, & stress but relieved with rest or GTN.
Unstable	Symptoms occur unpredictably, even at rest, & are resistant to GTN.

Q: What is Myocardial Infarction (MI)?

The progression of myocardial ischaemia to infarction & necrosis due to complete coronary artery occlusion.

Q: What are the risk factors for coronary artery disease?

Non-Modifiable	Modifiable
Increasing Age	Smoking
Male Gender	Hypertension
Previous MI	Hyperlipidaemia
Family History of IHD	Diabetes Mellitus
	Obesity
	Sedentary Lifestyle
	Stress

Q: How would you investigate a patient with ACS?

After assessing & managing the patient according to **ALS guidelines**, using an **ABC approach**, obtaining a **full history** & performing a **thorough clinical examination**, I would consider the following investigations as part of my simultaneous assessment & management.

Investigation	Interpretation
Blood Tests	• FBC, U&E, TFT.
	• Fasting glucose, cholesterol & lipid profile.
	• Cardiac enzymes (Troponin T / Troponin I, LDH, CK, AST).
ECG	• Tall T waves (initially) / inverted T waves (hours to days later).
(Fig 3.6)	• ST depression (indicative of cardiac ischaemia) / ST elevation (STEMI).
	• New LBBB.
	• Pathological Q waves.
CXR	• Cardiomegaly, pulmonary oedema, mediastinal widening (aortic dissection).
Other	• Stress testing.
	• Coronary angiography.

Fig 3.6: ECG indicating acute coronary syndrome with T wave changes, ST depression, LBBB & pathological Q-waves.

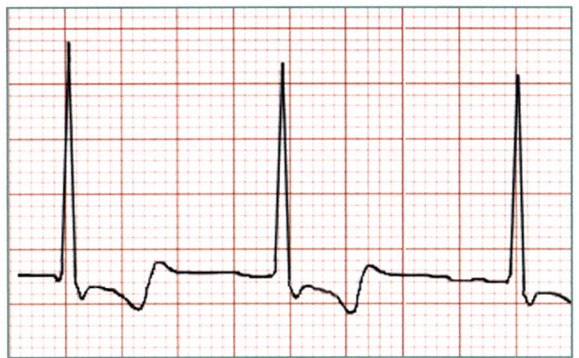

Q: What are the differential diagnoses for ACS?

Causes may be classified as follows:

Cardiac	Respiratory	Gastro-Oesophageal
Angina	PE	GORD
Aortic Dissection	Pneumonia	PUD
Pericarditis		Oesophagitis
Myocarditis		

Q: What are the treatment options for myocardial ischaemia/infarction in the acute phase?

 Memory: 'ROMANCE T'

Treatment	Interpretation
Reassure	Patients will be anxious
Oxygen	High flow at 15L/min via a non-rebreathing mask
Morphine	IV & titrate to patient's requirement
Aspirin	PO 300mg
Nitrates	SL GTN (spray or buccal tablets)
Clopidogrel	PO 300mg
Enoxaparin	SC 1mg/kg (treatment dose)
Thrombus	Consider **thrombolysis** (STEMI / new-onset BBB) or **percutaneous coronary intervention**

Q: What are the definitive treatment & secondary prevention options for myocardial ischaemia/infarction?

Conservative	Medical	Surgical
Smoking Cessation	Aspirin	Coronary Angiogram ± Angioplasty
Diet Modification	β-Blockers (if no contraindication)	Coronary Artery Bypass Graft
Weight Loss	ACE Inhibitors (if evidence of heart failure)	
Reduce Alcohol Intake	Statins	
Cardiac Rehabilitation (advice on exercise, stress reduction, driving & employment)	Diabetic Treatment	

Q: What are the contraindications to thrombolysis?

Absolute	Relative
Uncontrolled Hypertension (Systolic >180mmHg / Diastolic >110mmHg) Despite Medication	Severe Uncontrolled Hypertension (Systolic >180mmHg / Diastolic >110mmHg)
Active Haemorrhage	Anticoagulant Use / Bleeding Diathesis
Major Surgery (within last 2 weeks)	Recent Gastrointestinal / Genitourinary / Other Internal Haemorrhage (within past 6 months)
Suspected Aortic Dissection	Recent Trauma including Head Injury (within 2-4 weeks) or Traumatic/Prolonged (>10 minutes) CPR
Major Intracranial Events: • Previous cerebral haemorrhage • Known intracranial neoplasm • Known history of cerebral aneurysm/arteriovenous malformation • Intracranial Haemorrhage on CT • Recent thromboembolic stroke (within last 6 months)	Active Peptic Ulcer Disease
Suspected Aortic Dissection	Pregnancy

Aortic Dissection

Q: What is aortic dissection?

A tear in the intimal layer of the aorta with resultant stripping of the intima from the media to form a false lumen. This can result in occlusion of the true lumen, its branches, & propagate or result in aortic rupture.

Q: How does aortic dissection present?

- Classically with sudden onset, severe anterior chest or interscapular back pain secondary to intimal stripping from the aortic wall.
- Diagnosis may be missed without a high level of suspicion.
- Bilateral brachial BP recording may demonstrate a left-right discrepancy.
- CXR may demonstrate mediastinal widening.

Q: What are the causes of aortic dissection?

Causes	Pathology
Hypertension	• Chronic history
Trauma	• Acceleration-deceleration injuries
Iatrogenic	• Cardiac catheterisation
	• Intra-aortic balloon pump
	• Following cardiac surgery
Infective	• Untreated tertiary syphilis
Connective Tissue Disorders	• Marfan's syndrome
	• Ehlers-Danlos syndrome
Other	• Pregnancy
	• Coarctation of the aorta
	• Bicuspid aortic valve

Q: How is aortic dissection classified?

There are 2 commonly used classifications i.e. **DeBakey** (**Types I-III**) & **Stanford** (**Types A & B**). The Stanford classification is more commonly used & is described below:

Memory:	Type A	Affects Ascending Aorta & Arch
	Type B	Begins Beyond Brachiocephalic vessels

Type	Location	Preferred Management
Type A	Affects the ascending aorta & arch (within the initial 4cm of the ascending aorta in 90% of cases)	Surgical
Type B	Affects the descending aorta	Medical

Q: What are the complications of aortic dissection?

Complications depend on the type of dissection:

Stanford Type A	Stanford Type B
Death (rupture & haemorrhage)	**Death** (rupture & haemorrhage)
Cardiac Tamponade (pericardial involvement)	**Renal Failure** (renal artery occlusion)
MI (coronary artery occlusion)	**Bowel / Mesenteric Ischaemia** (coeliac / mesenteric artery occlusion)
Stroke (carotid artery occlusion)	
Aortic Regurgitation (aortic valve involvement)	**Lower Limb Ischaemia** (iliac / femoral artery occlusion)

Note: Type A may progress to type B.

Q: What are the treatment options for aortic dissection?

Treatment is either medical or surgical & dependent on the Stanford Classification:
- Stanford A: predominantly surgical management
- Stanford B: predominantly medical management

Surgical	Medical
Graft repair:	**BP control (MAP 60-75mmHg):**
• Open Resection ± AVR	• β-Blockers: *propranolol, labetalol, esmolol*
• Endovascular Stent Graft	• Calcium Channel Blockers: *diltiazem, verapamil*
	• Cardiac Vasodilators: *sodium nitroprusside* (as an adjunct to rate control & avoid reflex tachycardia)

Heart Failure

Q: What is heart failure?

- Heart failure occurs when the heart is unable to provide sufficient cardiac output in order to meet the demand of the body.
- It can be classified as High vs. Low Output Failure or anatomically as either Left vs. Right Ventricular Failure, or by duration of symptoms as Acute vs. Chronic heart failure.

Q: What is congestive cardiac failure (CCF)?

- Also known as Congestive Heart Failure (CHF).
- It usually occurs when the heart's function as a pump is inadequate for the body's demands.
- The resultant increase in venous pressure results in 'congestion' which is seen clinically as pulmonary & peripheral oedema.

Q: What is Low-Output heart failure & what are the causes?

- Cardiac output is insufficient to meet body demand, or in need of high filling pressures.
- They can be classified as follows:

Excess Preload	Pump Failure	Excess Afterload
Fluid Overload	MI	Aortic Stenosis
Mitral Regurgitation	Cardiomyopathy	Hypertension
	Constrictive Pericarditis	
	Cardiac Tamponade	
	Heart Block	

Q: What is High-Output heart failure & what are the causes?

- High-output failure is much less common than low-output failure.
- The Cardiac Output may be either normal or increased, but still unable to meet a pathological increase in demand.

Causes	Notes
Hyperthyroidism	Increased metabolism & hence demand
Paget's Disease of Bone	High vascularity of Paget's bone increases demand
Endotoxic Shock	Peripheral vasodilatation increases demand to supply vital organs
Anaemia	Increased cardiac work to increase systemic delivery of oxygenated blood
Arteriovenous Malformation (AVM)	Increased cardiac work due to either shunting or increased blood flow via the AVMs

Q: What are the symptoms & signs of chronic heart failure?

Heart Failure	Symptoms	Signs
Right	• Ankle Swelling • Nocturia • Abdominal Discomfort • Fatigue • Weight Gain • Fluid Retention	• Raised JVP • Hepatomegaly / Splenomegaly • Ascites • Ankle / Sacral Oedema • Left Parasternal Heave
Left	• SOB on Exertion / Rest • Orthopnoea • Paroxysmal Nocturnal Dyspnoea • Productive Cough (pink, frothy sputum) • Fatigue	• Tachypnoea • Tachycardia • Basal Crackles ± Pleural Effusion

Q: What are the long-term treatment options for chronic heart failure?

Lifestyle Modification	Medical
Patient Education	Treat Cause
Smoking Cessation	ACE Inhibitor / Angiotensin II Receptor Antagonist
Exercise	Diuretics
Weight Loss	β-Blocker
Reduce Dietary Salt Intake	Aldosterone Antagonists
Reduce Alcohol Intake	
Fluid Restriction	

Acute Left Ventricular Failure

Q: What is acute left ventricular failure?

- A sudden onset of cardiogenic pulmonary oedema secondary to left ventricular failure.
- This may be new or as a result of decompensated chronic heart failure.
- Patients can be in extremis with severe pulmonary oedema.

Q: What are the causes of acute left ventricular failure?

Myocardial	Valvular	Other
Acute Ischaemia	Acute Mitral Regurgitation	Cardiac Tamponade
Acute Infarction	Arrhythmias	Aortic Dissection
Myocarditis	Valve Destruction	Flash Pulmonary Oedema

Q: What are the clinical features of acute left ventricular failure?

Symptoms	Signs
Distress & Anxiety	Tachypnoea
Feeling of Impending Doom	Tachycardia
SOB at Rest	Gallop Rhythm
Orthopnoea (unable to lie flat)	Pulsus alternans
Preceding Nocturnal Cough (PND)	Signs of Cardiomegaly
Productive Cough (pink, frothy sputum)	Cardiac Wheeze
	Cyanosis
	Basal Crackles ± Pleural Effusion
	Signs of Pericardial Effusion

Q: What investigations assist with the diagnosis & management of left ventricular failure?

Investigation	Interpretation
Blood Tests	• FBC, U&E, LFTs, TFT. • Fasting glucose, cholesterol & lipid profile. • Cardiac enzymes (Troponin T / Troponin I, LDH, CK, AST). • ABG (looking for type 1 & 2 respiratory failure)
ECG	Look for signs of: • Cardiomegaly • Left ventricular strain • Prior MI • Arrhythmia • Ischaemia
CXR	• Signs of cardiomegaly & pulmonary oedema (Fig 3.7).
Echo	• Either TTE or TOE to ascertain ejection fraction & identify valvular abnormalities

Q: What are the radiological features of left ventricular failure?

- Cardiomegaly
- Pulmonary oedema
- Pleural effusion
- 'Bat wing' perihilar shadowing
- Kerley B lines with interstitial oedema
- Fluid within pulmonary fissures
- Splaying of the carina
- Prominent visible vasculature due to upper lobe blood diversion

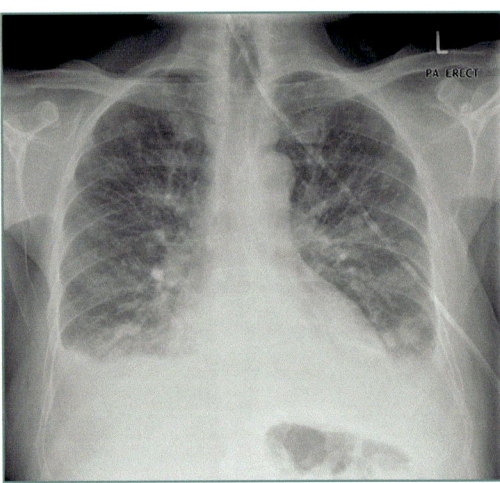

Fig 3.7: Acute left ventricular failure.

There is bilateral 'fluffy' shadowing throughout the lung fields indicating pulmonary oedema. There are bilateral pleural effusions with upper lobe venous congestion. The heart is enlarged (cardiomegaly) & oxygen tubing traverses the left side of the chest.

Q: How would you manage a patient in acute left ventricular failure?

- Acute left ventricular failure is a medical emergency & should be treated with continuous cardiac monitoring on either a coronary care or high dependency unit.

After **simultaneous assessment & management** according to **ALS guidelines**, using an **ABC approach**, obtaining a **full history** performing a **thorough clinical examination** & ordering **appropriate investigations**, I would implement the following treatment.

Memory: **'PROM-FUN'**

Treatment	Interpretation
Position	Sit upright to improve ventilation & oxygenation
Reassure	Patients will be anxious
Oxygen	15L/min via a non-rebreathing mask
	Note: Remember that hypoxia will kill your patient before hypercapnia.
Morphine	IV, titrated to patient requirement
Furosemide	40-80mg iv initially
	Note: Use caution in shock as a large diuresis can cause catastrophic hypovolaemia.
Urinary Catheter	Strict fluid balance & fluid restriction
Nitrates	Sublingual or continuous IV infusion if BP allows
Other	Treat causative features
	Escalate early as may require:
	• CPAP
	• Inotropes
	• Intra-aortic balloon pump (cardiogenic shock)

Valvular Heart Disease

Q: What is valvular heart disease?

- Any disease that affects any one of the 4 cardiac valves.
- This in turn affects cardiac blood flow due to a disruption in Virchow's triad.
- The type of disease can be classified as follows:

Disease Type	interpretation
Stenosis	• Narrowing of the valve due to calcification/foreign bodies
	• Difficulty opening
Regurgitation / Incompetence	• 'Leaky' valve allowing backflow of blood
	• Difficulty closing fully

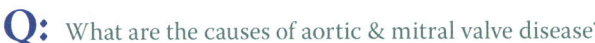

Q: What are the causes of aortic & mitral valve disease?

Causes may be classified as those which damage the valve itself & those that damage surrounding structures:

Disease	Valve Damage	Surrounding Structure Damage
Aortic Stenosis	• Calcification (commonest) • Congenital (bicuspid valve, subaortic membrane) • Rheumatic Fever	• Idiopathic Hypertrophic Subaortic Stenosis (rare) • William's Syndrome (rare)

Aortic Regurgitation	Acute:
	• Endocarditis
	• Trauma
	Chronic:
	• Rheumatic Heart Disease
	• SLE
	• Calcification
		• Aortic Root Dilation:
		  - Aortic aneurysm
		  - Aortic dissection
		  - Marfan's syndrome
		  - Ankylosing spondylitis
		  - Systemic hypertension
		  - Syphilis
		• Tetralogy of Fallot

Mitral Stenosis	• Rheumatic Heart Disease • Endocarditis (rare) • SLE (rare)	
Mitral Regurgitation	• Endocarditis • Mitral Valve Prolapse (idiopathic) • Rheumatic Fever • Chordal Rupture • Papillary Muscle Dysfunction / Rupture	• Cardiomyopathy • Functional: stretching of the valve ring in left ventricular dilatation

Q: What are the clinical features of valvular heart disease?

Disease	Signs	Symptoms
Aortic Stenosis	• Ejection systolic murmur	
	• Radiation to carotids	
	• Fourth heart sound	• SOB on Exertion
Aortic Regurgitation	• Early diastolic murmur	• Fatigue
	• Water-hammer pulse	• Exertional syncope
		• Dizziness
Mitral Stenosis	• Mid-diastolic murmur	• Angina
	• Right ventricular heave	• Palpitations
	• Malar flush	• Orthopnoea / PND
	• Raised JVP	• Nocturnal Cough
	• AF	• Ankle Swelling
	• Lateral displacement of apex beat	• Pulmonary Oedema
Mitral Regurgitation	• Pan-systolic murmur	
	• Radiation into axilla	

Q: What are the treatment options for valvular heart disease?

Risk Stratification	Medical	Surgical
• Avoid strenuous exercise	• Treat cause	• Valvuloplasty (AS)
• Smoking cessation	• Anti-hypertensives	- Balloon
• Diet modification	• Statins	- Surgical
• Weight loss	• Diuretics	• Valve Replacement
• Reduce alcohol intake	• β-Blockers / Calcium Channel Blockers	- Mechanical + anticoagulation
	• Anticoagulation (if VTE risk)	- Tissue (porcine, bovine, allograft, autograft)
		- Transcatheter (AVR)

Infective Endocarditis

Q: What is infective endocarditis (IE)?

- A condition in which the cardiac valves become infected.
- Vegetations form on valve leaflets resulting in valvular damage & septic embolisation.
- Presentation is insidious with malaise, fever, & a new murmur.

Q: What are the risk factors for infective endocarditis?

Cardiac	Other
Prosthetic Heart Valve	Dental Infection / Abscess
Mural Thrombus	Vascular Instrumentation (within last 60 days e.g. angiogram, central line, IVDU)
Previous Bacterial Endocarditis	Arterial Prosthesis
Existing Valvular Heart Disease	Immunosuppression
Congenital Heart Disease	
Cardiac Pacemaker	

Q: What signs may be evident in an individual with infective endocarditis?

Site	Signs
Hands & Skin	• Splinter Haemorrhages • Finger Clubbing • Janeway Lesions • Osler's Nodes • Petechial Haemorrhages
Eyes	• Conjunctival Haemorrhages • Roth Spots
Kidneys	• Microscopic Haematuria • Glomerulonephritis
Thorax / Abdomen	• Tachycardia • Cardiac Murmurs • Splenomegaly (secondary to infection)

Q: Which investigations would you consider in a patient with suspected infective endocarditis?

After taking a **thorough history** & **clinical examination** I would consider the following investigations:

Investigation	Interpretation
Blood Tests	• **FBC:** Normochromic normocytic anaemia, raised WCC
	• **CRP:** Good trend marker
	• **Blood Cultures:** >3 sets taken from different sites at different times
	Note: Also request a screen for atypical organisms & fungi.
	Note: Samples should be taken peripherally as well as from any existing lines.
Echo ± TOE	• Valvular vegetation
ECG	• Sinus tachycardia
Orthopantomogram (OPG)	• Assess dentition

Depending on the presence of septic emboli & site of embolisation, other investigations may include:

Investigation	Interpretation
Urinalysis	• Microscopic haematuria
	• Proteinuria (in glomerulonephritis)
CTPA	• Pulmonary infarction
Abdominal USS	• Splenomegaly
Contrast CT Abdomen & Pelvis	• Mesenteric ischaemia
CT Head	• Stroke

Q: How is infective endocarditis diagnosed?

- Diagnosis requires a high level of suspicion due to the insidious nature of presentation.
- The **Modified Duke Criteria** divides clinical signs into major & minor criteria.
- A definite diagnosis of Infective Endocarditis can be made in the presence of:
  - 2 major criteria   OR
  - 1 major & 3 minor criteria   OR
  - All 5 minor criteria

Major Criteria	Minor Criteria
Positive Blood Cultures: - 2 separate cultures positive for a typical IE micro-organism taken >12hrs apart - 3 positive cultures taken 1hr apart **Endocardial Involvement on Echo:** - Valvular vegetation - Abscess - New partial dehiscence of a prosthetic valve - New regurgitation murmur	**Pyrexia** >38°C **Predisposing Risk:** IVDU, predisposing cardiac condition **Vascular Phenomena:** - Major arterial emboli - Septic pulmonary infarcts - Intracranial haemorrhage - Conjunctival haemorrhages - Janeway's lesions - Mycotic aneurysm **Immunological Phenomena:** - Glomerulonephritis - Roth's spots - Rheumatoid factor - Osler's nodes **Microbiological Evidence:** - Positive blood cultures which do not meet the major criteria, or serological evidence of infection with organism consistent with IE

Q: Which micro-organisms cause infective endocarditis?

Bacteria	Fungi
Streptococcus -viridans (most common), -intermedius, -bovis	*Candida albicans*
Staphylococcus -aureus, -epidermidis	*Histoplasma capsulatum*
Pseudomonas aeruginosa	*Aspergillus*
Enterococcus	
HACEK (Haemophilus, Aggregatibacter, Cardiobacterium, Eikenella, Kingella)	

Q: How is infective endocarditis treated?

The mainstay of treatment is medical however early referral for surgery should be considered in patients with:

- Persistent bacteraemia
- Repeated embolisation
- Worsening LVF
- Fungal endocarditis
- Myocardial abscess
- Unstable infected prosthetic valves

Medical	Surgical
• Antibiotics	• Valve replacement
- Early microbiology input	
- Guided on cultures & sensitivities	
- Long course, high dose, intravenous	
• Treat complications (heart failure, emboli)	

Hypertension

Q: What is hypertension?

- A raised BP (systolic ≥140mmHg & diastolic of ≥ 90mmHg).
- Patients may be asymptomatic or present with symptoms secondary to target organ damage.

Q: What are the causes of hypertension?

Causes may be classified as primary / essential (no identifiable cause) & secondary (specific identifiable cause):

Cause	Interpretation
Primary	• 90% of all hypertension causes
/ Essential	• Genetic & environmental factors involved
Secondary	• **Renal:** Represents 80% of secondary causes
	- Intrinsic (75%): GN, PAN, PCKD
	- Renovascular (25%): RAS
	• **Endocrine:** Cushing's syndrome, hyperthyroidism, acromegaly, Conn's syndrome, hyperaldosteronism, hyperparathyroidism, phaeochromocytoma.
	• **Drugs:** Steroids, OCP, cyclosporin.
	• **Other:** Aortic coarctation, pregnancy, alcohol.

Q: What risk reduction advice would you give as part of hypertension management?

Lifestyle Modification	Dietary Modification
Smoking Cessation	Reduce Cholesterol & Saturated Fats
Exercise	Reduce Salt
Weight Loss	Reduce Alcohol
Stress Reduction	Increase Fruit, Vegetables & Oily Fish

Q: What are the complications of hypertension?

Site	Complication
Cerebral	• TIA
	• Intracerebral Haemorrhage e.g. CVA
	• Intracranial Haemorrhage e.g. SAH
	• Dementia
Ocular	• Hypertensive Retinopathy
Cardiac	• IHD, Angina, MI
	• Left Ventricular Hypertrophy
	• Heart Failure
	• Hypertensive Cardiomyopathy
Renal	• Hypertensive Nephropathy
	• CRF
	• ESRF
Vascular	• Peripheral Vascular Disease
	• Aortic Aneurysm
	• Carotid Artery Stenosis
	• Aortic Dissection

Q: What are the medical treatment options for hypertension?

The medical management of hypertension can be described, according to the British Hypertension Society (BHS), by the following algorithm:

Fig 3.8: The stepwise management of hypertension.

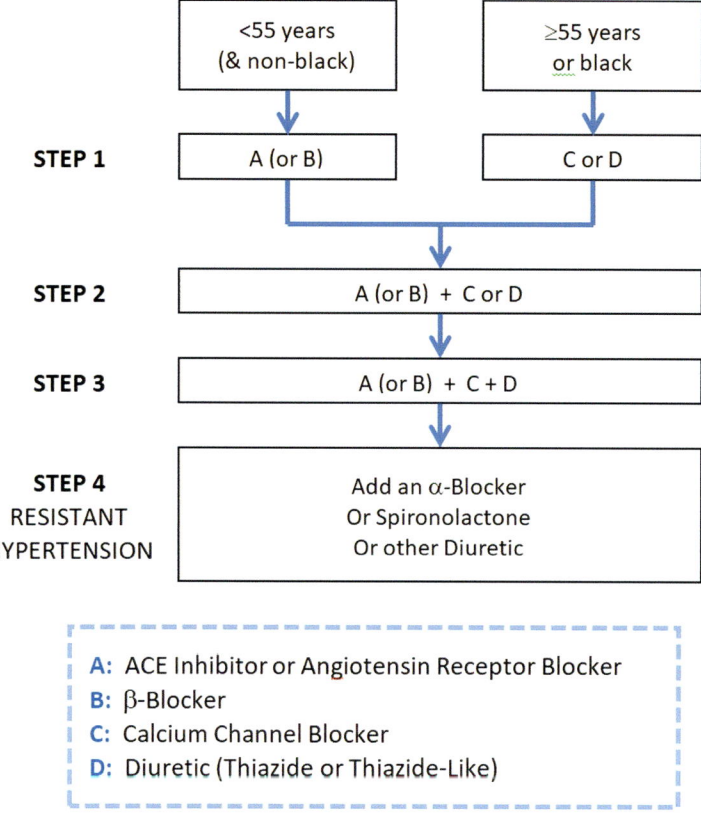

Atrial Fibrillation (AF)

Q: What is Atrial Fibrillation (AF)?

- AF is a cardiac arrhythmia.
- Regular electrical impulses from the sinoatrial node are disturbed by rapid irregular electrical discharges from the atria.
- Patients may be asymptomatic or complain of palpitations, SOB, chest pain, feeling faint or sudden collapse.
- ECG is usually diagnostic, revealing an irregularly irregular rhythm with no P waves (Fig 3.9).

Fig 3.9: ECG demonstrating Atrial Fibrillation.

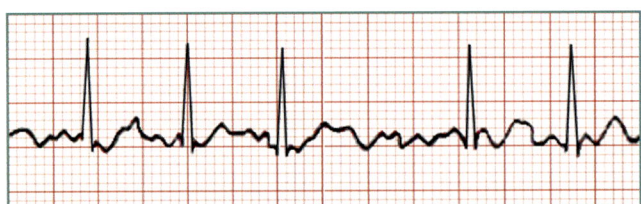

Q: What are the causes of AF?

Cardiac	Metabolic	Other
MI	Hyperthyroidism	Alcohol
Heart Failure	Hypokalaemia	Sepsis
Hypertension		Malignancy
Pericarditis		Pulmonary Embolus
Myocarditis		Trauma
Endocarditis		
Cardiomyopathy		
Cardiac Surgery		

Q: How would you investigate a patient found to be in AF?

After taking a **full history** & performing a **thorough clinical examination** I would consider the following:

Investigation	Interpretation
Observations	• Look for haemodynamic instability as this will affect management.
ECG **(Fig 3.9)**	• An irregularly irregular rhythm with no discernible P waves confirms diagnosis. • Atrial flutter (Fig 3.10) in contrast produces a characteristic 'saw-tooth' waveform on ECG with a tachycardia in the region of 300 beats per minute.
Blood Tests	• **FBC:** Infection = raised WCC. • **U&E:** Metabolic causes = deranged electrolytes. • **TFT:** Hyperthyroidism = low TSH. • **Thyroid Autoantibodies:** Graves' disease = anti-TSH receptor antibodies. • **Digoxin Levels:** If already on digoxin.
Septic Screen	Indicated in the presence of sepsis as a potential cause for AF.
Echo ± TOE	• Identify any valvular heart disease & mural thrombi which increase the risk of CVA.

Fig 3.10: ECG demonstrating Atrial Flutter.

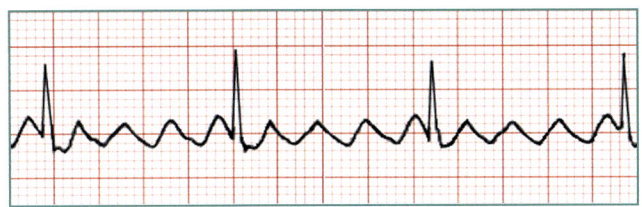

Q: What are the treatment options for AF?

AF with haemodynamic instability must be managed with immediate cardioversion, otherwise the following treatment options should be considered:

Management	Options
Rate Control	• β-Blockers • Cardiac Glycosides • Calcium Channel Blockers

Rhythm Control	• **Chemical Cardioversion**
	  - Amiodarone
	  - Flecainide
	• **Electrical Cardioversion**
	  - DC electrical shock (useful with associated hypotension)
	• **Catheter ablation of AV node**
	Note: There is a risk of embolisation unless the patient has been anticoagulated with heparin or warfarin

Anticoagulation	• Aspirin • Warfarin

Heart Block

Q: What is heart block?

A blockage, at any level, of cardiac electrical conduction:

- Sino-atrial (SA) node
- Atrio-ventricular (AV) node
- Bundle branches
- Fascicles

Q: How would you classify heart block?

1st Degree	2nd Degree	3rd Degree (Fig 3.13)
Prolonged PR interval on ECG	**Type 1 / Mobitz I / Wenckebach (Fig 3.11):** • Progressive PR interval prolongation resulting in a non-conducted P wave • Minimal haemodynamic disturbance • Asymptomatic patients do not usually require treatment	No electrical impulse transmission between the atria & the ventricles via the AV node (AV dissociation).
Does not normally cause haemodynamic disturbance	**Type 2 / Mobitz II (Fig 3.12):** • Intermittently non-conducted P waves not preceded by PR prolongation • May progress rapidly to complete heart block	Perfusing rhythm is usually maintained by a junctional or ventricular escape rhythm
		High risk of sudden cardiac death

Fig 3.11: ECG demonstrating second degree heart block (Mobitz I).

There is progressive PR interval prolongation resulting in a non-conducted P wave.

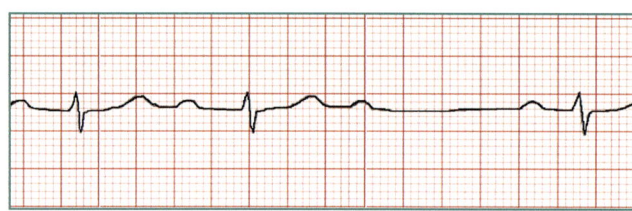

Fig 3.12: ECG demonstrating second degree heart block (Mobitz II).

There is intermittent P wave non-conduction without preceding PR prolongation.

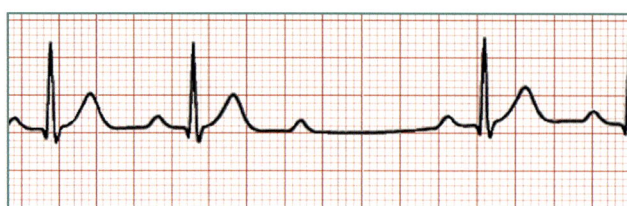

Fig 3.13: ECG demonstrating third degree heart block.

No electrical impulse transmission is seen between the atria & the ventricles via the AV node (AV dissociation).

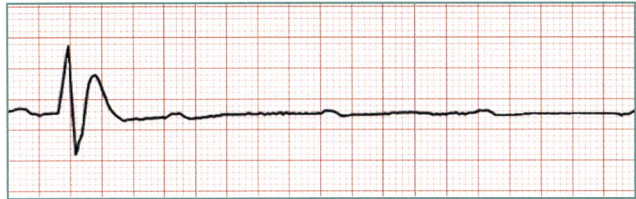

Q: What are the causes of heart block?

Acquired causes are more common than congenital causes.

Congenital	Acquired
All Heart Block Types	Acute MI
	Electrolyte Disturbances
	Infection
	Drugs e.g. β-Blockers, Calcium Channel Blockers, Digoxin
	Iatrogenic e.g. Open Heart Surgery

Q: How would you investigate a patient in heart block?

After taking a **full history** & performing a **thorough clinical examination** I would consider the following:

Investigation	Interpretation
Observations	Look for haemodynamic instability as this will affect management.
ECG	Looking for characteristic ECG features as described above.
Blood Tests	**FBC:** Infection = raised WCC.
	U&E: Metabolic causes = deranged electrolytes.
	Digoxin Levels: If already on digoxin.
Septic Screen	Indicated in the presence of sepsis.
Echo ± TOE	Indicated if there is suspicion of acute MI.

Q: What are the treatment options for heart block?

- Heart block does not always need treatment.
- Treat the underlying cause early.
- Transcutaneous pacing (TCP) if haemodynamically unstable followed by permanent pacemaker insertion.

Ventricular Tachycardia/Ventricular Fibrillation

Q: What is ventricular tachycardia (VT) (Fig 3.14)?

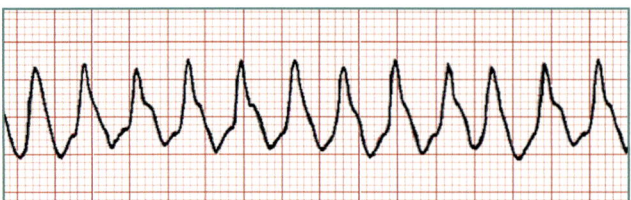

- VT is a broad complex tachycardia originating from a ventricular ectopic focus.
- It is defined as ≥3 successive ventricular extrasystoles at a rate of >120bpm.
- VT can be classified based by morphology or duration (i.e. sustained or non-sustained VT).
- Causes & treatment options include:

Cause	Treatment
Coronary Artery Disease	ALS guidelines
Structural Heart Disease	Electrical / chemical cardioversion
Electrolyte Disturbance: ↓K$^+$, ↓Ca^{2+}, ↓Mg^{2+}	
Sympathomimetic Agents: Caffeine, Cocaine	

Q: What is ventricular fibrillation (VF) (Fig 3.15)?

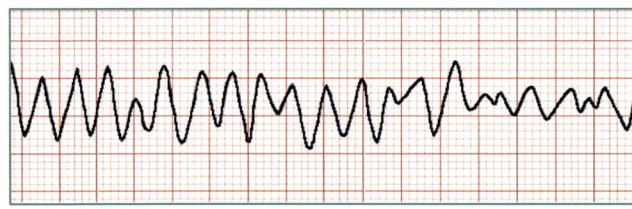

- VF is a condition in which there is uncoordinated contraction of the ventricular muscle fibres.
- This results in complete ventricular function failure, potential cardiac arrest & sudden death.
- Causes & treatment options include:

Cause	Treatment
Coronary Artery Disease (most common association)	Medical emergency & treatment as per ALS algorithm.
Acute MI / Ischaemia	Treat underlying cause.
Untreated VT	Implantable cardioverter defibrillator if high risk of recurrence.

Bradycardia

Q: What is bradycardia?

- Defined as a heart rate below 60 beats per minute (bpm).
- Absolute bradycardia is defined as a heart rate below 40 bpm.
- A relative bradycardia may be greater than 60 bpm if the rate is insufficient for haemodynamic requirements of a patient.

Q: What are the causes of bradycardia?

Cardio-Respiratory	Metabolic	Other
Acute MI	Hypothyroidism	Drugs e.g. β-Blockers, Calcium Channel Blockers, Digoxin
Hypoxia	Severe Obstructive Jaundice	Cushing's Reflex (systemic response to raised intracranial pressure)
Sick Sinus Syndrome	Adrenal Insufficiency	
Pericardial Tamponade		

Q: What are the treatment options for bradycardia?

Management is according to **ALS** guidelines:

Asymptomatic ± Haemodynamically Stable	Symptomatic ± Haemodynamically Unstable
Monitor & Observe	Give Atropine
	If ineffective:
	- Transcutaneous pacing
	- Dopamine or epinephrine infusion
	Consider:
	- Expert opinion
	- Transcutaneous pacing if efforts are ineffective

Cardiomyopathy

Q: What is cardiomyopathy?

- Disease of the cardiac muscle (myocardium).
- Often presents with heart failure.
- Classified as either:
  1. Dilated
  2. Hypertrophic
  3. Restrictive

Q: What are the aetiological, pathological & clinical features of cardiomyopathy?

	Dilated	Hypertrophic	Restrictive
Aetiology	• Idiopathic • Familial • MI • Drugs (cocaine, alcohol) • Infection (viral myocarditis, Chagas disease) • Pregnancy	• Genetic disorder (autosomal dominant) • May be a familial trait OR arise from *de novo* genetic mutation	• Amyloid • Sarcoid • Radiation • Haemochromatosis • Myocardial fibrosis
Pathology	• Most common cardiomyopathy • Presentation at 20-60 years • Progressive ventricular dilation = decreased ejection fraction	• Commonest cause of sudden death in young athletes • Affects sarcomere formation • Myocardium becomes abnormally thickened • LV dysfunction occurs due to stiffness & diastolic dysfunction ensues	• Least common cardiomyopathy • Progressive myocardial rigidity restricts diastolic filing
Clinical Features	• Fatigue • SOBOE • Orthopnoea & PND • Dysrhythmia (AF, SVT, VT) • S3 & S4 ± murmur • Ascites	• Often asymptomatic • Features of CCF • Sudden death	• CCF features • Decreased tissue perfusion

Q: How would you investigate cardiomyopathy?

After taking a **full history** & performing a **thorough clinical examination** I would consider the following:

Investigation	Dilated	Hypertrophic	Restrictive
CXR	• Cardiomegaly • Pulmonary oedema	• Normal / Cardiomegaly	• Normal / Cardiomegaly
ECG	• Sinus tachycardia • AF • LBBB & Right axis deviation	• ST / T wave abnormalities • AF	• Low voltage QRS complexes
Ambulatory ECG	• Ventricular arrhythmias	• Ventricular ectopics • Paroxysmal AF	• AF, ventricular arrhythmias
Echo	• Left ventricular dilatation (& thin walls) • Reduced ejection fraction • Mural thrombus • Left atrial enlargement • Mitral / tricuspid regurgitation	• Asymmetric ventricular & septal hypertrophy • Preserved systolic function	• Bi-atrial enlargement • Thickened ventricular walls • Moderate pulmonary venous hypertension
MRI	• Assess LVH severity	• Identify areas of infarction	• Not routinely performed
Cardiac Catheterisation	• Raised filling pressures	• Assess degree of outflow obstruction	• Raised diastolic pressures
Endomyocardial Biopsy	• Exclude differentials, e.g. amyloid	• Exclude differentials, e.g. amyloid	• Identify cause, e.g. amyloid, sarcoid
Radionucleotide Studies	• Assess left ventricular dilatation	• Not routinely performed	• Not routinely performed

Q: What are the treatment options for cardiomyopathy?

Treatment	Dilated	Hypertrophic	Restrictive
CONSERVATIVE	Education & counselling	Education & counselling	Education & counselling
MEDICAL	Treat CCF & arrhythmia	Treat CCF & arrhythmia, ventricular pacing	Treat CCF & arrhythmia
SURGICAL	Cardiac transplant in refractory cases	Septal ablation / myectomy, cardiac transplantation in refractory cases	Cardiac transplantation (poor prognosis)

Cardiac Tamponade

Q: What is cardiac tamponade?

- Cardiac tamponade is a medical emergency.
- Accumulation of fluid occurs in the pericardial space, causing mechanical ventricular obstruction. Diastolic filling is restricted, hence reducing end diastolic volume & subsequent stroke volume.
- Shock & death may occur rapidly, especially with trauma, if cardiac tamponade is not quickly diagnosed & treated.

Q: What are the causes of cardiac tamponade?

Mechanism	Cause

Iatrogenic	• Cardiac Instrumentation:
	  - Cardiac Pacing
	  - Cardiac Catheterisation
	• Cardiac Surgery

Cardiovascular	• Acute MI • Dissecting Thoracic Aortic Aneurysm • Acute Pericarditis
Trauma	• Penetrating Heart Trauma • Blunt Chest Wall Trauma
Other	• Renal Failure • SLE • Chest Wall Radiotherapy

Q: What are the clinical features of cardiac tamponade?

- There should be a high index of suspicion in chest trauma.
- It should always be considered in trauma patients presenting with PEA & no obvious cause of hypovolaemia or tension pneumothorax.
- The classic signs of cardiac tamponade are Beck's Triad, however other signs may be present:

Beck's Triad	Other Signs
Hypotension	Pulsus Paradoxus
Muffled Heart Sounds	Cyanosis
Raised JVP	Loss of Consciousness

Q: What specific investigations would you consider for cardiac tamponade?

Investigations	Examples
ECG	• Tachycardia
CXR	• Cardiomegaly
	• Globular Cardiac Shadow
Echo	• Pericardial Effusion

Q: How is cardiac tamponade treated?

After **simultaneous assessment & management** according to **ALS guidelines**, using an **ABC approach**, obtaining a **full history,** performing a **thorough clinical examination** & ordering **appropriate investigations**, I would consider the following treatment.

Medical	Surgical
High Flow Oxygen	Pericardiocentesis
IV Fluids	Pericardiectomy (pericardial window via thoracotomy)
Analgesia	

Pericarditis

Q: What is acute pericarditis?

- Acute occurrence of pericardial inflammation.
- As inflammation ensues, fluid accumulation occurs in the space between the visceral & parietal pericardial layers.
- Adhesion formation occurs between the pericardial layers & this may occasionally extend to involve the pleura & sternum.
- This space normally contains 20mls of fluid & can accommodate a further 120mls without significant haemodynamic compromise.

Q: What are the causes of acute pericarditis?

Classification	Interpretation
Neoplastic	• Accounts for 30%
Autoimmune	• Accounts for 25%
Infective	• **Viral:** Accounts for 20%
	• **Bacterial:** TB accounts for 5%, remaining bacteria account for a further 5%
Renal	• Uraemia accounts for 5%
Idiopathic	• Accounts for 5%
Other	Other causes account for 5-10% & include:
	• Trauma
	• Drugs e.g. hydralazine
	• MI
	• Myocarditis
	• Dissecting aortic aneurysm

Q: What are the clinical features of acute pericarditis?

Symptoms	Signs
Chest Pain: Commonest symptom. May be pleuritic in nature with concomitant pleural inflammation.	Tachycardia
Fever	Pericardial Rub
Fatigue	Pyrexia
SOB	Beck's Triad in Tamponade
Dry Cough	

Q: How would you investigate acute pericarditis?

After **simultaneous assessment & management** according to **ALS guidelines**, using an **ABC approach**, obtaining a **full history** performing a **thorough clinical examination** & ordering **appropriate investigations**, I would consider the following investigations:

Investigation	Interpretation
Blood Tests	• FBC
	• U&Es
	• Cardiac markers
	• Blood cultures
ECG	• Sinus tachycardia
	• ST elevation
	• PR depression
	• Low voltage QRS complexes
CXR	• Normal
	• Globular 'flask-shaped' cardiac shadow (with large effusions/ tamponade)
Echo ± TOE	• Identify a pericardial effusion
Cardiac MRI	• Pericardial inflammation
Pericardiocentesis	• MC+S

Q: What is the treatment of acute pericarditis?

Immediate	Short Term	Long Term
Pericardiocentesis (treat cardiac tamponade)	Analgesia	Corticosteroids
	NSAIDs	Colchicine (useful in recurring pericarditis)
	Corticosteroids	
	Antibiotics (if bacterial infection)	
	Stop Oral Anticoagulants (prevent tamponade)	

Q: What is constrictive pericarditis?

Pericardial inflammation resulting in a thickened, non-compliant pericardium. Ventricular filling & cardiac output is resultantly impaired.

Q: What are the causes of constrictive pericarditis?

Causes	
Infective	TB (in endemic areas)
Trauma	Post-traumatic/post-operative (following haemopericardium)
Neoplastic	Tumour related/post-radiotherapy
Idiopathic	Unknown cause

Q: What are the clinical features of constrictive pericarditis?

Symptoms	Signs
SOB on Exertion	Tachycardia
Worsening Fatigue	Raised JVP
	Kussmaul's Sign (JVP rises on inspiration)
	Pericardial Knock
	Right Heart Failure (hepatomegaly, ascites, fatigue & peripheral oedema)

Q: What are the treatment options for constrictive pericarditis?

Medical	Surgical
`First line treatment is symptomatic e.g. analgesia, diuretics	Definitive treatment is with pericardiectomy (high mortality 5-15%)

Cardiac Pericardiocentesis

Q: What are the indications for cardiac pericardiocentesis?

Indications for may be classified as:
- **Diagnostic** or **Therapeutic**.
- **Emergency** or **Non-Emergency:**

Emergency (Haemodynamically Unstable Patient)	Non-Emergency (Haemodynamically Stable Patient)
Cardiac Tamponade	Diagnostic
	Palliative
	Prophylactic

Q: How is percutaneous pericardiocentesis performed?

- Full pre-procedure assessment including history, examination & appropriate investigations.
- Explain procedure to patient & obtain informed consent.
- Ensure patient has supplemental O_2 & IV access.
- Position patient in semi-recumbent position (30°-45°).
- Attach cardiac monitor.
- Skin preparation & draping.
- Identify xiphoid process & infiltrate LA.
- Insert a wide bore needle just left of the xiphoid process at an angle of 45° to the skin.
- Aim the needle towards the tip of the left scapula.
- Watch for ectopic beats when the myocardium is touched.
- Aspirate whilst advancing the needle.
- If blood is aspirated attach a 3-way tap & syringe to remove larger amounts of blood.

Note: This is not a definitive procedure & blood has often already coagulated. Virtually all patients who require emergency pericardiocentesis for trauma will also require emergency thoracotomy. Ensure that cardiothoracic surgery & other relevant teams have been contacted well in advance.

Q: What are the complications of percutaneous pericardiocentesis?

Immediate	Early	Late
Arrhythmias	Fluid Re-Accumulation	Infectious Pericarditis
Coronary Vessel Injury	Coronary Artery Aneurysm	
Pneumothrax / Haemothorax		
Pneumopericardium		
MI		
Organ Perforation		
e.g. Lung, Liver, Stomach		

CHAPTER 4
RESPIRATORY

Ms Prita Daliya
Dr Christopher Lutterodt
Dr Emily McDonald
Dr Nicola Downer

CHAPTER CONTENTS

RESPIRATORY EXAMINATION

START: Start with the patient lying supine at 45°, exposed to underwear.
          Use sheet appropriately, to maintain patient dignity.

INSPECTION	Interpretation
GENERAL:	
General State	Assess for signs of breathlessness, cachexia, pain or distress.
Listen	Listen for stridor, wheeze, snoring & coughing.
Breathing Pattern	Look for signs of respiratory distress such as **nasal flaring**, **pursed-lip breathing**, **accessory muscle** use (sternocleidomastoid / abdominal muscles), **intercostal recession** or **tri-podding**.
Respiratory Rate (RR)	Observe/palpate over 1 minute. Normal = 12-14 breaths/min. **Note: Best performed whilst palpating the pulse, as making the patient aware that you are measuring the respiratory rate can cause it to change as they focus on their breathing.**
Scars (Fig 4.1)	Look at the anterior chest, back & under the axillae for scars indicative of previous surgery. • **Lateral thoracotomy:** Lobectomy, pneumonectomy. • **Sub-axillary:** Percutaneous lung biopsy, chest drain. • **Neck:** Lymph node biopsy.
HANDS:	
Tremor	• **Coarse tremor** e.g. CO_2 retention. • **Fine tremor** e.g. bronchodilator use.
Temperature	Warm & sweaty with pneumonia.
Peripheral Cyanosis	Blue discolouration of the fingertips e.g. hypoxia, low cardiac output & Raynaud's phenomenon.
Tar Staining	Yellow discolouration of the fingertips & nails from smoking.
Finger Clubbing (Fig 2.2)	Increased nail curvature *(also see abdomen chapter)*. The respiratory causes of which include fibrosing alveolitis, lung cancer & bronchiectasis.
Muscle Wasting	Intrinsic hand muscle wasting e.g. brachial plexus involvement with **Pancoast tumours.**
FACE:	
Horner's Syndrome	A combination of *ptosis, miosis* & *anhydrosis* due to an apical lung tumour invading the ipsilateral sympathetic chain.
Conjunctival Pallor	Anaemia.
Central Cyanosis	Bluish discolouration of the tongue & mucous membranes in hypoxia. This is a poor prognostic sign.

CHEST:	
Shape	May be associated with underlying lung pathology:
(Figs 4.2 - 4.4)	• **Pectus excavatum (funnel chest):** Restrictive lung disease.
	• **Pectus carinatum (pigeon chest):** Restrictive lung disease.
	• **Barrel chest:** Asthma, COPD.
	• **Scoliosis & Kyphosis:** Restrictive lung disease.
Chest Movement	Assess symmetry & depth. Asymmetrical movements may represent pathology on the side of reduced movement.

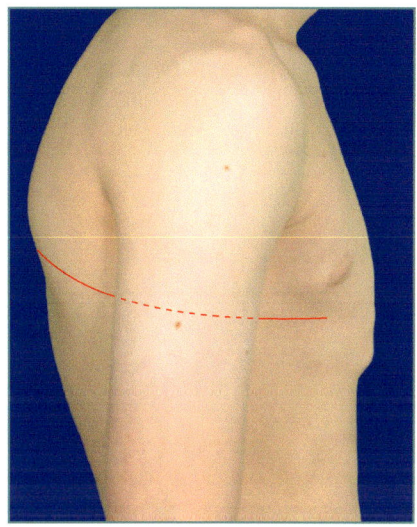

Fig 4.1: Right lateral thoracotomy scar.

Typically extends from the lateral chest under the nipple-areola complex, within the 5th intercostal space, then posteriorly to be in line with the scapula tip. This provides access for lobectomy, pneumonectomy & mediastinal structures e.g. oesophagus.

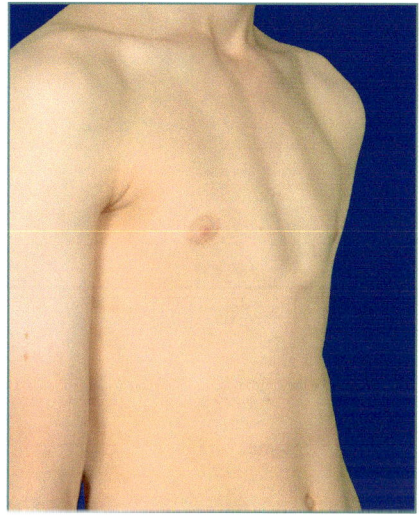

Fig 4.2: Pectus excavatum (funnel chest).

The most common congenital chest wall deformity. A sunken appearance of the sternum is noted. May be associated with restrictive lung disease.

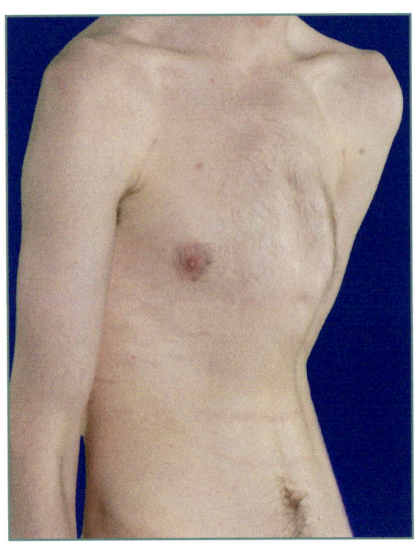

Fig 4.3: Pectus carinatum (pigeon chest).

Congenital protrusion of the sternum & ribs is noted, with characteristics resembling the chest wall of a pigeon. May be associated with restrictive lung disease.

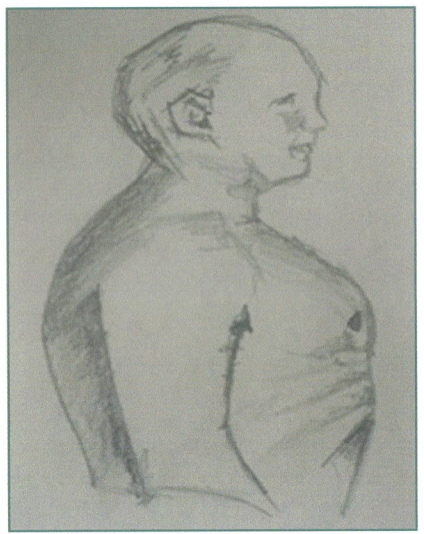

Fig 4.4: Barrel chest.

Increased AP diameter of the chest wall is illustrated. May result as a consequence of severe asthma / COPD.

Ask about pain.

PALPATION	Interpretation
Pulse Rate	A **bounding** radial pulse may be present in CO_2 retention & sepsis.
Supraclavicular Fossae	Palpate both supraclavicular fossae for enlarged **lymph nodes**, which may be associated with lung tumours or a **Pancoast tumour.**
Trachea Deviation (Fig 4.5)	With a ring & index finger on each sternoclavicular joint, use your middle finger on the same hand to assess for tracheal centrality.
	Tracheal deviation is **towards** a lobar collapse & **away from** a tension pneumothorax or massive pleural effusion.
Chest Expansion	Ask the patient to breathe in, then out fully. Quickly place your thumbs (facing up) on the patient parasternally, then place your index fingers in the line of the 5th intercostal spaces. Ask the patient to take a deep breath in. Normal expansion = 5-7cm. This is also grossly reduced in ankylosing spondylitis.
Tactile Vocal Fremitus	Place the ulnar border of the hand horizontally against the chest wall & ask the patient to say 'ninety-nine'. The transmitted vibrations are felt through the chest wall & will be increased (stronger) over areas of consolidation, & reduced (weaker or absent) over pleural effusions (Fig 4.6).
	Increased (stronger transmission) in consolidation.
	Reduced (weaker transmission) in pleural effusion (Fig 4.6), pneumothorax (Fig 4.7).

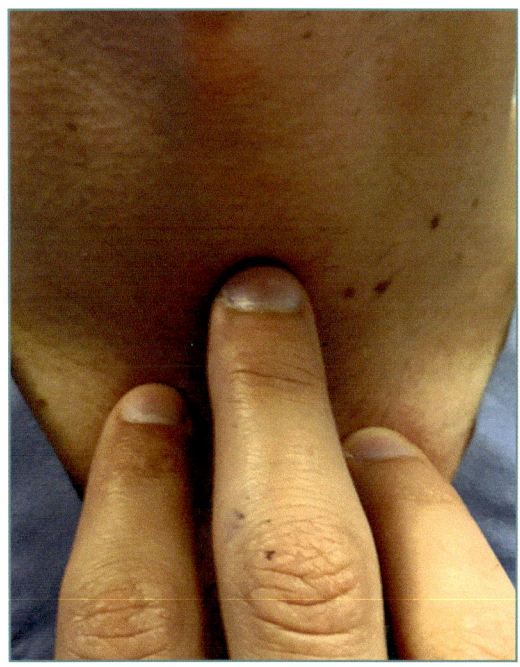

With a ring & index finger on each sternoclavicular joint, use your middle finger on the same hand to assess for tracheal centrality. **Tracheal deviation is towards a lobar collapse & away from a tension pneumothorax or massive pleural effusion**.

PERCUSSION	Interpretation
Chest	Percuss the anterior & posterior chest wall at 3 different levels. Remember to also percuss the lateral chest on each side (middle lobe on the right) & over the lung apices (over the clavicles/supraclavicular fossae). The percussion note helps to identify the underlying pathology:

- **Stony dull:**   Pleural effusion.
- **Dull:**   Consolidation, collapse.
- **Hyper-resonant:**   Pneumothorax

AUSCULTATION	Interpretation
Lung Fields	Use the stethoscope diaphragm to auscultate the anterior & posterior chest wall at 3 different levels. Remember to also auscultate the lateral chest on each side (middle lobe on the right), & over the supraclavicular fossae (lung apices).

Normal breath sounds will be **vesicular**.

Abnormal sounds include:

- **Bronchial breathing** in consolidation & lobar collapse. This is a coarse sound similar to breathing through a tube. It sounds similar to if you were to auscultate your own trachea & breathe deeply through your mouth.

- **Monophonic wheeze** in large airway obstruction.

- **Polyphonic wheeze** in small airway obstruction (e.g. asthma, COPD).

- **Crackles** in lung consolidation, fibrosis, bronchiectasis & pulmonary oedema.

Vocal Resonance	Using the stethoscope diaphragm, auscultate the chest whilst the patient **says** the phrase 'ninety-nine'.
	• **Increased resonance** (louder transmission) in consolidation.
	• **Reduced resonance** (quieter transmission) in pleural effusion (Fig 4.6), pneumothorax (Fig 4.7).
Whispering Pectoriloquy	Using the stethoscope diaphragm, auscultate the chest whilst the patient **whispers** the phrase 'ninety-nine'.
	• **Increased resonance** (louder transmission) in consolidation.
	• **Reduced resonance** (quieter transmission) in pleural effusion (Fig 4.6), pneumothorax (Fig 4.7).

COMPLETION	Interpretation
Peripheral Oedema	Pitting oedema of the legs / sacrum may be seen in cor pulmonale (see OSCE questions & answers section).
Abdominal Examination	Hepatomegaly & ascites in cor pulmonale.
Other Observations	O_2 saturations, BP, HR & temperature.
Sputum Sample	Assess colour, consistency, volume & for the presence of blood. Send for MC+S.
Further Investigations	PEFR, ABG, CXR, Spirometry / Lung Function Tests

FINISH:

OSCE QUESTIONS

Respiratory Clinical Features

Q: How would you clinically distinguish between pleural effusion, consolidation, lobar collapse & pneumothorax?

	Pleural Effusion (Fig 4.6)	Consolidation	Collapse	Pneumothorax (Fig 4.7)
Trachea Centrality	Central / Pushed Away from Affected Side	Central	Pulled Towards Affected Side	Central / Pushed Away from Affected Side
Chest Expansion	Reduced on Affected Side	Reduced on Affected Side	Reduced on Affected Side	Reduced on Affected Side
Percussion Note	Stony Dull	Dull	Dull	Hyper-Resonant
Breath Sounds	Reduced	Bronchial	Reduced	Reduced / Absent
Added Sounds	Crepitations & Bronchial Breathing Above Effusion	Bronchial, Coarse Crackles ± Rub	Crackles	None
Vocal Resonance	Reduced	Increased	Increased	Reduced
Whispering Pectoriloquy	Reduced	Increased	Increased	Reduced
Tactile Vocal Fremitus	Reduced	Increased	Reduced	Reduced / Absent

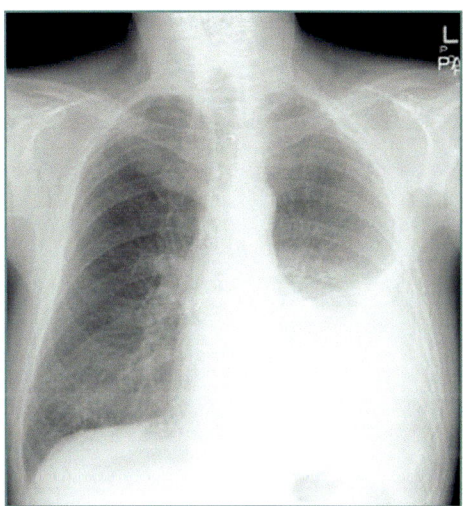

Fig 4.6: Left pleural effusion.

There is increased opacification of the left mid-lower lung with obscuration of the left hemidiaphragm & heart border. The left costophrenic angle is blunt & there is a meniscus at the superior border of the opacity. These features are in keeping with a left pleural effusion.

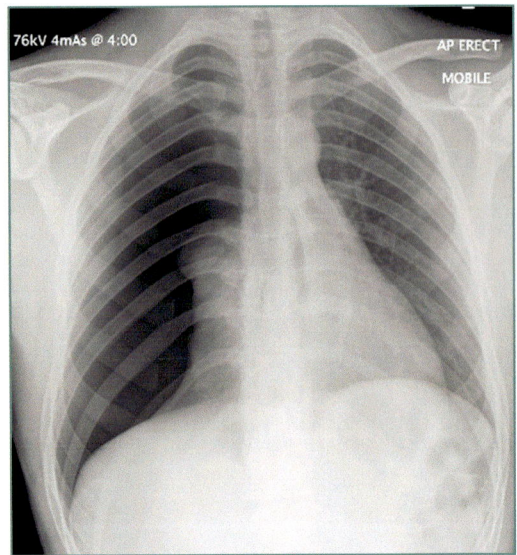

76kV 4mAs @ 4:00   AP ERECT
MOBILE

Fig 4.7: Right pneumothorax.

There is a sharp line (visceral pleura) outlining the edge of the right lung that is occupying a small volume of the right thoracic cavity. There are no lung markings beyond this line. The features are in keeping with a right pneumothorax.

Q: What is cor pulmonale?

- Right ventricular failure due to right ventricular hypertrophy from chronic pulmonary disease with associated pulmonary hypertension.
- Clinical features therefore relate to the underlying respiratory disease & right ventricular failure.

Pneumonia

Q: What is pneumonia?

- An inflammatory lung condition, usually of infective origin.
- It primarily affects the alveoli which become fluid-filled & impede adequate oxygenation & ventilation.

Q: What are the risk factors for the development of pneumonia?

Risk Factor	Notes
Age	• Younger Patients: <2 years
	• Older Patients: >65 years
Respiratory Disease	• Asthma
	• COPD
	• Bronchiectasis
	• Cystic Fibrosis
Lifestyle	• Smoking
	• Alcohol
Immunosuppression	• Diabetes Mellitus
	• HIV / AIDS
	• Immunosuppressants
	• Long-term Steroids
Drugs	• IVDU (*Staphylococcus aureus*)
Neurological	• CVA
	• Parkinson's Disease
Other	• Immobility
	• GI Stasis (vomiting, ileus, obstruction)
	• Following Intubation / GA
	• Post Major Surgery (following cardiothoracic / gastrointestinal surgery)

Q: How would you classify pneumonia?

Pneumonia may be classified by the **micro-organisms involved** e.g. viral, bacterial, atypical or as follows:

Classification	Interpretation
Community Acquired (CAP)	Unrelated to hospital admission.
Hospital Acquired (HAP)	≥2 days after hospital admission.
Immunocompromised	Immunocompromised patients are at greater risk e.g. DM, HIV, immunosuppressants & steroids.

Q: Which bacterial micro-organisms cause pneumonia?

- Bacterial pneumonia may be classified as community acquired, hospital acquired & atypical.
- Atypical pneumonia implies a less severe & gradual onset respiratory presentation, often consisting of a dry cough only.
- Extrapulmonary symptoms may be more troublesome to the patient e.g. diarrhoea, fatigue, headache, myalgia, nausea, sore throat & vomiting.

Community Acquired	Hospital Acquired	Atypical
Streptococcus pneumoniae (70%)	Pseudomonas	Mycoplasma
Haemophilus influenzae*	Klebsiella	Legionella
Chlamydia	Staphylococcus	Chlamydia
Legionella	Escherichia coli	
Mycoplasma		

* ***Haemophilus*** **is traditionally more common in children, however, HiB vaccination is resulting in a decreasing prevalence.**

Q: Aside from bacteria, which other micro-organisms cause pneumonia?

- Parasites, fungi & viruses may all cause pneumonia.
- HSV affects newborns & CMV classically affects immunosuppressed patients.

Parasites	Fungi	Viruses
Toxoplasma	Histoplasma	Adenovirus
Strongyloides	Cryptococcus	Influenza
	Pneumocystis	RSV
		HSV (newborns)
		CMV (immunosuppressed)

Q: Which micro-organisms are more likely to affect immunocompromised patients?

Bacteria	Viruses	Atypical
Streptococcus pneumoniae	CMV	Candida
Staphylococcus aureus	Adenovirus	Aspergillus
Haemophilus influenza		Pneumocystis carinii
		Mycobacteria

Q: What are the clinical features of pneumonia?

Pulmonary	Extra-Pulmonary
Cough	Fever / Rigors
Sputum	Malaise
SOB	Myalgia
Pleuritic Chest Pain	Nausea / Vomiting
Haemoptysis (uncommon)	Confusion (particularly in elderly)

Q: How would you investigate a patient with a suspected pneumonia?

After taking a **full history** & performing a **thorough clinical examination** I would consider the following investigations depending on the presentation & severity.

Investigation	Interpretation
Blood Tests	• FBC, U&E, LFT, CRP
	• ABG
	• Lactate (sepsis bundle)
	• Serology & Cold Agglutinins for Atypical Organisms
CXR	• Confirms Clinical Diagnosis
(Fig 4.8)	• Assess Complicating Features:
	- Infiltrates
	- Effusions
	- Consolidation
	- Cavitation
Microbiology	• Blood Cultures
	• Sputum Samples
	• Pleural Fluid Aspirate
	• ZN Staining for TB
	• PCR / Serology for Atypical Organisms
Other	• Bronchoscopy ± BAL
	• ECG, Echo & Cardiac Enzymes (exclude non-respiratory differential diagnoses)

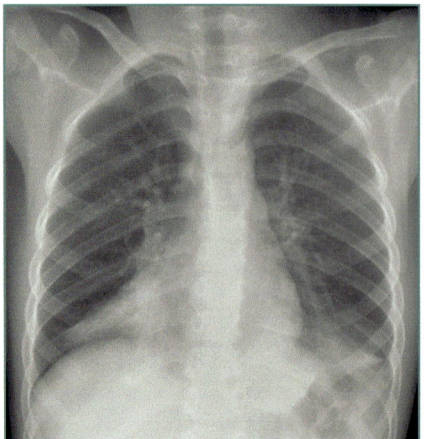

Fig 4.8: Right middle lobe pneumonia.

There is consolidation within the right lung field that obscures the right heart border, in keeping with a right middle lobe pneumonia.

Q: What are the complications of pneumonia?

These may be classified as pulmonary or extra-pulmonary as follows:

Pulmonary	Extra-Pulmonary
Empyema	**GENERAL:**
Lung Abscess	DVT (dehydration & immobility)
Pleural Effusion	Post-Streptococcus GN
Pneumothorax	**DUE TO SEPTICAEMIA:**
Post-Infective Bronchiectasis	Cerebral Abscess
	Endocarditis
	Meningitis
	Septic Arthritis

Q: What features are suggestive of a severe pneumonia with a high risk of mortality?

- **CURB-65** criteria help to predict mortality in Community-Acquired Pneumonia (CAP).
- Each risk factor scores 1 point (maximum 5).
- Mortality risk increases with score.

Feature	Interpretation
Confusion	New confusion (secondary to sepsis)
Urea	Serum urea ≥7mmol/L
Respiratory Rate	Tachypnoea ≥30 breaths/min
Blood Pressure	Systolic blood pressure <90mmHg
	Diastolic blood pressure <60mmHg
65	Age ≥65 years

- **Score 0-1:** Low mortality risk.
- **Score 2:** Moderate mortality risk.
- **Score ≥3:** High mortality risk, consider escalation to Level-2 care (critical care).

Q: How would you manage community acquired pneumonia (CAP) in adults?

- Initial assessment & management according to **ALS guidelines**, using an **ABC approach**, obtaining a **full history** & performing a **thorough clinical examination**.
- Initial antibiotic therapy is empirical but should subsequently be tailored to microbiological findings. Empirical treatment is based on severity of pneumonia as follows:
  - **Low Severity:** *Amoxicillin (PO)
  - **Moderate Severity:** *Amoxicillin + Clarithromycin (PO/IV)
  - **High Severity:** **Co-amoxiclav + Clarithromycin (IV)
    *Replace for doxycycline in penicillin allergy
    **Replace with cephalosporin in penicillin allergy
- Venous thromboprophylaxis.
- Nutritional optimisation.
- Respiratory physiotherapy including encouraging deep breathing, expectoration, postural drainage & mobilisation.

Tuberculosis (TB)

Q: What is TB?

- Common bacterial infection caused by *Mycobacteria spp.,* commonly *Mycobacterium tuberculosis.*
- Affects many parts of the body but is seen primarily affecting the lungs due to its transmission
- It is estimated that ⅓ of the world's population has been infected.
- Usually asymptomatic, however 10% result in active disease.
- Left untreated, active disease results in death in 50% of cases.

Q: What is the pathogenesis of TB?

- Highly infectious **granulomatous inflammatory disease**.
- Transmission is via aerosol droplet spread (sneezing, coughing, spitting).
- **Ghon focus** = primary lung infection, usually sited in the upper part of the lower lobe / lower part of the upper lobe.
- **Simon focus** = lung infection due to haematogenous spread, usually sited in the upper lobe.
- Immunocompromised individuals more likely to develop active disease.
- Granulomas form by aggregation of macrophages, T-cells, B-cells & fibroblasts.
- Granulomas may undergo central caseous necrosis giving them the texture of soft, white cheese.

- Infection often 'peaks & troughs', with healing by **fibrosis** & replacement of normal tissue with **scarring** & **cavitation** (Fig 4.9).
- Bacteria within granulomas may become **dormant,** resulting in latent infection.
- **Miliary TB** = haematogenous dissemination of multiple small white tubercles throughout body tissues. Occurs most commonly in young / immunocompromised patients. 30% mortality even with treatment (Fig 4.10).

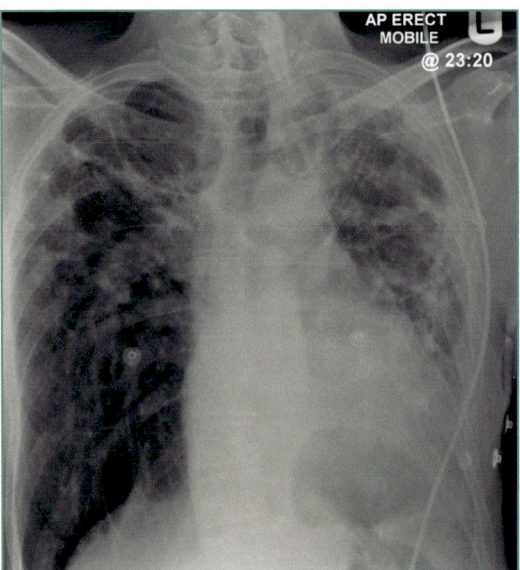

Fig 4.9: Chronic pulmonary TB.

Scarring, fibrosis & cavitation is seen throughout the upper lung fields.

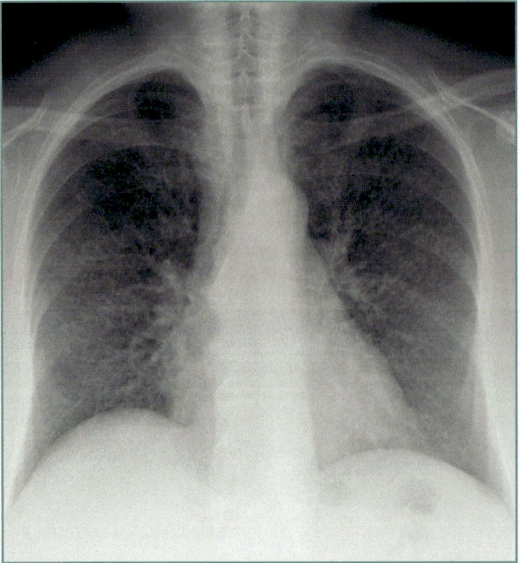

Fig 4.10: Miliary pulmonary TB.

Multiple small white 'millet seed like' nodules are seen throughout the lung fields in keeping with miliary pulmonary TB. This is due to haematogenous dissemination of multiple small white tubercles throughout body tissues. It occurs most commonly in young / immunocompromised patients. There is a 30% mortality even with treatment.

Q: What are the clinical features of TB?

- These may be classified as general features, those related to pulmonary disease (90% of infections develop in lungs) & extrapulmonary disease (20% of active disease spreads to other organs, particularly in immunocompromised individuals):

General Features	Pulmonary Disease	Extrapulmonary Disease
• Fever	• 25% Asymptomatic	• Meningitis
• Night Sweats	• Prolonged Productive Cough	• Neck Scrofula
• Appetite Loss	• Chest Pain	• Urogenital TB
• Weight Loss	• Haemoptysis	• Pott's Disease of Spine
• Fatigue	• Chronicity	• Osteomyelitis
• Clubbing	• Rasmussen's Aneurysm: *Erosion of infection into pulmonary artery = massive haemorrhage*	• Miliary TB

Q: How is TB investigated?

Screening	Investigation
Mantoux Test	**Microbiology:**
	• Blood, sputum & body fluids may be sent for MC+S.
	• ZN staining reveals acid-fast bacilli.
Heaf Test	**CXR**

Q: How is TB treated?

Prevention	Antibiotics	Epidemic Prevention
Bacillus Calmette–Guérin Vaccine (BCG)	Isoniazid & Pyridoxal Phosphate (6 months)	Notifiable Disease
	Rifampicin (6 months)	Contact Tracing
	Pyrazinamide (2 months)	
	Ethambutol (2 months)	

Q: What are the side effects of TB medication?

- Drug-resistant TB is an increasing public health concern.
- Specific drug side effects include:
  - **Isoniazid:** Peripheral neuropathy (pyridoxal phosphate is protective) & hepatotoxicity.
  - **Rifampicin:** Red-orange staining of body fluids & hepatotoxicity.
  - **Pyrazinamide:** Arthralgia & hepatotoxicity.
  - **Ethambutol:** Optic neuritis & red-green colour blindness.

Cystic Fibrosis (CF)

Q: What is CF?

- The most common chronic suppurative lung condition in Caucasians (1/2500 births).
- The name refers to the cysts (cystic) & scarring (fibrosis) commonly found in the pancreas.
- Due to autosomal recessive mutation in cystic fibrosis transmembrane conductance regulator gene (CFTR) on chromosome 7.
- The most common mutation (ΔF508) results in phenylalanine loss at position 508 on the protein. It is present in ⅔ of cases.
- Results in ciliated epithelial cells with defective chloride ion transport = sodium & water consequently also have decreased transport = thickened secretions.
- Clinical features include cough, SOB, production of dehydrated & viscous respiratory secretions.
- Lung parenchymal damage occurs due to recurrent chest infections.
- Respiratory failure may ensue.
- Non-respiratory clinical features are common. Many are related to thickened & altered secretions e.g. gastrointestinal malabsorption due to thickened, altered exocrine pancreas secretions.

Q: How is CF diagnosed?

Diagnosis is centred on a **full history** & **thorough clinical examination**, with any of the following parameters:

- **2 x Positive Sweat Tests:** The most common diagnostic investigation. Pilocarpine is administered to increase sweating & iontophoresis is used to detect increased sodium & chloride in the patient's sweat.
- **2 x Gene Mutations**
- **Nasal Eosinophilic Cationic Protein** (can be used for monitoring)

Q: What are the clinical features / complications of CF?

Respiratory	Gastrointestinal	Endocrine	Urogenital
Thick Sputum	Meconium Ileus (10 % of neonates)	Cystic Fibrosis Related Diabetes	Male Infertility (congenital absence of vas deferens)
Cough	Poor Growth & Failure to Thrive (children)	Osteoporosis	Female Infertility (thickened cervical mucus)
SOB	Intussusception		
Recurrent Chest Infections	Malabsorption & Weight Loss		
Bronchiectasis	Biliary Stasis (thickened secretions)		
Difficulty / Inability to Expectorate	Pancreatitis (thickened exocrine secretions)		
Respiratory Failure	General: Constipation, Abdominal Pain		

Q: What are the treatment options for CF?

Pulmonary	Extra-Pulmonary
MEDICAL:	Support Groups
Bronchodilators	Genetic Counselling
Steroids	Nutritional Supplementation
Chest Physiotherapy (postural drainage)	Nebulised Recombinant DNase
Mucolytic Medication e.g. Pulmozyme (Neb)	Pancreatic Enzyme Replacement
Antibiotics (for acute exacerbations & prophylaxis)	Diabetes Treatment
Immunisations (including influenza & pneumovax)	Bisphosphonates (to counteract steroid-related osteoporosis)
SURGICAL:	
Lung Transplantation	

Q: What is the prognosis for CF?

- Although prognosis is much better these days CF remains incurable.
- Treatment is aimed at improving quality of life, preventing & treating complications.
- Mean reported survival is approximately 30-50 years.

Bronchiectasis

Q: What is bronchiectasis?

- Obstructive lung disease characterised by irreversible bronchial tree dilation & destruction.
- This results in an excessive build-up of mucus which can be prone to infection.
- Usually results from recurrent pneumonia e.g. *Staphylococcus, Klebsiella, Bordetella pertussis.*
- Characteristic features include cough, excessive sputum production & SOB.
- Diagnosis is based on clinical history relating to cause (e.g. recurrent pneumonia) & CT.

Q: What are the causes of bronchiectasis?

Cause	Features
Congenital	• **α1-Antitrypsin Deficiency**
	• **CF**
	• **Kartagener's Syndrome:** *Primary ciliary dyskinesia, situs inversus, chronic sinusitis & bronchiectasis.*
	• **Young's Syndrome:** *Rhinosinusitis, reduced fertility & bronchiectasis.*
Infective	• **Bacterial:** Pneumonia / TB
	• **Fungal:** Aspergillosis
	• **Viral:** Measles / RSV / HIV
Inflammatory	• **RA**
	• **SLE**
	• **Ulcerative Colitis / Crohn's Disease**

Q: How is bronchiectasis treated?

- Treatment should address the cause:

Conservative	Medical	Surgical
Respiratory Physiotherapy (including postural drainage to clear secretions)	Oxygen	Lobectomy (medically resistant localised disease)
	Antibiotic Treatment (prophylaxis & acute exacerbations)	Lung Transplant (end stage disease)
	Bronchodilators (Inh)	
	Steroids (Inh & PO)	
	Immunoglobulin (IVI)	
	Immunisations (against pneumonia, influenza, pertussis)	

Pulmonary Embolism (PE)

Q: What is PE?

- An embolus passes from the venous circulation into the pulmonary circulation.
- The embolus commonly originates from a DVT.
- Other emboli could include air, fat, amniotic fluid or other foreign material.
- Once lodged in the pulmonary circulation, a ventilation-perfusion (V/Q) mismatch occurs = respiratory compromise & right ventricular strain.

Q: What clinical features would raise suspicion of PE?

- Taking a **full history** will demonstrate **relevant risk factors** e.g. DVT history, recent travel, recent surgery, co-existent malignancy.
- A **low-grade fever** may be present with associated pulmonary haemorrhage / infarction.
- 15% of all **sudden death** cases are due to PE.
- Remaining clinical features may be classified as follows:

Classification	Symptoms	Signs
Respiratory	· SOB	· Tachypnoea
	· Cough	· Pleural Rub
	· Pleuritic Chest Pain	· Pleural Effusion
	· Haemoptysis	· Cyanosis
Cardiac	· Palpitations	· Tachycardia
		· Hypotension
		· Raised JVP
DVT	· Painful Calf	· Tender & Swollen Calf

Q: What is the Well's score?

- Calculates the probability that a PE is present.
- Utilises a series of parameters, which are allotted points as follows:

Well's Parameters	Points
PE = Most Likely Diagnosis	3.0
DVT Clinically Suspicious	3.0
DVT / PE History	1.5
Immobilisation for ≥3 Days / Surgery Within Previous 4 Weeks	1.5
HR >100bpm	1.5
Haemoptysis	1.0
Malignancy	1.0

- **Score >6:** High PE Risk
- **Score 2-6:** Moderate PE Risk
- **Score <2:** Low PE Risk

Q: What investigations would you consider for suspected PE?

Investigations	Interpretation
Blood Tests	• **FBC, U&E, LFT, CRP, ESR, Coagulation Screen**
	• **D-Dimer:** *High negative predictive value for DVT / PE = a normal D-dimer excludes DVT/ PE.*
	• **ABG**
ECG	• **Sinus Tachycardia:** *Commonest abnormality seen.*
	• **RBBB / RAD**
	• $S_1Q_3T_3$**:** *S wave in Lead I, Q wave in Lead III, T wave inversion in Lead III.*
CXR	• **Wedge Shaped Shadows:** *From pulmonary infarction.*
	• **Excludes Differential Diagnoses**
V/Q Scan	• **V (ventilation) / Q (perfusion) Mismatch**
CTPA	• **Identify Embolus Site & Size**
Echo / TOE	• **Exclude Cardiac Differentials**
Doppler USS Legs	• **Look for DVT**

Q: How would you treat PE?

- Initial assessment & management is according to **ALS guidelines**, using an **ABC approach**, obtaining a **full history** & performing a **thorough clinical examination**.
- Specific treatment options include:

Treatment	Interpretation
Resuscitation	• A full resuscitative approach is necessary:
	- **Airway:** *High flow oxygen (15 L/min).*
	- **Breathing:** *Sit the patient up.*
	- **Circulation:** *Ensure IV access (2 large bore cannulae), IV fluids to maintain systolic BP at 100mmHg.*
Anticoagulation	• SC low molecular weight heparin (1.5mg/kg).
	• Change to warfarin prior to discharge (target INR=2.5, range=2-3).
Thrombolysis	• Indicated in haemodynamic instability secondary to massive PE.
Surgery	• Pulmonary thrombo-endarterectomy (rarely performed) carries a high mortality risk (25-30%), but may be required with thrombolysis failure / contraindications.
IVC Filter	• Useful if high risk of further embolisation / recurrent PE, or when anticoagulation is ineffective / contraindicated.

Asthma

Q: What is asthma?

- Classically, a type I hypersensitivity condition (classically extrinsic type).
- Bronchial inflammation, bronchospasm & reversible airways obstruction ensues.

Q: What types of asthma do you know of?

Classification	Interpretation
Extrinsic	• Atopic Association e.g. Asthma/ Hay Fever
	• Type I Hypersensitivity Reaction (IgE Mediated) to Allergen e.g. Pollen / Dust
	• Familial Trait
	• Presents in Childhood
Intrinsic	• Non-Atopic
	• Non-IgE Mediated Response
	• Adult Onset
	• 'Hyper-Reaction' of Airways to 'Irritant'
	• Precipitated by:
	- Emotional Extremes e.g. Laughing / Crying
	- Chemicals e.g. Smoke / Aspirin / Cleaning Agents
	- Chest Infection
	- Exercise e.g. Exercise-Induced Asthma

Q: What pathophysiological processes occur in type I hypersensitivity conditions such as extrinsic asthma?

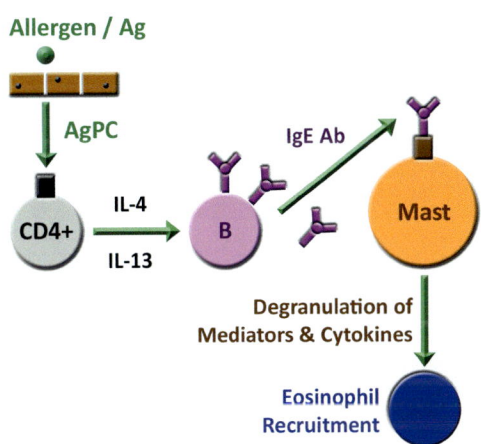

Fig 4.11: Type I hypersensitivity.

Allergen / Ag & APC

CD4+ Helper T-Lymphocytes release IL-4 & IL-13

B Cells release IgE Ab

Mast Cells Degranulate Mediators & Cytokines after Binding IgE Ab

Eosinophil Recruitment Occurs

1. Allergens are inhaled (or ingested).
2. These allergens / antigens are recognised by dendritic antigen presenting cells.
3. CD4+ T-helper cells are targeted by antigen presenting cells.
4. T-helper cells release IL-4 & IL-13.
5. B-cells produce IgE antibodies that are antigen-specific, in response to IL-4 & IL-13 release.
6. IgE antibodies bind to mast cells & basophils which degranulate & release mediators & cytokines.
7. Mediators & cytokines result in symptoms & recruitment of cells e.g. IL-5 & eosinophils.

Q: What are the clinical features of asthma?

- Expiratory polyphonic wheeze is characteristic.
- Cough, SOB, chest tightness.
- Acute attacks characteristically develop over minutes, although may develop over hours, days or more chronically following a gradual decline in respiratory function.

Q: What investigations would you consider for asthma?

Investigation	Interpretation
ACUTE ASTHMA:	
PEFR	Assess severity of acute attack.
	PEFR <33% of predicted / best recording = severe life threatening attack.
Blood tests	FBC, CRP, ESR to exclude infection.
CXR	Exclude pneumothorax (Fig 4.7) / pneumonia (Fig 4.8).
ABG	Type I respiratory failure in early stages of an acute attack, but may progress to type II once the patient becomes exhausted.
CHRONIC ASTHMA:	
PEFR	Patients with diurnal variation, in particular a reduction in early morning PEFR are at risk of sudden acute attacks.
CXR	Exclude chest infection.
Spirometry	FEV_1/FVC ratio <70% = obstructive lung disease pattern (normal range = 70-75%).

Q: What are the features of acute severe & life threatening asthma?

Acute Severe	Life Threatening
PEFR 33-50% of predicted or best	PEFR <33% of predicted or best
Tachypnoea ≥25 breaths/min	SpO_2 <92% or P_aO_2 <8kPa
Tachycardia ≥110bpm	Normal P_aCO_2 (4.6-6.0kPa)
Unable to complete a sentence in one breath	Silent chest
	Central cyanosis
	Poor respiratory effort
From British Thoracic Society Guidelines 2011	Arrhythmia
	Exhaustion, altered conscious level

Q: What are the treatment options for acute asthma?

Treatment	Interpretation
Oxygen	• Sit the patient up.
	• High flow oxygen (15L/min) to maintain SpO_2 between 94%-98%.
β₂-Agonist Bronchodilator	• 5mg salbutamol nebuliser, repeated as required.
Ipratropium Bromide	• 0.5mg ipratropium bromide nebuliser.
	• Repeat 4-6 hourly if necessary.
Sterolds	• 200mg IV prednisolone.
	• Then oral prednisolone (40-50 mg daily) for at least 5 days.
Magnesium Sulphate	• Consider IV infusion in patients with a poor response to β₂-agonist treatment / life threatening asthma.
	Note: Consider only after discussion with a specialist.
Intravenous Bronchodilator	• Consider IV infusion of salbutamol / aminophylline if no improvement on nebulisers.
Antibiotics	• Start empirical treatment with signs of infective exacerbation.
	• Routine administration is not indicated.
Escalation of Care	• Consider early referral to ITU in the presence of worsening hypoxia, exhaustion, type 2 respiratory failure or failure of treatment.

Memory: Nebulisers should be oxygen-driven not air-driven.

Q: What is the stepwise approach to the management of chronic asthma?

Fig 4.12: Asthma medical treatment.

Based on BTS Guidelines. Patients should be started on the step required for their asthma severity & stepped up/down as necessary. SAβA: short acting β_2-agonist, LAβA: long acting β_2-agonist.

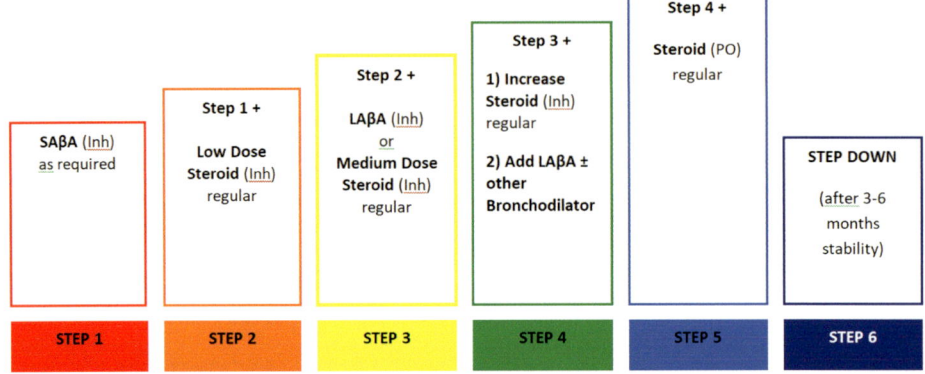

Chronic Obstructive Pulmonary Disease (COPD)

Q: What is COPD?

- COPD is a chronic progressive obstructive airways condition.
- It is mostly irreversible.
- It encompasses emphysema & chronic bronchitis.
- There is often a history of smoking ≥20 pack years.
- Affects 15-20% of smokers.

Q: What are the differences between chronic bronchitis & emphysema?

Chronic Bronchitis   **Symptomatic Definition:** *Cough productive of sputum for ≥3 months & for ≥2 consecutive years.*

Memory: 'Blue Bloater'

- Cyanosis   (Blue)
- Overweight   (Bloater)
- Hypoventilation
- Chronic CO_2 Retention Features e.g. Bounding Pulse, Warm Peripheries, Tremor

Emphysema   **Pathological Definition:** *Permanent dilation & destruction of the tracheobronchial tree, distal to the terminal bronchioles, with destruction of alveolar septae.*

Memory: 'Pink Puffer'

- No Cyanosis
- Thin & Polycythaemia   (Pink)
- Hyperventilation   (Puffer)

Q: What are the clinical features of COPD?

Clinical Features	Chronic Bronchitis		Emphysema	
SOB	Intermittent		Progressive	
Cough	Persistent & Severe		Absent / Mild	
Sputum	Copious		Absent / Mild	
Central Cyanosis	Present	(Blue)	Absent	
Body Habitus	Overweight	(Bloater)	Thin + Polycythaemia	(Pink)
Respiration	Hypoventilation		Hyperventilation	(Puffer)
Plethoric Face	Present		Absent	
Barrel Chest	Absent		Present	
Percussion Note	Normal		Hyper-Resonant	
Auscultation	Wheeze		Decreased Breath Sounds	

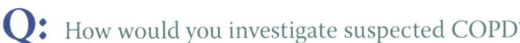

Q: How would you investigate suspected COPD?

After taking a **full history** & performing a **thorough clinical examination**, I would consider the following investigations:

Investigation	Interpretation
FBC	Polycythaemia.
	WCC may be elevated in infective exacerbations.
ABG	To measure degree of hypoxia, monitor hypercarbia & distinguish between type I / type II respiratory failure.
CXR	• **Chronic Bronchitis:** Increased bronchovascular markings, cardiomegaly.
	• **Emphysema:** Hyperinflated lungs, flat hemidiaphragms, bullae.
	• Identify infective exacerbation.
	• Exclude a complicating pneumothorax (Fig 4.7).
PEFR	In contrast to asthma there is little variability in COPD.
Spirometry	A FEV_1/FVC ratio <70% = obstructive airways disease (normal range = 70-75%).
	<15% response to reversibility is significant.

Q: What are the treatment options for COPD?

Conservative	Medical (Fig 4.13)	Surgical
• Smoking Cessation	Bronchodilators (Inh)	Bullectomy
- Support Groups		
- Nicotine Replacement Therapy		
• Chest Physiotherapy	Corticosteroids (Inh)	Lung Transplant
• Dietician Input	Mucolytic Therapy	
	Vaccination:	
	- Influenza	
	- Pneumococcus	
	Antibiotics (acute exacerbations)	
	Ambulatory / Long-Term Oxygen Therapy	
	ITU & Ventilation (respiratory failure)	

Fig 4.13: COPD medical treatment.

Based on BTS guidelines.

* SAβA as required may continue at all stages. ** Discontinue SAMA.

SAβA: Short-acting β₂ agonist, SAMA: Short-acting muscarinic antagonist, ICS: Inhaled corticosteroid, LAβA: Long-acting β₂ agonist, LAMA: Long-acting muscarinic antagonist.

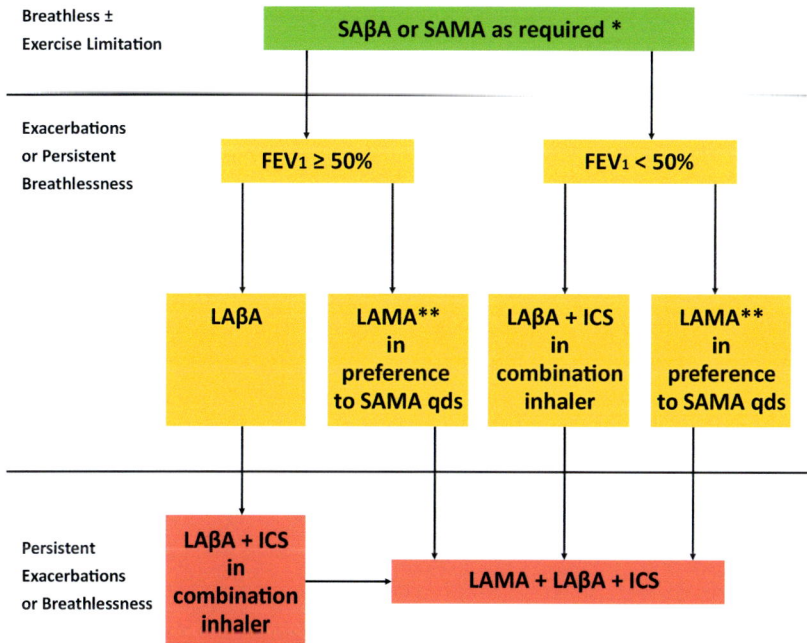

Q: What are the complications of COPD?

Pulmonary	Extra-Pulmonary
Pneumonia	**Polycythaemia**
Cor Pulmonale (pulmonary hypertension & right heart failure)	**Osteoporosis** (Secondary to multiple courses of PO steroids)
Pneumothorax	**Depression / Anxiety**
Respiratory Failure	

Lung Cancer

Q: What is lung cancer?

- Malignant tumour of the lung parenchyma.
- Leading cause of cancer-related death in western countries.

Q: What are the risk factors for developing lung cancer?

Environmental	Respiratory
Smoking	COPD
Passive Smoking	Idiopathic Pulmonary Fibrosis
Asbestos Exposure	TB
Radon Gas Exposure	
Arsenic Exposure	

Q: How may lung cancer present?

- The majority of patients are symptomatic at diagnosis (90%).
- Constitutional symptoms include fatigue, anorexia, weight loss.
- Respiratory symptoms include cough, breathlessness, haemoptysis, pleuritic chest pain.
- Metastatic symptoms are due to local invasion e.g. Horner's syndrome due to a Pancoast tumour, or distant spread e.g. liver, bone, brain.
- Paraneoplastic syndromes may be present e.g. hypercalcaemia (PTHrP), SIADH (ADH), Cushing's syndrome (ACTH).

Q: What types of lung cancer do you know of?

Classification	Interpretation
Non Small Cell	• 75% of all lung cancers
	• **Squamous Cell:** Commonest, associated with smoking, commonly affects main airways (right/left bronchus)
	• **Adenocarcinoma:** Prevalence increasing, affects respiratory mucosa
	• **Large cell:** Grows rapidly, cells look large & round at microscopy
Small Cell	• 20% of all lung cancers
(oat cell cancer)	• Cells look small, with large nuclei at microscopy (oat cells)
	• Related to smoking
	• Early metastases to liver, bone, brain
Secondary	• <5% of all lung cancers
	• Metastases from elsewhere
	• Common primary sites include colorectal & breast
Mesothelioma	• <5% of all lung cancers
	• Pleural tumour
	• Related to previous asbestos exposure

Q: What are the investigations for lung cancer?

Investigation	Interpretation
Blood Tests	FBC, U&E, LFT, CRP
CXR (Fig 4.14)	Initial diagnosis & complicating features e.g. pneumonia, effusion, collapse
Chest CT / PET-CT	High-resolution imaging for detail on local spread
Bronchoscopy ± Biopsy	Direct visualisation & tissue sampling for histopathology
Sputum Cytology	If histological biopsy not possible
CT-Guided Biopsy	Guided percutaneous biopsy
Videothoracoscopy (VATS) / Mediastinoscopy	Guided percutaneous biopsy
Identify Metastases	**CT abdomen / pelvis:** liver, adrenal metastases
	CT head: brain metastases
	Bone scan: bone metastases
Identify Primary	Immunostaining tissue biopsy (immunohistochemistry / immunocytochemistry)

The following investigations may also be required for Paraneoplastic Syndromes related to lung carcinomas:

Paraneoplastic Syndrome	Investigation
Hypercalcaemia	PTHrP
Hypoglycaemia	Insulin-like growth factor
SIADH	ADH
Carcinoid	Serotonin
Cushings	ACTH

Fig 4.14: Cavitating bronchogenic carcinoma.

There is opacification in the left lung field with central cavitation, associated hilar lymphadenopathy & blunting of the left costophrenic angle in keeping with a pleural effusion. These features are in keeping with a left cavitating bronchogenic carcinoma.

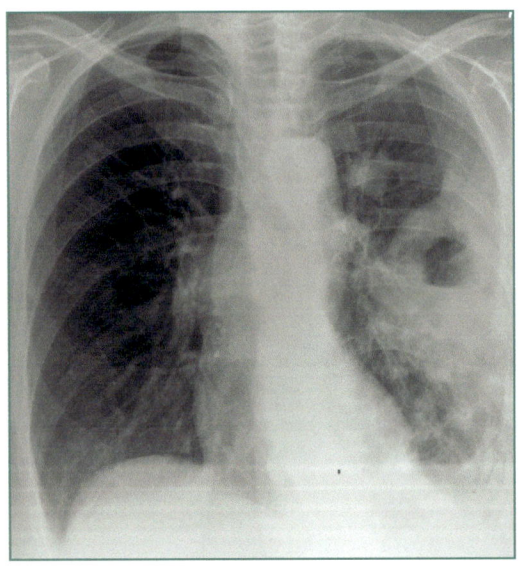

Q: How is lung cancer treated?

Treatment is managed within a MDT environment, depending on stage & respectability. Treatment options include:

Conservative	Medical	Surgical	Palliative
Support Groups	Chemotherapy	Lobectomy (lung partly removed)	Symptom Relief: - Analgeia - Nebulisers - Oxygen
Counselling	Radiotherapy	Pneumonectomy (lung completely removed)	Radiotherapy (bone pain)
	Biological Therapy: - Erlotinib - Gefitinib - Crizotinib		

Interstitial Lung Disease (ILD) / Diffuse Parenchymal Lung Disease (DPLD)

Q: What is ILD / DPLD?

- ILD / DPLD refers to a group of lung diseases that affect the lung interstitium.
- These diseases are distinguished from obstructive airways disease.
- The 3 most common diseases are asbestosis, chronic silicosis & coal worker's pneumoconiosis.
- Alveolar epithelium, pulmonary capillary endothelium, basement membrane, perivascular & perilymphatic tissues are involved.
- Prolonged ILD usually results in pulmonary fibrosis.
- Patients present with SOB, but may have an associated cough, wheeze or chest pain.

Q: What are the causes of ILD / DPLD?

Causes may be classified as:

Causes	Interpretation
Idiopathic	• Sarcoid
	• Idiopathic Pulmonary Fibrosis
Inhaled Substances	• Silicosis
	• Asbestosis
	• Coal Workers' Pneumoconiosis (CWP)
	• Berylliosis
Drugs	• Antibiotics
	• Chemotherapeutics
	• Antiarrhythmics
	• Statins
Connective Tissue Disorders	• Systemic Sclerosis
	• Dermatomyositis / Polymyositis
	• SLE
	• RA
Infective	• Atypical Pneumonia
	• PCP Pneumonia
	• TB
	• *Chlamydia trachomatis*
	• RSC
Malignant	• Lymphangitic Carcinomatosis

Q: Which investigations would be useful to aid diagnosis?

Investigation	Result
CXR	• Pulmonary fibrosis in CWP
	• Pleural plaques & calcification in asbestosis (Fig 4.15)
	• Eggshell calcification in silicosis
	• Pulmonary shadowing in cryptogenic fibrosing alveolitis
	• Ground glass appearance in ARDS
Lung Function Tests	• Restrictive picture
	• Impaired gas transfer
Blood Tests	• FBC
	• ESR
	• TFTs
	• Autoimmune profile
Urinalysis	• Proteinuria
	• Haematuria
High Resolution CT	• The most accurate imaging method
Transbronchial Lung Biopsy **BAL**	• May give further information e.g. if malignancy cannot otherwise be excluded

Fig 4.15: Asbestosis.

Left pleural thickening & calcification (pleural plaques) & diaphragmatic calcification is seen. The features are in keeping with left pulmonary asbestosis.

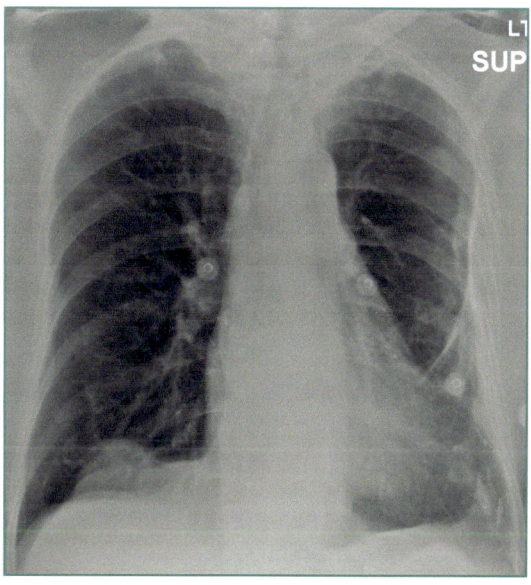

Q: What is the treatment in symptomatic individuals?

Conservative	Medical
Removal / Avoidance of Causative Factors	Analgesia
	Antibiotics (infective exacerbations)
	Corticosteroids
	Supplemental Oxygen (with hypoxaemia)

Sleep Apnoea

Q: What is sleep apnoea?

- Periods of disordered breathing during sleep.
- Patients experience *apnoea* (pauses in respiration) or *hypopnoea* (shallow breathing / reduced respiratory rate), while sleeping.
- Patients experience daytime somnolence (feeling tired during the day) due to restless sleep.
- Partners may witness extremely vigorous snoring & periods of apnoea such that patients may present on their partner's advice!

Q: How is sleep apnoea classified?

Classification	Features
Obstructive	• Decreased pharyngeal tone & excess soft tissue = airway constriction.
	• Risk factors include: males, age >65, obesity, excess ETOH, smoking.
Central	• Failure in the brain's respiratory control centre = normal respiratory drive suppression.
	• More prevalent in males >65 years.
	• Also associated with serious illness e.g. IHD, CVA, CNS trauma.
Mixed	• Mixture of obstructive & central sleep apnoea.

Q: What investigations would you consider in sleep apnoea?

After taking a **full history** & performing a **thorough clinical examination** I would consider the following investigations:

Investigation	Features
Sleep Diary	• Indicates patterns of sleep, including number of times patient wakes at night & if they feel rested in the morning.
	• The patient's partner can also record episodes of apnoea / snoring if observed.
Polysomnography	• Sleep cycle studies are diagnostic & correlated with oximetry but are expensive.
	• O_2 saturations fall during periods of apnoea.

 Q: How is sleep apnoea treated?

Treatment should be focused on conservative measures with surgical options reserved as a last resort.

Conservative	Medical	Surgical
Weight Loss	**Acetazolamide** (reduces pH for respiration)	**Relieve Nasal Congestion:** Septoplasty / Turbinate Surgery
Appropriate Sleeping Environment	CPAP	**Reduce Pharyngeal Obstruction:** Tonsillectomy / Uvulopalatopharyngoplasty / Maxillomandibular Advancement
Appropriate Sleeping Schedule		**Stiffen Soft Tissues:** Pillar Procedure (insertion of Dacron pillars into the soft palate) / Hyoid Bone Myotomy
Mandibular Advancement Device		

CHAPTER 5
BREAST

BH Miranda
DT Sharpe
V Ramakrishnan

CHAPTER CONTENTS

BREAST EXAMINATION

START: Patient exposed from the waist upwards, lying at 45°.

Maintain the patient's dignity using e.g. bed sheet.

Chaperone is vital.

When asked to examine the breasts, remember to systematically examine as follows:

1. Lumps should be considered as any other lump & should be addressed first.

2. Features of breast disease should be considered next.

3. The above points should be considered both with the patient's hands behind their head (to accentuate lumps, asymmetry & tethering) & pushing against their hips (to accentuate lumps attached to the pectoralis muscle). It is additionally possible to inspect the breasts with the patient leaning forward over the side of the bed (to accentuate abnormalities in large breasts).

4. Once all the above points are addressed for the 'good' breast first, remember afterwards to compare with the 'diseased' breast i.e. inspect for lumps & breast features of the good breast, then the diseased breast; then palpate for lumps & breast features of the good breast, then the diseased breast.

If you are asked to examine a breast lump that you are unable to identify, you may wish to ask the patient if they have noticed any lumps anywhere.

INSPECTION	Interpretation
6 x S's	Describe lump site, size, shape, symmetry, overlying skin & associated scars (*see lumps 'n' bumps chapter*).
Fungation	Comment on presence of fungating carcinoma. It is important to **check the inframammary fold** that may hide a fungating carcinoma & other breast signs.
Asymmetry	Carcinoma may be present in the higher breast (Fig 5.1).
Tethering	Due to infiltration of the ligaments of Astley-Cooper.
Peau D'Orange	Due to micro-oedema.
Lymphoedema	May indicate lymphatic infiltration by carcinoma, or previous surgery with lymph node removal.
Nipple Signs	**Memory:** **Remember the 6 x D's of nipple disease:** • Paget's **D**isease (Fig 5.2) • **D**ischarge • **D**epression • **D**eviation • **D**isplacement • **D**estruction

Ask about pain.

Remember to examine the good breast first, then the diseased breast, according to the system described above.

Check for temperature changes, using the back of your hand.

PALPATION	Interpretation
SEC FFP TR	Palpate lump surface, edge, consistency, fixity to skin & underlying structures, fluctuance, pulsatility & expansility, transilluminability & reducibility.
Breast	Palpate the breast using the palmar surfaces of the index, middle & ring fingers of both hands in succession, sweeping down the clock face positions of the good breast first, then the diseased breast. Remember to thoroughly examine each breast with the patient's hands behind their head, then pressing against their waist. **Note: Most carcinomas present in the upper, outer quadrant of the breast.**
Inframammary Fold	This is often forgotten & must be specifically palpated.
Axillary Tail of Spence	This is often forgotten & must be specifically palpated.
Nipple Discharge	Explain to the patient that it is important for you to check for a discharge by gently squeezing the nipple & gain permission to do so.
Axillary Lymphadenopathy	Palpate for axillary lymphadenopathy, facing the patient, by supporting their arm with your corresponding arm. You will then be able to use your free hand to palpate for lymphadenopathy i.e. support the patient's right arm with your right arm, then examine the right axilla with your left hand. It may be easier to examine the left axilla with the patient sitting on the edge of the bed. Remember to examine the anterior, posterior, medial & lateral walls in addition to the apex.
Supraclavicular Lymphadenopathy	This is often forgotten & must be specifically palpated

COMPLETION	Interpretation
Surgical Complications	Consider the nerves that may have been damaged in a post-mastectomy patient e.g. long thoracic nerve of Bell (winging of the scapula) & intercostobrachial nerve (loss of sensation in the distribution of T2).
Respiratory Exam	May indicate metastases.
Abdominal Exam	May indicate metastases.
Spinal Exam	Spinal tenderness in particular may indicate metastases.
Encourage Self Exam	Encourage the patient to regularly monitor their breasts, using a simple examination technique in front of the mirror.
Triple Assessment	If a lump is suspected / detected, complete triple assessment (*see below*).

FINISH:

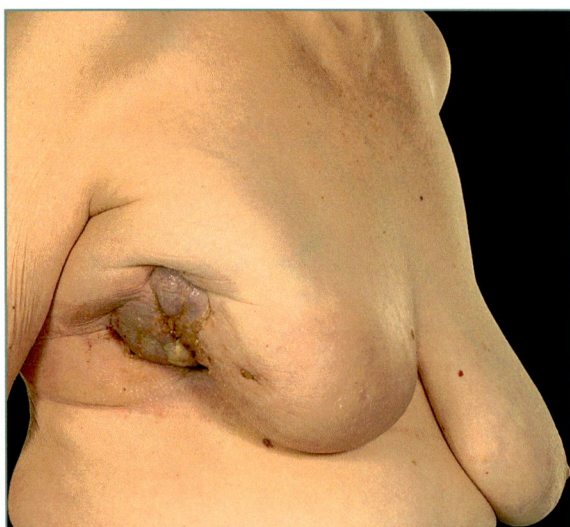

Fig 5.1: Carcinoma of the right breast (recurrence) & marked breast asymmetry, with the right breast lying higher than the left.

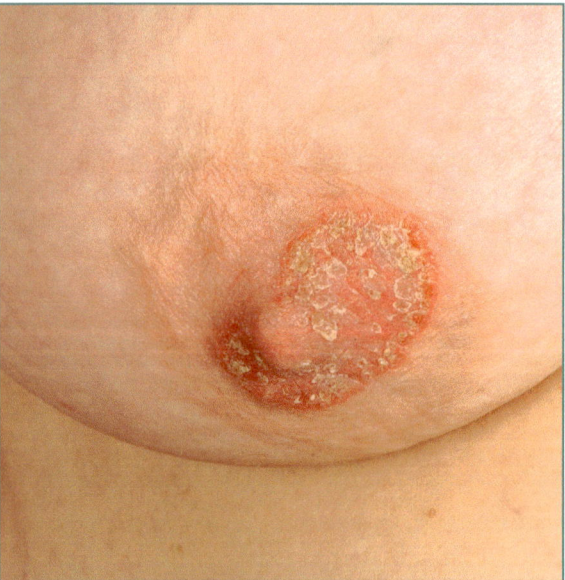

Fig 5.2: Paget's Disease of the nipple.

OSCE QUESTIONS

Breast Disease

Q: How would you classify breast disease?

Breast disease may be classified as **benign** or **malignant**. The aetiology of benign breast disease may be classified as aberrations of normal development & involution (ANDI). ANDI was first introduced at an international breast conference in Cardiff & describes abnormal processes of development, involution & cyclical hormonal activity as follows:

Peak Age (years)	Process		Aberration
15–25	Development		Fibroadenoma & Excessive Breast Development
25–40	Cyclical Hormonal		Cyclical Nodularity & Mastalgia
35–55	Involution	Lobular:	Cysts
		Ductal:	Duct Ectasia & Periductal Mastitis
		Epithelial:	Hyperplasia & Fibrosis

Note: Malignancy is more prevalent in females over the age of 55 years.

Q: What is a fibroadenoma?

The most common benign neoplasm in females. It is a fibroepithelial tumor, composed of glandular tissue & stroma. The peak age of onset is 15–25 years. Clinically, it presents as a painless, smooth, firm & rubbery lump that is highly mobile. Approximately 10% will resolve spontaneously within 1 year.

Q: What is excessive breast development?

Excessive enlargement of the breast due to glandular & stromal proliferation. Minor degrees may be seen in infants due to the effect of maternal oestrogens. Females with excessive breast development may have a hormonal imbalance or hormone-secreting tumour. Males with excessive breast development have gynaecomastia. The causes of excessive breast development are classified as follows:

Classification	Cause
Physiological	Puberty & Pregnancy
Pathological	Hormone-Secreting Tumours, Hypogonadism & Liver Cirrhosis
Pharmacological	Cimetidine, Digoxin, Spironolactone & THC

Q: What are cyclical nodularity & mastalgia?

These affect pre-menopausal females & are hormone dependent. Cyclical breast changes occur, resulting in lumps (nodularity) & pain (mastalgia) related to the menstrual cycle. Treatment options may be classified as follows:

Conservative	Medical	Surgical
Reassurance	Evening Primrose Oil	Mastectomy (for treatment resistant severe mastalgia)
Firm Supporting Bra	Analgesia	
Evening Primrose Oil	Oral Contraceptive Pill	
	Danazol	
	Bromocriptine	
	Tamoxifen	

Q: What are breast cysts?

Breast cysts are fluid-filled, distended & involuted lobules. They present as smooth lumps that may be painful & have a peak age of onset of 35–55 years. Fine needle aspiration may relieve symptoms by drainage of cystic fluid that may then be analysed by microbiology & cytology.

Q: What is duct ectasia?

Duct ectasia is characterised by involution & dilation of the subareolar ducts. Clinical features may include nipple inversion, nipple discharge (may be blood stained), subareolar mass & mastalgia.

Q: What is periductal mastitis?

Periductal mastitis refers to inflammation, often with associated infection, of the subareolar ducts. It may present in a similar manner to duct ectasia, with a subareolar mass, pus discharge from the nipple & mastalgia. When bacterial infection is involved, broad spectrum antibiotics will almost always resolve the issue.

Q: What is epithelial hyperplasia?

Epithelial hyperplasia is characterised histologically by an increase in the number of epithelial lining cells of the terminal duct lobular unit. When atypical dysplasia is present, there is an increased risk of progression to carcinoma.

Q: What is fat necrosis?

Fat necrosis often occurs after trauma to the fatty breast tissue e.g. during breastfeeding or surgery. Inflammation, fibrosis & calcification may ensue. Clinically fat necrosis may be difficult to distinguish from carcinoma as it presents as a hard, irregular lump, sometimes tethered to skin or associated with axillary lymphadenopathy. Most cases resolve spontaneously.

Breast Tumours & Cancer

Q: How would you classify breast tumours?

Tumours of the breast may be classified as benign, pre-malignant or malignant as follows:

Benign	Pre-Malignant / *in situ*	Malignant / Invasive
Fibroadenoma	Ductal Carcinoma *in situ*	Invasive Ductal Carcinoma (80% of invasive)
Intraductal Papilloma	Lobular Carcinoma *in situ*	Invasive Lobular Carcinoma (10% of invasive)
Lipoma		Invasive Medullary, Mucinous, Tubular & Papillary Carcinomas (10% of invasive)

Q: What is Paget's Disease of the nipple?

Paget's Disease of the nipple (Fig 5.2) is an eczematous nipple presentation that, when present, is almost always associated with underlying carcinoma. 2% of all carcinomas are associated with Paget's Disease. Clinical features include persistent nipple erythema, crusting, paraesthesia & pain.

Q: What investigations should be ordered to guide management of breast disease?

Investigations must be tailored towards the suspected underlying aetiology, however, employing the concept of **triple assessment** is vital:

Triple Assessment Stage	Interpretation
1. **Clinical Examination**	Clinical examination is the first part of triple assessment.
2. **Imaging**	Mammogram (Fig 5.3) / USS
3. **Tissue Sampling**	FNAC / Core Biopsy / Open Biopsy

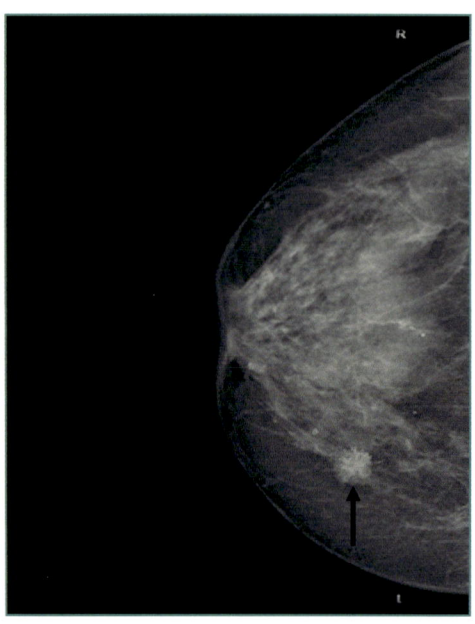

Fig 5.3: Mammogram of a malignant breast tumour with spiculated calcification (arrow

To assess metastasis, the following investigations are useful:

- **LFTs & Liver USS**   (liver)
- **CXR**   (chest)
- **Radioisotope Bone Scan**   (bone)
- **CT Brain**   (brain)

Q: What is the epidemiology of breast cancer?

- Commonest cancer in females (after skin).
- 500,000 deaths / year worldwide.
- 1% occurs in males.

Q: What are the risk factors for breast cancer?

General	Oestrogen Exposure Related
Age	Early Menarche & Late Menopause
Family History	1st Pregnancy >30 years
BRCA1 & BRCA2 Genes	Non-Breast-Feeding Mothers
Previous Breast Malignancy	OCP / HRT

Q: What types of breast cancer do you know of?

Non-Invasive Lesions	Invasive Carcinoma
Ductal Carcinoma *in situ.*	Invasive Ductal Carcinoma (70%).
Lobular Carcinoma *in situ.*	Invasive Lobular Carcinoma (20%).
	Other (10%): Microinvasive, Tubular, Medullary, Mucinous, Papillary.

Q: How is breast cancer staged clinically?

Breast cancer is staged according to the AJCC TNM classification system. There are 2 classifications in relation to nodal involvement; clinical classification is based on clinical examination (cN) & test/scan results, pathological classification (pN) is based on post-operative pathological findings.

Primary Tumour Extent (T)		Regional Lymph Nodes (N)		
Tx	Primary tumour cannot be evaluated.	**cNx**	Regional nodal status cannot be evaluated.	
T0	No evidence of primary tumour.	**cN0**	No regional lymph node involvement.	
Tis	Carcinoma *in situ.*	**cN1**	Mobile ipsilateral level I / II axillary node(s).	
T1	**Primary tumour longest axis ≤2cm:**	**cN2**	cN2a:	Fixed / matted ipsilateral level I / II axillary node(s).
	T1a: ≤0.5cm.		cN2b:	Internal mammary node(s) only.
	T1b: >0.5cm & ≤1cm.			
	T1c: >1cm & ≤2cm.			
T2	Primary tumour longest axis >2cm & ≤5cm	**cN3**	cN3a:	Ipsilateral infra-clavicular node(s).
			cN3b:	Ipsilateral internal mammary & axillary node(s).
T3	Primary tumour longest axis >5cm.		cN3c:	Ipsilateral supra-clavicular node(s) .
T4	**Primary tumour extension:**	**Metastasis & Distant Lymph Nodes (M)**		
	T4a: Extension to chest wall.	**Mx**	Distant metastasis & lymph nodes cannot be evaluated.	
	T4b: Oedema, skin ulceration or satellite nodes present.			
		M0	No distant metastasis.	
	T4c: T4a & T4b together.	**M1**	Distant metastasis or contralateral lymph node involvement.	
	T4d: Inflammatory carcinoma.			

CHAPTER 5

CARDIOLOGY

143

Q: What are the medical / surgical treatment options for breast cancer?

This depends on the site & size of tumour, patient co-morbidities, patient wishes & must be discussed with an MDT environment.

Treatment	Notes
Hormonal Therapy	• Tamoxifen (selective oestrogen receptor modulator for receptor positive cases). • Aromatase Inhibitors e.g. Anastrozole.
Chemotherapy	• Neo-Adjuvant (shrinks tumour before surgery). • Adjuvant (reduces recurrence risk post-operatively). • To Treat Recurrence. • Drugs Include: Fluorouracil, Cyclophosphamide, Doxorubicin
Surgical	• Breast Conserving Surgery. • Mastectomy (including prophylactic contralateral mastectomy). • Sentinel Lymph Node Biopsy (staging). • Axillary Lymph Node Sampling / Dissection. • Breast Reconstruction. **Note: Breast cancer surgery is mostly undertaken for curative purposes.**
Radiotherapy	• Primarily used after surgery to decrease recurrence risk.

CHAPTER 6
ABDOMEN

BH Miranda
MJ Portou
MC Winslet

CHAPTER CONTENTS

Abdominal Examination

OSCE Questions

ABDOMINAL EXAMINATION

START: Patient lying flat & exposed to underwear ideally, to allow for hernia & PR examinations. This also allows for thorough examination e.g. the chest wall for spider naevi or gynaecomastia & both legs for oedema.

Use sheet covers appropriately, to maintain patient dignity.

INSPECTION	Interpretation
Moving Abdomen	No guarding. Guarding is the maintenance of a rigid abdomen, to reduce pain.
Cough	May reveal a hernia.
Head off Bed	Asking the patient to lift their head off the bed may reveal divarification of the rectus abdominis at the linea alba. This may also reveal a hernia.
Caput Medusa	Distended periumbilical veins *(later in chapter)*.
Scars	Previous surgery.
HANDS:	
Hepatic Asterixis	A *'liver flap'* is often encephalopathy associated. It occurs due to delivery of toxins, usually metabolised by the liver, to the brain.
Leukonychia	Nail whitening due to hypoalbuminaemia.
Koilonychia	Nail spooning due to Fe deficiency.
Clubbing	*(later in chapter)*
Palmar Erythema	Localised vasodilation due to decreased oestrogen.
Dupuytren's Contracture	This may be idiopathic, familial, associated with chronic liver disease or Peyronie's Disease *(see hand chapter)*.
WRIST / ARM:	
Excoriations	Pruritis.
Needle Marks	IVDU is associated with HBV & HCV transmission.
Tattoos	HBV & HCV transmission from tattoo needles.
Bruising	Clotting abnormality.
Pulse	Check Rate & Rhythm. Rate increases in acute pancreatitis, perforation & 3rd space fluid loss.
FACE:	
Pale Conjunctiva	Anaemia sign.
Yellow Sclera	Jaundice.
Corneal Arcus	May be congenital or associated with chronic cholestasis & hypercholesterolaemia. It may also develop inconsequentially after the age of 50.

Xanthelasma	Fleshy, yellow, subcutaneous deposits of cholesterol, often around the eyelids & eyes.
Kayser-Fleicher Rings	Copper deposits present in Wilson's Disease. **Note: These are only truly seen with the use of a slit lamp, so mention this!**
MOUTH:	
Glossitis	Vitamin B12 deficiency.
Angular Stomatitis	Fe & Vitamin B12 deficiency.
Aphthous Ulcers	Crohn's Disease, Behcet's Disease & HSV.
Pigmentation	**Peutz-Jegher's Syndrome** is an autosomal dominant condition associated with mucosal pigmentation & gastrointestinal hamartomatous polyps. Mucosal pigmentation is also seen in Addison's Disease.
Telangiectasia	**Osler-Weber-Rendu Syndrome** is an autosomal dominant condition associated with haemorrhagic telangiectasia of the mucous membranes e.g. oral & nasal, gastrointestinal tract & lungs. Epistaxis & gastrointestinal bleeding are common features.
NECK:	
Troisier's Sign	*The presence of a left supraclavicular lymph node, also known as Virchow's Node.* Associated with gastrointestinal carcinomas, particularly gastric carcinoma.
CHEST:	
Gynaecomastia	Due to decreased oestrogen metabolism by damaged hepatocytes.
Spider Naevi	*Branched, dilated arterioles that blanch with pressure & refill from the centre outwards; >5 = abnormal.* Due to decreased oestrogen metabolism.
Axillary Hair Loss	Due to decreased oestrogen metabolism.
ABDOMEN:	
6 x S's	Describe lump / mass site, size, shape, symmetry, overlying skin & associated scars (Fig 6.1).
Distension	**Memory:** **The 5 x F's of Abdominal Distension.** Fat Fluid Faeces Flatus Foetus
Visible Peristalsis	Kneel down & look across the abdomen for peristalsis due to bowel obstruction.
Aortic Pulsations	Kneel down & look across the abdomen for AAA pulsations.
Scars	Ensure you roll the patient to check for more posterior scars *(later in chapter)*.

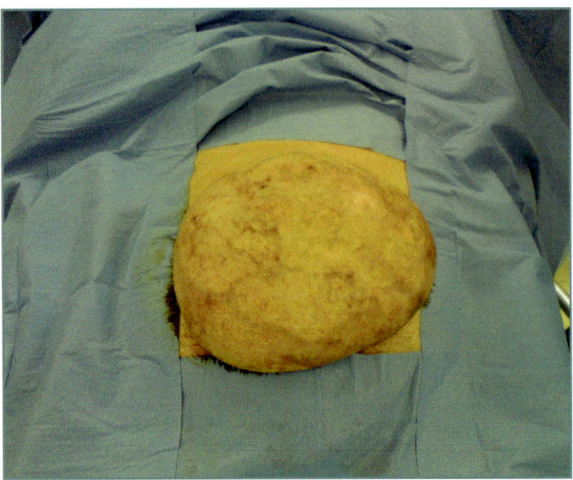

Fig 6.1: Large abdominal mass.

Ask about pain.

Look at the patient's face throughout the examination.

Warm your hands by rubbing them together & warn the patient that they may be cold.

 Memory: The 9 x regions of the abdomen: 1 x epigastric, 2 x hypochondrium, 1 x umbilical, 2 x lumbar, 1 x suprapubic & 2 x iliac (Fig 6.2).

PALPATION	Interpretation
9 Regions SOFT	Localising tenderness & superficial lumps / masses.
	Guarding may be palpated as the patient tenses their abdominal muscles to *'guard'* inflamed abdominal organs from pain upon pressure. Guarding may be classified as voluntary or involuntary as follows:
	• **Voluntary:** A conscious & deliberate contraction of anterior abdominal wall muscles to prevent deeper palpation. Relaxation occurs once pressure is released.
	• **Involuntary:** Reflex anterior abdominal wall muscle spasm caused by peritoneal inflammation which cannot be wilfully suppressed.
9 Regions DEEP	Localising deep lumps / masses.
SEC FFP TR	Palpate lump / mass surface, edge, consistency, fixity to skin & underlying structures, fluctuance, pulsatility & expansility, transilluminability & reducibility.
Liver	Use the radial border of your right index finger, thumb & fingers extended, to palpate from right iliac fossa to right hypochondrium. Describe the distance below the costal margin (cm).
Spleen	Use the tips of your right index, middle & ring fingers to palpate from right iliac fossa to left hypochondrium. Rolling the patient towards you may assist palpation. The spleen has a notch, you can't get above it, it enlarges to the right iliac fossa & is not ballotable.
Kidneys	Ballot the kidneys. Kidneys have no notch, you can get above them, they enlarge vertical-inferior & are ballotable.
Gall Bladder	Where the right border of rectus crosses the costal margin.
Abdominal Aortic Aneurysm	Palpate for expansility, with thumbs & fingers extended, running your index fingers parallel to the abdominal aorta. This is usually best localised above the umbilicus, just left of midline.

PERCUSSION	Interpretation
Liver	Delineate extension (cm) beyond the costal margin.
Spleen	Delineate extension (cm) beyond costal margin.
Ascites	Demonstrate **shifting dullness**. Start percussion from the umbilicus away from you. Demonstrate the resonant (air) to dull (fluid) interface at the flanks & leave your finger at that point. Roll the patient towards you & maintain that position for a few minutes, allowing gravity to drain peritoneal fluid. Continue percussion in the same direction, demonstrating that what once was dull, has now *'shifted'* to resonant! The presence of fluid may be further confirmed by demonstrating a **percussion thrill**.

AUSCULTATION	Interpretation
Bowel Sounds	Describe frequency & quality e.g. hyperdynamic & tinkling.
Hepatic Bruit	Hepatocellular carcinoma.
Aortic Bruit	AAA.
Renal Bruit	Renal artery stenosis.

COMPLETION	Interpretation
Lymphadenopathy	Check inguinal lymph nodes.
Hernial Orifices	Inguinal hernias.
External Genitalia	Full examination.
Digital Rectal Exam	Identify mass, blood or mucus.
Urine Dipstick	Glycosuria.
Fluid Chart	If available.
Stool Chart	If available.
Ankle Oedema	Hypoalbuminaemia *(see vascular chapter for other causes)*.

FINISH:

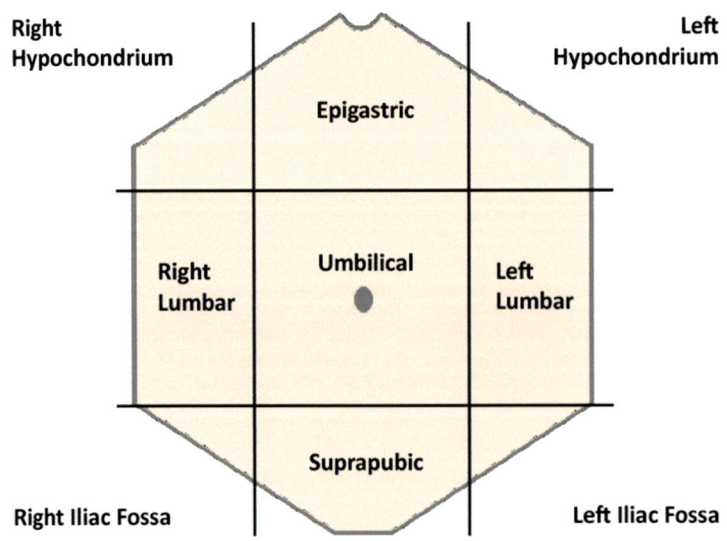

Fig 6.2: The 9 abdominal regions.

OSCE QUESTIONS

Clubbing

Q: What are the stages of clubbing (Fig 2.2)?

1. Congestion / Fluctuation of Nail Fold / Nail Bed
2. Loss of Lovibond's Angle (normally = 165°) Between Nail Plate & Nail Fold
3. Increased AP Diameter & Convexity of Nail Bed & Nail Plate = Parrot Beaking
4. Increased Lateral Diameter of Finger Tip = Drum Stick Appearance
5. Hypertrophic Osteoarthropathy

Q: What are the causes of clubbing?

Clubbing may be **idiopathic**. Other causes are classified as follows:

Gastrointestinal	Respiratory
Cirrhosis	Bronchial Carcinoma
Inflammatory Bowel Disease	Chronic Suppurative e.g. Abscess, Bronchiectasis & Empyema
Malabsorption Diseases	Fibrosing Alveolitis
Lymphoma	Mesothelioma
Cardiovascular	**Rare**
Infective Endocarditis	Graves' Disease (thyroid acropachy)
Cyanotic Congenital Heart Disease	Familial

Upper Gastrointestinal

Q: What is dysphagia?

Difficulty swallowing.

Q: What are the causes of dysphagia?

These may be classified as follows:

Congenital		
Oesophageal Atresia		
Acquired		
LUMINAL	**INTRAMURAL**	**EXTRAMURAL**
Food Bolus	Achalasia*	Hilar Lymphadenopathy
Foreign Body	Carcinoma	Pharyngeal Pouch
Oesophageal Web	GORD	Retrosternal Goitre
Plummer-Vinson Sydrome*	Oesophagitis	Lung Carcinoma
	Oesophageal Dysmotility	
	Scleroderma	
	Stricture e.g. Radiation*	
NEUROLOGICAL	**OTHER**	
Stroke	Stomatitis	
Myasthenia Gravis	Glossitis	
Motor Neurone Disease	Tonsillitis & Pharyngitis	

* Associated with an increased risk of developing malignancy. Plummer-Vinson Syndrome is the presence of an oesophageal web, associated with Fe deficiency anaemia.

Q: What is odynophagia?

Pain on swallowing.

Q: Can you give a spot diagnosis for the 3 conditions depicted in the barium swallows below?

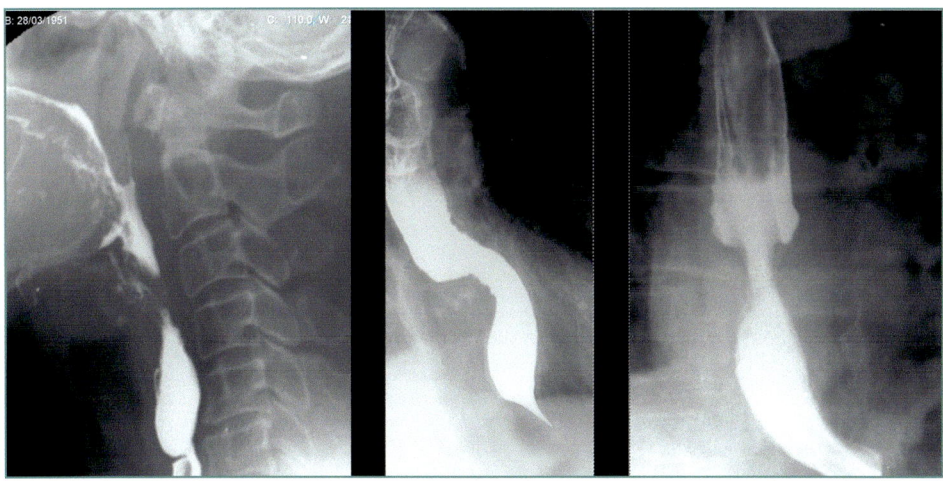

Fig 6.3: Barium swallows of patients with different causes of dysphagia.

Left = oesophageal web. Middle = achalasia (bird's beak / rat's tail sign). Right = oesophageal carcinoma (shouldered stricture)

Q: What are the causes of odynophagia?

Many causes of dysphagia also result in odynophagia. Below are some of the common causes:

Cause	Examples
Trauma	Pharyngeal Trauma, Radiation, Oesophageal Burn, Mallory-Weiss Syndrome & Ruptured Oesophagus
Foreign Body	Oropharyngeal & Oesophageal
Infection	Pharyngitis, Tonsillitis, Oesophagitis (HSV & Candida) & Abscess
GORD	Oesophagitis & Ulceration
Neoplasia	Pharyngeal, Laryngeal & Oesophageal Carcinoma
Motility	Achalasia & Oesophageal Dysmotility Syndromes
Neurological	Stroke, Myasthenia Gravis & Motor Neurone Disease
Other	Plummer-Vinson Syndrome, Pharyngeal Pouch & Scleroderma

Q: What are the causes of an epigastric mass?

Skin & Soft Tissue	Gastrointestinal	Vascular
Cyst	Epigastric Hernia	AAA
Lipoma	Gastric Carcinoma	Lymphadenopathy
Sarcoma	Pancreatic Carcinoma	
	Pancreatic Pseudocyst	

Hepatobiliary

Q: What are the causes of hepatomegaly?

Physiological	Alcohol Related
Riedel's Lobe	Cirrhosis
Hyperexpanded Chest	Fatty Liver
Infective	**Metabolic**
Hepatitis, EBV & CMV (virus)	Amyloid
TB & Abscess (bacteria)	Hereditary Haemochromatosis (HHC)
Malaria & Schistosomiasis (protozoa)	Wilson's Disease
Malignant	**Congestive**
Primary / Secondary	Right Heart Failure
Lymphoma	Tricuspid Regurgitation (pulsatile liver)
Leukaemia	Budd-Chiari Syndrome

Q: What are the most common causes of hepatomegaly in the UK?

Cause	Explanation
Malignancy	This may be primary or secondary & includes haematological malignancies e.g. CML.
Alcohol Related	Fatty Liver Disease & Alcoholic Hepatitis.
Infective	Viral e.g. HAV, HBV, HCV & EBV.
	Bacterial e.g. Liver Abscess.
	Parasitic e.g. Malaria (following foreign travel).

Q: What is Budd-Chiari Syndrome?

Budd-Chiari Syndrome is due to hepatic vein obstruction from e.g. thrombosis or carcinoma. The clinical picture includes upper abdominal pain, jaundice, hepatomegaly & ascites. LFTs are often deranged & progression to encephalopathy may occur.

Q: What are the causes of cirrhosis?

Congenital	Cardiac
HHC	Congestive Cardiac Failure (CCF)
Wilson's Disease	**Drugs**
α1-Antitrypsin Deficiency	Alcohol*
Autoimmune	**Infective**
Hepatitis	HBV / HCV*
Biliary	Schistosomiasis**
Primary Biliary Cirrhosis (PBC)	**Other**
Primary Sclerosing Cholangitis (PSC)	Sarcoid

* Common causes

** Important in Asia, Africa & South America

Q: What is portal hypertension & what are the causes?

Portal hypertension is defined as a portal vein pressure >10mmHg. Causes may be classified as pre-hepatic, hepatic or post-hepatic as follows:

Pre-Hepatic	Hepatic	Post-Hepatic
Portal Vein Thrombosis	Cirrhosis	Budd-Chiari Syndrome
Splenic Vein Thrombosis	Sarcoid	Constrictive Pericarditis
Splenic Arteriovenous Fistula	Schistosomiasis	Right Heart Failure

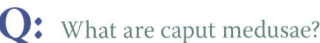

Q: What are caput medusae?

Distended, engorged periumbilical veins, due to severe portal hypertension with porto-systemic shunting of blood through the umbilical veins.

Causes of distended umbilical veins may be:

1. Physiological
2. Portal hypertension leading to porto-systemic shunting
3. IVC obstruction

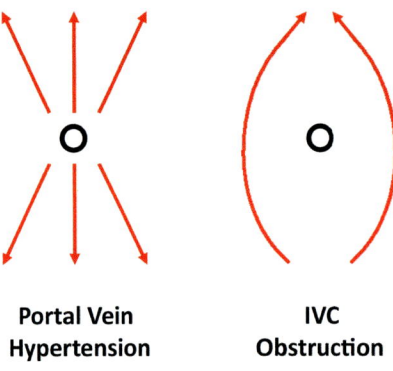

Fig 6.4: Diagram showing direction of blood flow with causes of umbilical vein distension.

Note direction of blood flow in diagram.

Portal Vein Hypertension   **IVC Obstruction**

Q: What is ascites?

Fluid in the peritoneal cavity.

Q: What are the causes of ascites?

These may be classified as transudate or exudate as follows:

TRANSUDATE (Protein < 30g/L)	EXUDATE (Protein > 30g/L)
Cirrhosis	Inflammation e.g. Pancreatitis
Nephrotic Syndrome	Infection e.g. TB
CCF	Malignancy (Primary / Secondary)
Pericarditis	

Q: How would you investigate ascites?

Investigation	Examples
Blood Tests	FBC, U&E, LFT, CRP & Coagulation.
Diagnostic Paracentesis	Note appearance of fluid. Send for: MICROBIOLOGY: MC+S CYTOLOGY: Malignant Cells BIOCHEMISTRY: Protein / Glucose / Amylase
Serum Ascites Albumin Gradient	Better clinical indicator than protein content alone. If the difference between the serum & ascites albumin concentrations is <1.1, an exudate is present. If >1.1, a transudate is present.
USS	Diagnostic USS may be used to assess intra-abdominal organs & extent of ascites. It may also be used to guide drainage procedures.
Doppler	May demonstrate portal vein flow, Budd-Chiari Syndrome & portal vein thrombosis.
Abdominal CT	Further imaging of intra-abdominal organs.

Q: What are the treatment options for ascites?

Classification	Treatment	Explanation
CONSERVATIVE	**Salt Restriction**	Assists production of urine to off-load fluid.
	Weight Monitoring	Quantifies diuresis. The weight loss goal is no more than 0.5kg/day for ascites alone. If patients have additional peripheral oedema, the weight loss goal is no more than 1kg/day.
	Water Restriction	If hyponatraemia is present.
MEDICAL	**Cause**	Treating the underlying cause will prevent progression of ascites.
	Diuretics	Spironolactone is the drug of choice. Otherwise a loop diuretic e.g. furosemide.
SURGICAL	**Paracentesis**	This may be diagnostic & therapeutic.
	TIPS	Transjugular intrahepatic portosystemic shunts, between the portal & hepatic veins, may be used in patients with advanced cirrhosis & recurrent ascites.
	LeVeen Peritoneovenous Shunt	Peritoneovenous shunts drain ascites directly into the venous circulation. They connect the peritoneal cavity to the SVC / IJV via a one-way valve to prevent back flow of blood. Short-term complications include fluid overload, long-term complications include shunt blockage, bacterial colonisation & infection.
	Liver Transplant	For end stage liver disease.

Q: What are the causes of gall bladder enlargement?

Causes may be classified according to the associated presence or absence of jaundice as follows:

Jaundiced	Not Jaundiced
Pancreas Carcinoma (Head)	Mucocoele
Cholangiocarcinoma	Empyema
	Gall Bladder Carcinoma
	Acute Cholecystitis

Note: Gallstones may cause chronic inflammation of the gallbladder. This results in fibrosis & thickening of the wall which does not become distended. Hence, painless jaundice in the presence of a palpable gallbladder is unlikely to be due to gallstone disease (the principle behind Courvoisier's Law).

Pancreatitis

Q: What is pancreatitis & what are the classical clinical features?

Inflammation of the pancreas, which may be an acute process, or develop into a chronic condition. Clinical features include severe epigastric pain that radiates through to the back, nausea & vomiting. Other clinical features may include ascites, abdominal guarding, or those related to the underlying cause / associated complications e.g. obstructive jaundice (gallstones), pyrexia (infection / sepsis), absent bowel sounds (paralytic ileus), **Cullen's Sign** (peri-umbilical bruising in acute haemorrhagic pancreatitis), **Grey Turner's Sign** (flank bruising in acute haemorrhagic pancreatitis).

Q: What are the causes of acute pancreatitis?

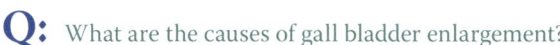

Memory: **I GET SMASHED**

Idiopathic   Steroids

                                    Mumps

Gallsones   Autoimmune

Ethanol   Scorpion Venom

Trauma   Hyper-calcaemia / lipidaemia

                                    ERCP

                                    Drugs e.g. azathioprine / furosemide

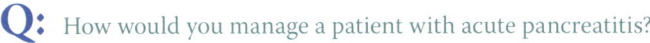

Q: How would you manage a patient with acute pancreatitis?

- **ALS Approach** & **Fluid Resuscitation**
- Full **History**
- Thorough Clinical **Examination**
- Serum Amylase or Lipase ≥3 times the upper limit of normal range.
- Prognostic **Blood Tests** & **ABG** (Modified Glasgow Criteria):

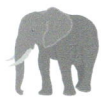

Memory: **PANCREAS** for Modified Glasgow Criteria

P_aO_2	<8kPa
Age	>55
Neutrophils	>15 x 10⁹/L
Corrected Calcium	<2mmol/L
Raised Urea	>16mmol/L
Enzymes (LDH)	>600U/L
Albumin	<32g/L
Sugar (Glucose)	>10mmol/L

Note: Presence of the above criteria should be assessed on admission, then daily for at least 48 hours. Presence of ≤2 criteria = severe pancreatitis unlikely. Presence of ≥3 criteria = severe pancreatitis more likely. CRP>100mg/L within the first 48 hours is suggestive of severe pancreatitis. Mortality rates are; 1–2 criteria = <1%, 3–4 criteria = 15% & >4 criteria = approaching 100% mortality.

- **AXR: Sentinel Loop Sign** may be present; this is a localised segment of isolated paralytic ileus (often duodenum) that appears to be dilated & gas filled.
- **USS:** Assessment of pancreatic inflammation extent, presence of causal gallstones (may require urgent ERCP & sphincterotomy), presence of dilated CBD.
- **Contrast CT Abdomen & Pelvis:** Usually performed at 6-10 days to delineate anatomy, haemorrhage & necrosis, especially with persisting clinical features. May also be performed on admission if there is diagnostic uncertainty e.g. normal amylase, exclude AAA, exclude visceral perforation.

Q: What are the treatment strategies for acute pancreatitis?

- Initial treatment is with fluid resuscitation, opioid analgesia (pethidine is least likely to cause Sphincter of Oddi spasm), metabolic correction (especially Ca), PPI (gastroprotection), nutritional support (early oral feeding favoured if tolerated) & treatment of the underlying cause.
- Severe cases require HDU / ITU management for organ failure support, drainage of pancreatic necrosis & antibiotic therapy ± surgical necrosectomy for infected necrosis.

Q: What are the complications of acute pancreatitis?

Classification	Complications
Local	Abscess, Ascites, Haemorrhage, Necrosis, Phlegmon, Pseudocyst
Gastrointestinal	Paralytic Ileus
Haematological	DIC
Hepatobiliary	CBD Stricture, Jaundice, Portal Vein Thrombosis
Metabolic	Hypoalbuminaemia, Hypocalcaemia, Hypomagnesaemia, Hypoxaemia Hyperglycaemia
Renal	Acute Renal Failure
Respiratory	ARDS, Pleural Effusion
Other	Chronicity (more common if ETOH is the cause) Overall Mortality =10%

Liver Tumours & Cancer

Q: What is the epidemiology of liver cancer?

- 1% of all cancers in the UK.
- Highest incidence in Africa & Asia.
- Lowest incidence in America & Europe.
- Hepatic metastases are the most common type in the UK.

Q: What benign hepatic tumours do you know?

Tumour	Description
Haemangioma	• Most common benign liver tumour.
	• Vascular neoplasm of endothelial cells.
	• Mainly affects middle-aged females.
	• Often small & solitary.
	• Usually incidental finding.
	• Treatment is conservative & monitoring.
	• Surgical excision indicated if rupture / rapid change in size occurs.
Focal Nodular Hyperplasia	• 2nd most common benign liver tumour.
	• Solitary stellate lesion.
	• Numerous small bile ducts within fibrous tissue.
	• May become vascular & enlarge.
	• No malignant potential.
	• Often resected as difficult to distinguish from hepatic adenoma.
Adenoma	• Well differentiated & circumscribed nodule.
	• Mainly affects females aged 20–40 years.
	• Increased risk with oestrogenic medications & anabolic steroids.
	• May spontaneously bleed.
	• Large lesions may present with hepatomegaly.
	• Small risk of malignant transformation.
	• Treatment is surgical excision.

Q: What malignant hepatic tumours do you know?

Tumour	Example	Description
PRIMARY	**Hepatocellular Carcinoma (HCC)**	• More common in Africa & Asia, with a younger presentation. • Large, heterogeneous, vascular & haemorrhagic malignancy. • Risks include HBV, HCV, cirrhosis & aflatoxin. • Produces α-fetoprotein tumour marker. • Never biopsy HCC as there is a risk of seeding. • Treatment is preventative e.g. HBV vaccination or curative e.g. partial hepatectomy / liver transplant.
	Cholangiocarcinoma	• Rare. • Aggressive adenocarcinoma of bile duct epithelium. • May present with obstructive jaundice. • Risks include liver fluke infestation & PSC. • Treatment is surgical excision ± chemotherapy & radiotherapy.
	Angiosarcoma	• Rare endothelial vascular malignancy. • Highly malignant.
	Hepatoblastoma	• Uncommon malignancy. • Occurs in infants & children. • Presents with abdominal mass. • Prognosis poor unless associated with α-fetoprotein production. • Treatment is neoadjuvant chemotherapy & surgical excision.
SECONDARY	**Metastasis**	• The most common hepatic malignancy. • Underlying primary tumour is frequently breast, gastrointestinal, lung, ovarian, prostatic or renal. • Features are of hepatic involvement & of the underlying primary. • Prognosis is generally poor & related to the underlying primary. • Treatment is surgical resection & of the underlying primary.

Pancreas Tumours & Cancer

Q: What is the epidemiology of pancreatic carcinoma?

- 3rd most common gastrointestinal cancer.
- Increasing incidence in developed countries.
- Accounts for approximately 5% of all cancer deaths.
- Uncommon in patients aged <50 years.
- 3 times more prevalent in males.
- 1 year survival = 10%.

Q: What are the pathological features of pancreatic carcinoma?

- 80% are adenocarcinomas of the exocrine pancreas.
- 60% occur at the head of the pancreas.
- Rarely due to endocrine tumours e.g. insulinoma & glucagonoma.

Q: What are the risks for pancreatic adenocarcinoma?

Congenital	Acquired
Male	Smoking
Family History	High Fat Diet
	Chronic Pancreatitis
	DM

Q: How does pancreatic carcinoma present?

- Often presents late.
- Painless jaundice (if carcinoma obstructs CBD).
- Anorexia & weight loss.
- Epigastric mass.
- Epigastric pain radiating to back.
- Ascites.

Q: What is Trousseau's Sign?

Thrombophlebitis migrans associated with malignancy e.g. lung & pancreas. This occurs due to a malignant hypercoagulable state. Clusters of tender blood clots appear in succession, along & within the lumen of the affected vessel(s) e.g. superficial veins throughout the body, deep limb veins & portal vein.

Note: Trousseau also described carpal spasm, caused by arm compression above systolic pressure, as a sign of hypocalcaemia.

Q: What specific treatments are available for pancreatic adenocarcinoma?

- 15% are resectable & therefore potentially curable.
- The most common procedure is Whipple's Procedure (pancreaticoduodenectomy) for carcinoma of the head of the pancreas.
- Other procedures include distal pancreatectomy (tail carcinoma) & total pancreatectomy (diffuse carcinoma).
- Patients may develop diabetes or require pancreatic supplements post-operatively.
- Chemotherapy has some role as adjuvant, neo-adjuvant or palliative therapy.
- Radiotherapy is only useful for palliative therapy.

Q: What endocrine tumours of the pancreas do you know?

Endocrine pancreatic tumours are associated with MEN I & may be classified as follows:

Tumour	Description
Insulinoma	• Tumour of β-islets of Langerhans.
	• 75% of all endocrine pancreatic tumours & 10% are malignant.
	• Presents with episodic hypoglycaemia, increased appetite & weight gain.
	• Curative treatment is with surgery & chemotherapy.
Glucagonoma	• Tumour of α-islets of Langerhans.
	• Hypersecretion of glucagon ensues.
	• 75% are malignant & 90% have hepatic / lymphatic metastases at presentation.
	• Presents with hyperglycaemic attacks, anaemia, rash & diarrhoea.
	• Also causes secondary diabetes mellitus.
	• Curative treatment is with surgery & chemotherapy.
	• Insulin & octreotide may be useful.
VIPoma	• Tumour of PP (pancreatic polypeptide producing) cells.
	• Hypersecretion of vasoactive intestinal polypeptide ensues.
	• Causes profuse watery diarrhoea, hypokalaemia, achlorhydria.
	• Curative treatment is surgical.
	• Corticosteroids & octreotide may be useful.
Gastrinoma	• Often found in pancreas but also gastric antrum & small intestine.
	• 60% are malignant & 10% are multiple.
	• Clinical features are due to overproduction of gastrin e.g. peptic ulcer disease.
	• Can result in Zollinger-Ellison syndrome.
	• Curative treatment is surgical.
	• Proton pump inhibitors & octreotide may be useful.

Spleen

Q: What are the functions of the spleen?

Function	Explanation
Reticuloendothelial System	Filters & removes RBCs, WBCs & platelets.
Storage	Holds 35% of body platelet stores.
Immunological	The destruction, via phagocytosis, of encapsulated organisms e.g. *Haemophilus influenzae, Streptococcus pneumoniae & Neisseria meningitidis.*
Synthesis	Synthesises antibodies & opsonin (enhances phagocytosis).

Q: What are the causes of splenomegaly?

Haemolytic Anaemia	Neoplastic
Sickle Cell	Leukaemia e.g. Chronic Myeloid*
Thalassaemia	Myelofibrosis*
Elliptocytosis	Non Hodgkin's Lymphoma
Spherocytosis	Tumour (Primary / Secondary)
Infective	**Splenic Vein Hypertension**
Abscess, TB & Endocarditis (bacteria)	Cirrhosis
HIV, IM & Hepatitis (virus)	Budd-Chiari Syndrome
Malaria* & Schistosomiasis (protozoa)	Portal Vein Thrombosis
Hydatid Cyst (parasite)	**Other**
Inflammatory	Amyloid
Rheumatoid Arthritis	CCF
Sarcoid	Felty's Syndrome

* These are causes of massive splenomegaly.

Q: What is hypersplenism?

Hypersplenism is defined by the presence of the following:

1. Splenomegaly
2. Cytopaenia*
3. Normal or Hyperplastic Bone Marrow
4. Response to Splenectomy**

* Cytopaenia may take the form of anaemia, leukopaenia, thrombocytopaenia or pancytopaenia.
** Response to splenectomy implies that hypersplenism is a retrospective diagnosis.

Kidneys

Q: What are the causes of a kidney mass?

Congenital	Neoplastic
Simple Solitary Cyst	Adenoma
Polycystic Kidney Disease (PCKD)	Renal Cell Carcinoma
Horseshoe Kidney	Wilms' Tumour
Hypertrophic Single Kidney	2° Metastasis
Infective	**Vascular**
Abscess	Infarction
Hydatid Cyst	Renal Vein Thrombosis
TB	**Other**
Inflammatory	Amyloid
Sarcoid	Hydronephrosis

Q: What is PCKD?

Polycystic kidney disease is characterised by the presence of bilateral renal cysts. It is an important cause of renal failure & may be classified as infantile or adult, with the following characteristics:

Characteristics	Infantile	Adult
Genetics	Autosomal recessive.	Autosomal dominant.
Presenting Years	Commonly at birth / infancy (prenatal USS now picks this up *in utero*).	Commonly in adults (although may present at any time).
Presenting Symptoms	Renal mass & poor renal function.	Usually in 5th decade with declining renal function. Also mass, loin pain, haematuria & hypertension.
Associations	Hepatic fibrosis, leading to portal hypertension & splenomegaly.	40% have berry aneurysms with risk of subarachnoid haemorrhage.
Prognosis	Survival without transplantation is usually until childhood only.	End stage disease usually between 50-70 years old. Good prognosis with dialysis.

Q: What are the clinical features of chronic renal failure?

Features may be considered as follows:

Features	Examples
Cardiovascular	Heart Failure, Hypertension, Pericarditis* & Peripheral Vascular Disease
Dermatological	Pale Yellow Skin & Pruritis*
Endocrine	Amenorrhoea, Impotence & Infertility
Fluid Overload	JVP Increase, Peripheral Oedema & Pulmonary Oedema
Gastrointestinal	Anorexia, Diarrhoea, Nausea & Vomiting*
Haematological	Anaemia, Ecchymosis & Epistaxis
Neurological	Confusion, Coma, Fits & Peripheral Neuropathy*
Respiratory	Halitosis & Pleural Effusion*
Surgical	Fistula & Nephrectomy Scar

* These features are commonly associated with uraemia.

Renal Tract Tumours & Cancer

Q: How are renal tumours classified?

Benign	Malignant	
Fibroma	*Primary:*	*Secondary:*
Cortical Adenoma	Renal Cell Carcinoma (RCC)	Metastases
Oncocytoma	Nephroblastoma / Wilms' Tumour	
Angiomyolipoma	Transitional Cell Carcinoma (TCC)	

Q: How would you investigate a patient with a suspected renal tract tumour?

After taking a **full history** & performing a **thorough clinical examination**, I would consider the following investigations:

Investigation	Notes	
Blood Tests	FBC, U&E, LFT & CRP.	
Urine Dipstick	Haematuria.	
Histology	May be USS guided e.g. RCC (although in RCC, biopsy is rarely required for diagnosis). May be taken at cystoscopy e.g. TCC bladder.	
Imaging	**Radiography:**	AXR / KUB may show malignant opacity.
		CXR may show cannonball metastases.
	USS Renal Tract:	Defines solid / cystic lesions.
		Defines local invasion e.g. RCC into IVC.
	IVU:	Space occupying lesions & filling defects visible.
		Distortion of renal tract outline.
	Flexible Cystoscopy:	Direct vision of bladder & urethra.
		Histological biopsy obtainable e.g. TCC bladder.
		Treatment possible e.g. TCC bladder.
	CT:	Assess local spread & metastasis e.g. RCC into IVC.
	Bone Scan:	Assess bone metastasis.

Renal Cell Carcinoma (RCC)

Q: What is RCC?

- Most common primary malignancy of the kidney parenchyma.
- Histologically an adenocarcinoma.
- Uncommon in patients aged <50 years.

Q: What are the risk factors for developing RCC?

- Male : Female (2:1)
- Family History
- Smoking
- Von Hippel-Lindau Syndrome.

Q: What are the clinical features of RCC?

- Classically presents with a triad of haematuria, abdominal mass & loin pain.
- May be an incidental finding on CT.
- May present with paraneoplastic syndromes e.g. hypertension (renin), polycythaemia (EPO) & hypercalcaemia (PTHrP).
- May present with features of metastasis e.g. bone pain, hepatomegaly, respiratory symptoms & confusion.

Q: How is RCC staged?

Either by TNM or Robson's Staging. Robson's Staging is as follows:

Stage	Explanation
I	Tumour Confined to Kidney.
II	Extension to Perinephric Fat.
III	Metastasis to Renal Vein.
IV	Metastasis to Adjacent / Distance Organs.

Q: Why may RCC present as a left varicocoele?

The tumour may invade the left renal vein & obstruct the left testicular vein (which drains into the left renal vein). This is uncommon with a right-sided RCC as the right testicular vein drains directly into the IVC.

Q: What are the treatment options for RCC?

Chemotherapy	Surgery	Radiotherapy
Progesterone	Nephrectomy	Palliative e.g. Bone Metastasis Pain
IFNα		
IL-2		
VEGF / PDGF Inhibitors		

Transitional Cell Carcinoma (TCC)

Q: What types of bladder carcinoma do you know?

- **TCC:** Most common type in the UK.
- **SCC:** Develops due to chronic inflammation from e.g. calculi / schistosomiasis.
- **Adenocarcinoma:** Also develops in remnants of the urachus.

Note: Schistosomiasis is the most common cause of bladder cancer worldwide.

Q: What is TCC of the renal tract?

- Malignant tumour of the transitional epithelium of the renal tract.
- 4 times more prevalent than RCC.
- Uncommon in patients aged <50 years.

Q: How does TCC of the renal tract present?

- Classically with painless haematuria.
- May present with features of metastasis.

Q: What are the risk factors for renal tract TCC?

- Male : Female (3:1).
- Smoking.
- β-Naphthylamine e.g. Dye & Rubber Industries.
- Nitrosamines e.g. Smoked Fish.

Q: What is field change?

Transitional cell epithelium lines the renal tract from the renal pelvices to the proximal urethra. Exposure to a carcinogen will increase the risk of TCC throughout this entire 'field' of transitional cell epithelium. This is the concept of field change.

Q: By what common routes may renal tract TCC spread?

Spread	Examples
Local	Prostate & Rectum (males), Uterus & Vagina (females).
Lymphatic	Iliac & Para-Aortic Lymph Nodes.
Haematogenous	Bone, Brain, Liver & Lungs.

Q: What are the treatment options for renal tract TCC?

Treatment options depend on site, grade & stage of disease. This should be discussed within an MDT environment. Treatment options include:

Chemotherapy	Radiotherapy	Surgery
Intravesical Cytotoxic Chemotherapy (bladder)*	Curative (early presentation)	Nephroureterectomy & Bladder Cuff Removal (ureter)
Intravesical BCG Immunotherapy (bladder)*	Palliative (late presentation)	Cystectomy (bladder)
		Cystoscopic Excision (urethra)

*Note: These require regular cystoscopy follow up.

Wilms' Tumour

Q: What is the epidemiology of Wilms' Tumour?

- Most common renal malignancy in children.
- Most common intra-abdominal malignancy in patients aged <10 years.
- Peak incidence ages 1–4 years.

Q: What is the pathology of Wilms' Tumour?

- Also known as a mixed nephroblastoma.
- Composed of metanephric blastema, stroma & epithelium elements with varying differentiation.
- Histology reveals abortive glomeruli & tubules surrounded by stroma.
- Stroma may contain bone, cartilage, fat & muscle.
- Aggressive & rapidly growing.

Q: How does Wilms' Tumour present & what is a common surgical treatment option?

- Abdominal mass, haematuria, hypertension, abdominal pain & intestinal obstruction.
- <5% are bilateral.
- Treatment depends on stage & involves nephrectomy ± chemotherapy & radiotherapy.

Lower Gastrointestinal

Q: What is Inflammatory Bowel Disease (IBD)?

Inflammatory bowel disease is an idiopathic inflammatory disease with a genetic predisposition & probable auto-immune component against the gastrointestinal tract. IBD is comprised of ulcerative colitis (UC) & Crohn's Disease (CD). Both are more prevalent in Ashkenazi Jews, followed by white Caucasian populations. Age of presentation peaks at around 20–30 years. Crohn's Disease is more prevalent in smokers, however ulcerative colitis is more prevalent in non-smokers.

Q: What are the intestinal presenting features of IBD?

Many features e.g. diarrhoea & mucus PR are similar, although UC features tend to be more severe than CD. Presenting features of CD may include growth retardation in children, anaemia, occult blood loss, low-grade fever & weight loss. UC often presents more acutely with abdominal pain, diarrhoea & frank blood loss PR. Severe acute exacerbations are also more prevalent in UC. Remember that CD features may be present throughout the entire gastrointestinal tract, whilst UC is limited to the colon.

Q: What features are characteristic of an acute exacerbation of UC?

- Abdominal Pain & Distension (may indicate perforated toxic megacolon)
- Bloody Stool
- Diarrhoea (>10 episodes in 24h)
- Faecal Urgency
- Pallor
- Pyrexia
- Tachycardia

Q: What investigations would assist in diagnosing IBD?

Investigation	Examples
Bloods	FBC, U&E & CRP
Radiology	AXR, Barium Enema & Small Bowel Follow Through
Procedures	Colonoscopy
Histology	Biopsy at Colonoscopy

Q: What differences may be seen between CD & UC on a barium enema?

Crohn's Disease	Ulcerative Colitis
String Sign (terminal ileum stricture)	Lead Piping (scarred, rigid colon)
Cobblestones / Skip Lesions	Loss of Haustration
Rose Thorn Ulcers	Toxic Megacolon

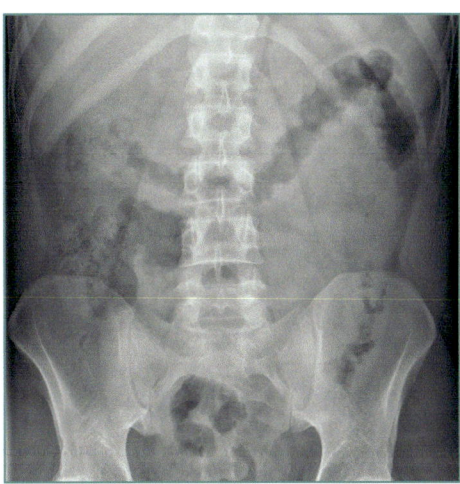

Fig 6.5: Ulcerative colitis radiography.

'Thumbprinting' is seen throughout the colon. This is due to thickening of the large bowel wall related to inflammation, with the normal haustra becoming thickened & projecting into the aerated lumen.

Q: What condition is shown in this barium enema & what is A, B & C?

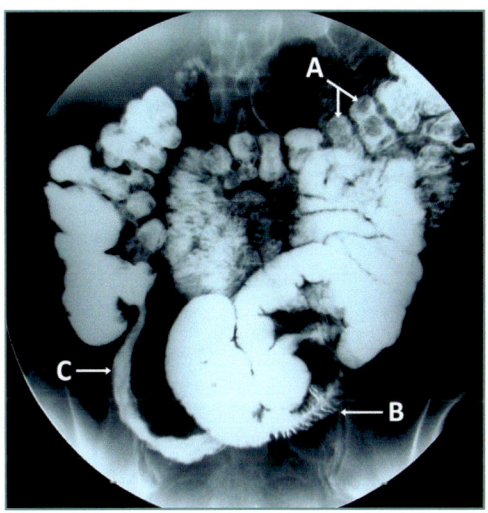

Fig 6.6: Barium enema of a patient with Crohn's Disease.

A: Cobblestones
B: Rose Thorn Ulcers
C: String Sign

Q: What are the pathological differences between CD & UC?

Features	Crohn's Disease	Ulcerative Colitis
MACROSCOPIC		
Pseudopolyps	√	√
Fistula	√	X
Stricture	√	X
Thick Wall	√	X
MICROSCOPIC		
Crypt Abscess	X	√
Granuloma	√	X
Inflammation	Patchy & Transmural	Continuous & Mucosal

Q: What are the complications of IBD?

These may be broadly classified according to IBD type as follows:

Crohn's Disease	Ulcerative Colitis
Infection	Infection
Failure to Thrive	Toxic Megacolon
Gastrointestinal Fistula	Primary Sclerosing Cholangitis*
Subacute Intestinal Obstruction	Colorectal Carcinoma

* PSC is present in 6–7% of patients with UC. UC is present in 60–70% of patients with PSC.

Q: What are the extra-intestinal associations of IBD?

- Mouth Ulcers (CD only)
- Perianal Skin Tags (CD only)
- Ankylosing Spondylitis
- Arthritis
- Iritis
- Erythema Nodosum
- Pyoderma Gangrenosum

Q: What are the treatment options for IBD?

Treatment	Crohn's Disease	Ulcerative Colitis
CONSERVATIVE	• Diet Modification • Psychological • Support Groups	• Psychological • Support Groups
MEDICAL	• Systemic Steroids • Immunosuppressants e.g. Azathioprine • Anti TNFα e.g. Infliximab	• Topical Steroids e.g. Predfoam Enemas • Systemic Steroids • 5-Aminosalicylic Acid e.g. Mesalazine
SURGICAL	• Drainage of Perianal Sepsis • Seton Fistulotomy • Strictureplasty • Segmental Resection • Defunctioning Loop Ileostomy	• Proctocolectomy & End Ileostomy • Ileo-Anal Pouch Formation

Q: Is surgery for IBD curative?

UC may be cured by surgery, as the disease is limited to the colon. CD affects the entire gastrointestinal tract, so relapses may occur even after surgical intervention. Approximately 70% of CD patients & 30% of UC patients require surgery at some time.

Q: What are the indications for surgery in IBD?

Indication	Explanation	
Medical Treatment Complications	Patients who experience severe side effects from medical treatment.	
Medical Treatment Failure	Patients with IBD resistant to medical treatment.	
Disease Process Complications	**Acute:**	Abscess
		Fistula
		Toxic Megacolon
	Chronic:	Strictures
		Colonic Dysplasia (leading to carcinoma)

Q: What are the causes of an iliac fossa mass?

Skin & Soft Tissue	Gastrointestinal		Vascular
Cyst	*Right Iliac Fossa:*	*Left Iliac Fossa:*	Iliac Aneurysm
Lipoma	Caecal Carcinoma	Diverticulitis	Lymphadenopathy
Sarcoma	IBD	Faeces	
	Appendix		
Testicular	**Gynaecological**		**Urological**
Incomplete Descent	Benign Ovarian Tumour		Transplant Kidney
Ectopic Testis	Malignant Ovarian Tumour		
	Fibroids		

Intestinal Polyps & Colorectal Carcinoma

Q: What are intestinal polyps?

Benign protuberant neoplasms in the intestinal lumen, most commonly affecting the colon / rectum.

Q: How are intestinal neoplasms classified?

Type	Example	
Epithelial	*Benign:* • Tubular Adenoma • Tubulovillous Adenoma • Villous Adenoma	*Malignant:* • Polypoid Adenocarcinoma • Carcinoid Polyp
Mesenchymal	*Benign:* • Fibroma • Leiomyoma • Lipoma	*Malignant:* • Sarcoma • Lymphomatous Polyp
Hamartomatous	• Juvenile Polyp • Peutz-Jegher's Syndrome • Haemangioma • Neurofibroma	
Inflammatory	• Ulcerative Colitis Pseudopolyp	

Q: What is the malignant potential of a colorectal adenoma?

Most colorectal adenocarcinomas arise within benign adenomas. Malignant potential relates to degree of dysplasia, adenoma type & size as follows:

Type	Malignant Change
Tubular Adenoma	5%
Tubulovillous Adenoma	20%
Villous Adenoma	40%

Size	Malignant Change
<1cm	1%
1–2cm	10%
>2cm	40%

Q: What is the epidemiology of colorectal cancer?

- Represents 10% of all cancers.
- 3rd most common cause of cancer related death.
- Uncommon in patients aged <50 years.
- More common in the western world.

Q: What are the risk factors for colorectal cancer?

Congenital	Acquired
Family History	Age
Familial Adenomatous Polyposis (FAP)	Western Diet (high fat & low fibre)
Hereditary Non-Polyposis Colorectal Carcinoma (HNPCC)	Colorectal Polyps
	Ulcerative Colitis

Q: What is familial adenomatous polyposis (FAP)?

- Rare autosomal dominant condition.
- Mutations of APC gene on chromosome 5q21.
- Patients develop hundreds of colorectal polyps that carpet the colon & rectum (seen at endoscopy), around the age of 20–30 years.
- Colorectal carcinoma develops in patients aged <40 years if untreated.
- Screening high risk patients from their early teens involves 6–12 monthly colonoscopy.
- Treatment is by colectomy.

Q: What is hereditary non-polyposis colorectal carcinoma (HNPCC)?

- Rare autosomal dominant condition.
- 80% lifetime risk of developing colon cancer.
- Mutations of genes involved in the DNA mismatch repair pathway.
- 90% of mutations occur in MLH1 (3p21) & MSH2 (2p21) genes.
- Amsterdam criteria identifies patients suitable for genetic testing.
- Screening high risk patients aged >25 years involves 6-12 monthly colonoscopy.
- Treatment is by colectomy.

Q: What is the adenoma-carcinoma sequence?

The stepwise pattern of mutational activation of oncogenes & inactivation / loss of tumour suppressor genes, resulting in the transition from normal epithelium to adenoma, then carcinoma (Fig 6.7).

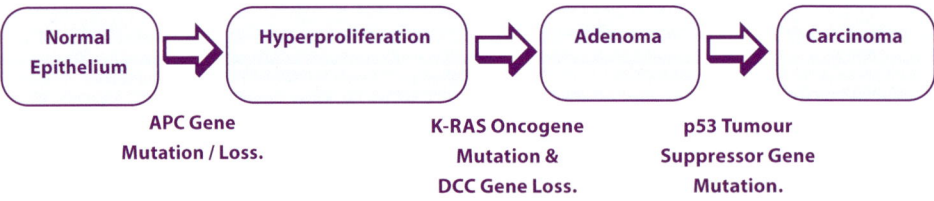

Fig 6.7: Diagram illustrating the steps of the adenoma-carcinoma sequence.

This also explains the **multi-hit hypothesis** as progression to carcinoma is due to the accumulation of multiple genomic alterations. The order of events that occur in the adenoma-carcinoma sequence may not be as important as the accumulation of genomic alterations.

Q: What are the clinical features of colorectal carcinoma?

Most are clinically silent for years. Features depend on the site of the cancer & may be classified as local, systemic or metastatic as follows:

Local	Systemic	Metastatic
Abdominal / Rectal Mass	Anorexia	Hepatomegaly
Abdominal Pain (unlikely if left sided)	Weight Loss	Jaundice
Altered Bowel Habit	Anaemia	Respiratory Symptoms
PR Bleeding	Paraneoplastic Syndromes	
Bowel Obstruction		
Bowel Perforation		
Tenesmus (rectal involvement)		

Q: What investigations would you order for a patient with suspected colorectal cancer?

Modality	Tests
Blood Tests	• FBC, U&E, CEA
Imaging	• CXR
	• USS Liver
	• CT Abdomen / Pelvis
	• Double Contrast Barium Enema
Procedures	• Rigid Sigmoidoscopy
	• Flexible Sigmoidoscopy / Colonoscopy
	Note: Biopsies should also be taken.

Q: How is colorectal carcinoma staged?

Dukes' Staging:

Stage	Description	5 Year Survival
A	Tumour confined to intestinal wall & no invasion into muscle layer.	90%
B	Invasion into muscle layer.	60%
C	Lymph node involvement.	40%
D	Distant metastasis.	<5%

TNM Staging:

Primary Tumour Extent (T)		Regional Lymph Nodes (N)	
Tx	Primary tumour cannot be evaluated.	Nx	Regional nodal status cannot be evaluated.
T0	No evidence of primary tumour.	N0	No regional lymph node involvement.
Tis	Carcinoma *in situ*.	N1	1–3 regional lymph nodes involved.
T1	Primary tumour confined to submucosa.	N2	≥4 regional lymph nodes involved.
T2	Primary tumour invades muscularis propria.	**Metastasis & Distant Lymph Nodes (M)**	
T3	Primary tumour invades subserosa.	Mx	Distant metastasis & lymph nodes cannot be evaluated.
T4	Primary tumour invades through bowel wall into adjacent tissues / organs.	M0	No distant metastasis or lymph node involvement.
		M1	Distant metastasis present.

Q: What are the surgical options for a patient with colorectal cancer?

Surgery for colorectal cancer may be palliative, e.g. faecal diversion procedures, or curative. Curative surgery depends on the site of the cancer (Fig 6.8). The aim is to get clear resection margins 5cm proximal & 2cm distal to the cancer. Surgical procedures therefore include:

Site	Operation
Caecum to Hepatic Flexure	Right Hemicolectomy
Transverse Colon	Extended Right Hemicolectomy
Splenic Flexure to Sigmoid Colon	Left Hemicolectomy
Sigmoid Colon	Sigmoid Colectomy
Upper Rectum (>5cm from anal verge)	Anterior Resection
Lower Rectum (≤5cm from anal verge)	Abdominoperineal (AP) Resection

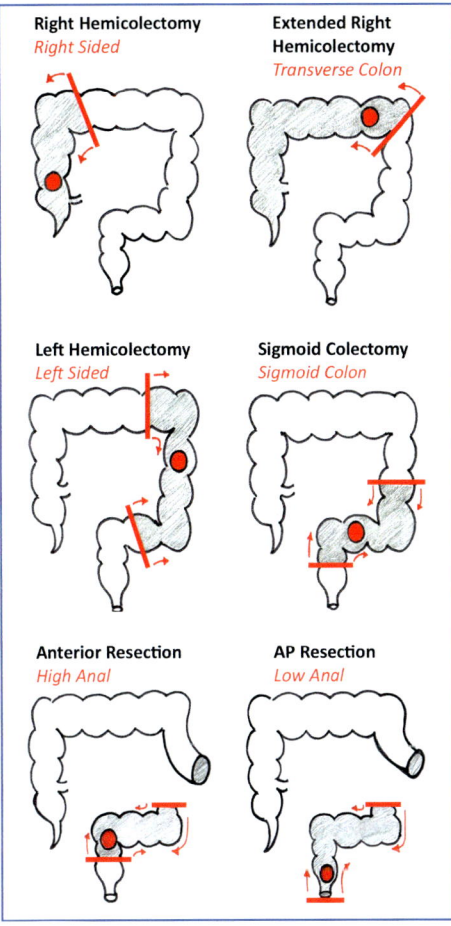

Right Hemicolectomy
Right Sided

Extended Right Hemicolectomy
Transverse Colon

Left Hemicolectomy
Left Sided

Sigmoid Colectomy
Sigmoid Colon

Anterior Resection
High Anal

AP Resection
Low Anal

Fig 6.8: Surgical treatment options for colorectal carcinoma, according to tumour location.

Rectum & Anus

Q: What is a sinus?

A blind ending tract extending from an epithelial defect. This may be normal e.g. cardiac, or pathological e.g. pilonidal sinus.

Q: What is a fistula & how can fistulae be classified?

An abnormal communication between 2 epithelial surfaces. The most common fistula is traumatically acquired as an ear piercing! Fistulae may be classified as follows:

Iatrogenic	Congenital	Acquired
Trauma e.g. Bowel Resection	Parkes-Weber Syndrome	Trauma e.g. Ear Piercing
Cimino-Brescia Fistula	Tracheo-Oesophageal	Infective e.g. TB / Perianal
		Inflammatory e.g. CD
		Neoplastic

Q: What is the cryptoglandular sepsis theory?

An anorectal abscess is a discrete soft tissue infection around the anus. The severity & depth is highly variable. The cavity of the abscess may discharge in a manner associated with formation of a fistulous tract. The cryptoglandular sepsis theory attributes a particular level of anal fistula development from a particular level of anorectal abscess as follows:

Anorectal Abscess	Corresponding Anal Fistula
Perianal	Subcutaneous / Submucous
Intersphincteric	Intersphincteric
Ischiorectal	High Anal (involves both anal sphincters)
	Low Anal (involves internal anal sphincter only)
Supralevator	Pelvirectal (above anorectal ring)

Q: How would you manage a patient with a perianal abscess?

- **Full History:** Is there as history of IBD, previous abscesses or immunosuppression e.g. diabetes, steroids, immunosuppressants or HIV?
- **Thorough Clinical Examination** including PR examination.
- **Proctoscopy / Sigmoidoscopy:** To seek internal fistula opening if present.
- **Surgery:** GA incision & drainage, sending pus for MC+S. Once deroofed, irrigate, deloculate, wash & pack the abscess to assist healing by secondary intention. Do not explore for a fistula acutely.
- **Clinic Follow-up:** If MC+S confirms presence of intestinal bacteria, suspect a fistula & arrange further investigation e.g. MRI, or treatment as necessary.

Q: You order an MRI of a patient with gastrointestinal flora at MC+S from a sample of pus taken at incision & drainage of an anal abscess. This demonstrates an anal fistula. What surgical treatment options are available?

These depend on the level & severity of the fistula as follows:

Procedure	Fistula
Lay Open	Subcutaneous, Submucous & Low Anal
Seton	High Anal & Intersphincteric
Fistulotomy & Flap	Complicated Fistulae

Q: What is Goodsall's Rule?

This describes the predictable course of an anal fistula, governed by its external opening (Fig 6.9). The patient is put in the lithotomy position & a line is imagined through 3 & 9 o'clock. Fistulae with external openings above this line form a radial tract directly to the same position internally. Fistulae with external openings below this line open in the posterior midline by horseshoeing through an unpredictable course.

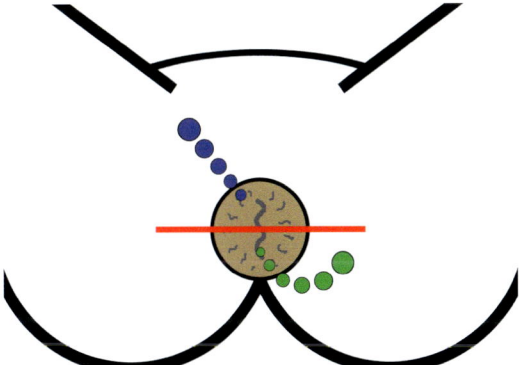

Fig 6.9: Goodsall's Rule.

Imagine line through 3 & 9 o'clock in lithotomy position.

External opening above line = direct course to internal opening.

External opening below line = horseshoeing course to midline internal opening.

Common Abdominal Scars

Q: Can you draw some common abdominal scars?

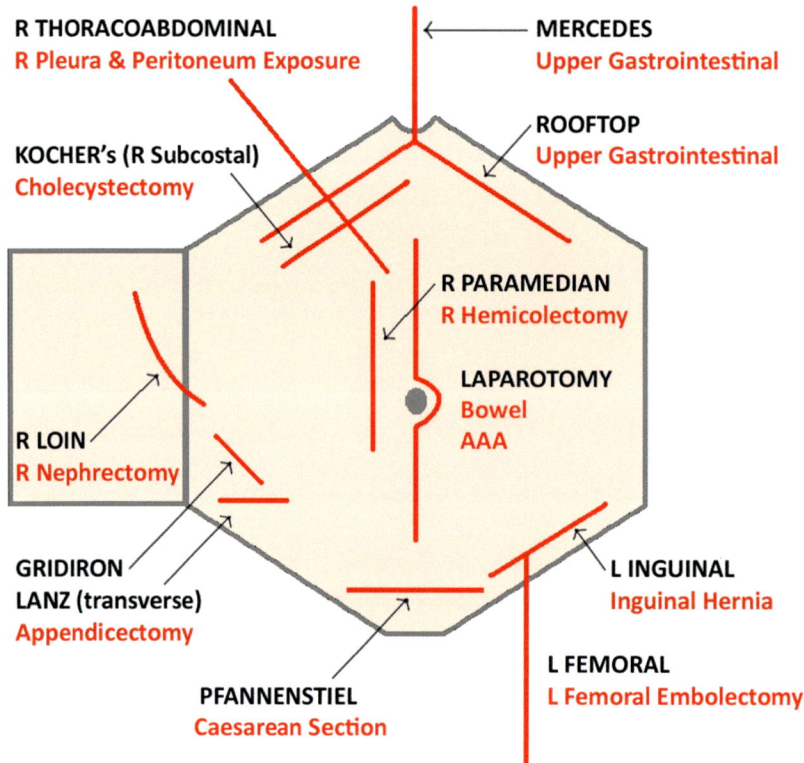

R THORACOABDOMINAL
R Pleura & Peritoneum Exposure

MERCEDES
Upper Gastrointestinal

ROOFTOP
Upper Gastrointestinal

KOCHER's (R Subcostal)
Cholecystectomy

R PARAMEDIAN
R Hemicolectomy

LAPAROTOMY
Bowel
AAA

R LOIN
R Nephrectomy

GRIDIRON
LANZ (transverse)
Appendicectomy

L INGUINAL
Inguinal Hernia

L FEMORAL
L Femoral Embolectomy

PFANNENSTIEL
Caesarean Section

Fig 6.10: Diagram of common abdominal scars. Note the right thoracoabdominal, midline laparotomy & left femoral incisions are labelled but not arrowed. **Red labelling indicates the potential reason for making the incision.**

CHAPTER 7
HERNIAE & SCROTUM

BH Miranda
MJ Portou
MC Winslet

CHAPTER CONTENTS

HERNIA EXAMINATION

START: The patient should be standing, fully exposed from umbilicus to knees.

Chaperone is vital.

Examine the groin lump / hernia, kneeling at the side of the patient.

Inspection	Interpretation
6 x S's	Describe lump site, size, shape, symmetry, overlying skin & associated scars.
Cough Impulse	Ask the patient to cough & check for an impulse.

Ask about pain.

Check for temperature changes, using the back of your hand.

Ask the patient if the lump is reducible.

If reduction of the hernia is not possible with the patient standing, assist them with lying down so they may reduce the hernia, then continue the examination with the patient standing again.

Palpation may be divided into 4 steps:

Palpation	Interpretation
Step 1 *'SEC FFP TR'*	Palpate lump surface, edge, consistency, fixity to skin & underlying structures, fluctuance, pulsatility & expansility, transilluminability & reducibility.
Step 2	Delineate anatomy (Fig 7.1). • Inguinal herniae emerge above & medial to the pubic tubercle. • Femoral herniae emerge below & lateral to the pubic tubercle.
Step 3	Ask the patient to reduce the lump & place the palmar surfaces of 2 fingertips over the superficial ring. Ask the patient to cough, then note if an 'impulse' is felt. Next remove your fingertips & ask the patient to cough again. • Indirect inguinal herniae will be contained at the superficial ring. • Direct inguinal herniae will reappear lateral to the controlled superficial ring.
Step 4	Ask the patient to reduce the lump & assist the patient in 'milking' the inguinal canal from the superficial to deep ring. Place the palmar surfaces of 2 fingertips over the deep ring & ask the patient to cough. Note if an 'impulse' is felt. Now remove your fingertips & ask the patient to cough again. • Indirect inguinal herniae will be controlled at the deep ring. • Direct inguinal herniae will reappear medial to the controlled deep ring.

Ausculation	Interpretation
Bowel Sounds	Herniae may contain bowel. This includes indirect inguinoscrotal herniae so do not forget to auscultate a scrotal lump!

Completion	Interpretation
Lymphadenopathy	Palpate for inguinal lymphadenopathy.
Contralateral Side	There may be an associated lesion.
Scrotum	There may be an associated lesion.
Abdominal Exam	Full abdominal examination is important, particularly in the acute stage, where incarceration & strangulation may precipitate abdominal pain & change in bowel habit.

FINISH:

SCROTAL LUMP EXAMINATION

START: The patient should be standing, fully exposed from umbilicus to knees.

                Chaperone is vital.

                Examine the scrotal lump, kneeling at the side of the patient.

Inspection	Interpretation
6 x S's	Describe lump site, size, shape, symmetry, overlying skin & associated scars.
Cough Impulse	Ask the patient to cough & check for an impulse. This may indicate an indirect inguinal-scrotal hernia rather than a true scrotal lesion.

Ask about pain.

Check for temperature changes, using the back of your hand.

Ask the patient if the lump is reducible.

Palpation	Interpretation
SEC FFP TR	Palpate lump surface, edge, consistency, fixity to skin & underlying structures, fluctuance, pulsatility & expansility, transilluminability & reducibility.
Get Above The Lump?	This is a vital step in the examination. If one can't get above a scrotal lump, it is likely to be an indirect inguinal-scrotal hernia. If one can get above the lump, it is likely to be a true scrotal lump.
Testicle	The testicle should be palpated as a separate structure.
Epididymis	The epididymis should be palpated as a separate structure.
Vas Deferens	The vas deferens should be palpated as a separate structure.

If you can't get above the lump, continue palpation as for a groin / hernia lump from STEP 2.

If you can get above the lump, continue the scrotal lump examination as outlined below.

Completion	Interpretation
Lymphadenopathy	Palpate for lymphadenopathy. Remember that the penis & skin of the scrotum drain to inguinal nodes. Remember that the testes drain to retroperitoneal para-aortic nodes that may be enlarged but not palpable.
Contralateral Side	There may be an associated lesion.

FINISH:

OSCE QUESTIONS

Herniae

Q: Can you delineate the hernia relevant anatomy of the inguinal region?

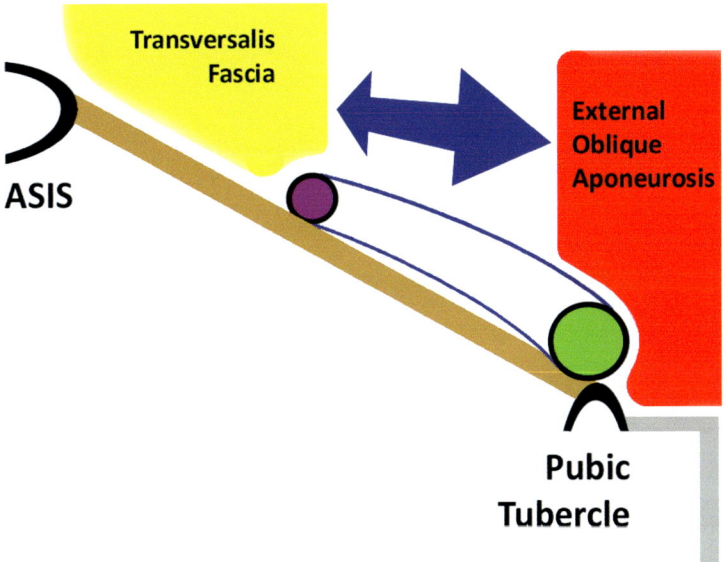

Fig 7.1: Hernia relevant anatomy of the right inguinal region *(see colour coding below).*

Anatomy	Notes
ASIS & Pubic Tubercle	The anterior superior iliac spine (ASIS) & pubic tubercles must be identified first.
Inguinal Ligament	Delineate the inguinal ligament which has attachments to both the anterior superior iliac spine (ASIS) & pubic tubercle.
Deep Ring	Point out the location of the deep ring which lies just above the midpoint of the inguinal ligament. It is formed by an aperture through the **transversalis fascia**. Mention that the femoral artery may be palpated below the inguinal ligament at the mid-inguinal point, halfway between the ASIS & pubic symphysis.
Superficial Ring	Point out the location of the superficial ring which lies just above the pubic tubercle. It is formed by an aperture through the **external oblique aponeurosis**.
Inguinal Canal	Finally, explain that the inguinal canal is an oblique communication between the deep & superficial inguinal rings, formed by the arching fibres of the **transversus abdominis** & **internal oblique** muscles.

Q: What are the borders of the inguinal canal?

Border	Anatomy
Posterior Wall	Transversalis Fascia
Anterior Wall	External Oblique Aponeurosis
Floor	Inguinal Ligament
Roof	Arching Fibres of Transversus Abdominis & Internal Oblique

Q: What are the differential diagnoses of a groin lump?

These include the differential diagnoses of any lump *(see lumps 'n' bumps chapter)* & those specific to the groin as follows:

Above the Inguinal Ligament	Below the Inguinal Ligament
Inguinal Hernia	Femoral Hernia
Testicular Maldescent	Testicular Maldescent
	Saphena Varix
	Femoral Artery Aneurysm

Q: What are the differential diagnoses of a scrotal lump?

These include the differential diagnoses of any lump *(see lumps 'n' bumps chapter)* & those specific to the contents of the scrotum. With respect to scrotal contents, differential diagnoses may be classified according to findings on palpation as follows:

Can't Get Above Lump	
Indirect Inguinal-Scrotal Hernia	
Congenital / Infantile Hydrocoele	
Can Get Above Lump & Palpable Separately to Testis	**Can Get Above Lump & Palpable With the Testis**
Epididymal Cyst	Haematocoele
Epididymitis	Hydrocoele
Spermatocoele	Orchitis
Varicocoele	Torsion
	Tumour

Q: What is an inguinal hernia?

An abnormal protrusion of abdominal contents through the inguinal region (Fig 7.2). It is the most common groin hernia & may be classified as direct / indirect as follows:

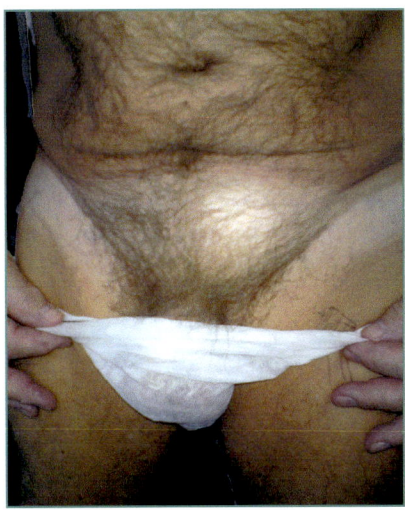

Fig 7.2: Left-sided indirect inguinal hernia.

Classification	Notes
Direct	Due to an acquired weakness in the transversalis fascia. Increased incidence with age, COPD, obesity & smoking. The hernia protrudes directly through the weakness (Hesselbach's Triangle), without traversing the inguinal canal.
Indirect	Due to a patent processus vaginalis. This is a congenital defect which allows for the hernia to traverse the deep ring, inguinal canal & superficial ring. If extension into the scrotum is observed, an indirect inguinoscrotal hernia is present.

Q: What are the treatment options for an inguinal hernia?

Treatment	Examples
Conservative	A truss is a device that may be used to help contain an easily reducible inguinal hernia within the abdomen, however it is not curative & rarely required.
Medical	Optimise COPD medication & treat pneumonia to prevent coughing which increases intra-abdominal pressure & may worsen the hernia.
Surgical	This is the gold standard treatment. It involves surgical herniotomy & herniorrhaphy that may be performed laparoscopically or open. **Lichtenstein's Repair** involves the use of a polypropylene mesh to reinforce the repair. If there is any concern about associated infection, **Shouldice's Repair** may be preferred as this does not involve the use of a mesh. Instead, a 4 layer overlapping muscle repair is undertaken.

Q: What is a femoral hernia?

An abnormal protrusion through the femoral canal. It is less common than an inguinal hernia. It is seen more commonly in females due to stretching of the femoral canal during pregnancy, or fat regression within the femoral canal after menopause.

Q: What are the treatment options for a femoral hernia?

There is no place for conservative management of a femoral hernia due to the high risk of incarceration & strangulation. All femoral herniae should therefore be operated on as soon as possible. Asymptomatic, reducible femoral herniae may be operated on using a low approach e.g. **Lockwood's Repair**. Symptomatic, strangulated femoral herniae may be operated on using a high approach e.g. **McEvedy's Repair**, which may easily be extended to a laparotomy to resect dead bowel if necessary.

Q: Do you know of any other herniae?

Hernia	Notes
Littre's	Containing a Meckel's Diverticulum.
Maydl's	Containing a 'W' shaped loop of bowel, such that the middle arm of the 'W' becomes compressed & strangulated.
Richter's	Containing only one side of the bowel wall, which may become strangulated.
Sliding	Part of the hernia sac wall is composed of bowel. This is also known as a hernia *'en glissade'*.
Epigastric	Abnormal protrusion of abdominal contents through the epigastric region of the linea alba. Surgery includes herniotomy & herniorrhaphy, with repair of the defective linea alba either directly or with a reinforcing mesh.
Incisional	Abnormal protrusion of abdominal contents through a weakness in the abdominal wall, at a site of previous surgery. The underlying aetiology is therefore iatrogenic. It is rarely symptomatic & risk of strangulation is low, so conservative treatment is often all that is required. Surgical options include tension free mesh repair either laparoscopically or open.
Spigelian	Abnormal protrusion of abdominal contents through the linea semilunaris. Open or laparoscopic mesh repair is advocated due to the risk of strangulation.

Hernia	Notes
Umbilical	Abnormal protrusion of abdominal contents through a defect of / near the cicatrix. It may be congenital or acquired (Fig 7.3). If congenital, it is due to a congenital defect of closure & includes the following: 1. **Exomphalos:** Herniation of abdominal contents, covered by a transparent membrane composed of 3 layers. The outer layer is amniotic membrane, the middle layer Wharton's Jelly & the inner layer peritoneum. There is a risk of perforation & peritonitis, so surgical repair is required. 2. **Gastroschisis:** Herniation of abdominal contents just lateral to the cicatrix, without a covering membrane. Hypothermia, hypovolaemia & sepsis may occur due to the presence of eviscerated bowel. Immediate treatment involves placement of a NGT, fluid resuscitation & protection of bowel with sterile packs & bags. Surgical repair is then required.
Paraumbilical	Abnormal protrusion of abdominal contents through a defect in the *linea alba* near the umbilicus. There is a high risk of strangulation. Surgical options include a Mayo repair, or repair of the defect using a reinforcing mesh. A Mayo repair involves herniotomy & herniorrhaphy, repairing the defect by suturing the upper part of rectus over the lower part of rectus in a *'vest over pants'* fashion.
Brainstem	Due to increased intracranial pressure e.g. post head injury.
Diaphragmatic	Hiatus hernia. (Fig 7.4)

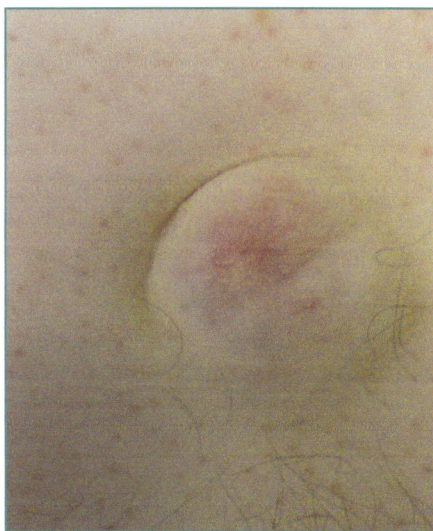

Fig 7.3: Umbilical hernia.

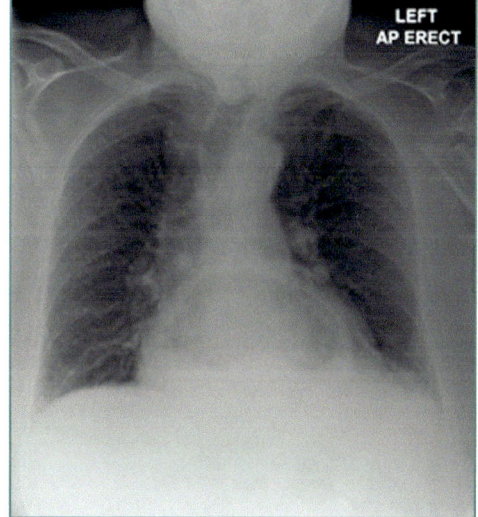

Fig 7.4: Hiatus hernia radiograph

A supra-diaphragmatic 'mass' is visible with an air-fluid level. This represents a hiatus hernia. There is also a left humerus fracture noted.

Testicular Maldescent

Q: What is testicular maldescent?

This terminology encompasses 3 abnormalities of descent of the testis as follows:

Abnormality	Notes
Retractile	This is due to an overactive cremasteric reflex & affects children. The testis appears to be incompletely descended, but may be noticed within the scrotum after a warm bath. Treatment is conservative as the testis becomes less retractile with age.
Ectopic	The testis descends to an abnormal position after exiting the superficial inguinal ring. Common locations include the superficial inguinal pouch, perineum, root of penis & within the femoral canal.
Undescended Testis	The undescended testis prematurely stops its descent anywhere along the normal path of descent as guided by the gubernaculum.

Q: What are the complications of an undescended testis?

Complications include an increased risk of:

- Trauma
- Torsion
- Tumour
- Infertility
- Psychological Distress

Undescended testes confer a 30X risk of developing a testicular tumour, most commonly a seminoma. Treatment consists of early orchidopexy.

Q: What is the treatment for an undescended testis?

Orchidopexy is the treatment of choice & this should be undertaken at the age of 1 year to prevent complications. If an undescended testis is noticed in an older child, a short course of hCG or GnRH may help in approximately 15% of cases.

Benign Scrotal Lumps

Q: What is a hydrocoele?

This is a scrotal swelling due to fluid accumulation within the tunica vaginalis & may be classified as follows:

Classification	Explanation
Primary	Due to a patent processus vaginalis.
Secondary	Occurs in response to underlying disease e.g. infection, torsion & tumour.

Q: What types of primary hydrocoeles do you know of?

Primary Hydrocoele	Notes
Vaginal	This is the most common primary hydrocoele. Accumulation of fluid is limited to the tunica vaginalis & neither extends to the vas deferens, nor communicates with the peritoneal cavity.
Congenital	Accumulation of fluid extends to surround the vas deferens. There is also communication with the peritoneal cavity as the processus vaginalis is not obliterated.
Infantile	Accumulation of fluid extends to surround the vas deferens. The processus vaginalis is obliterated at the level of the deep ring, so there is no communication with the peritoneal cavity.
Hydrocoele of the Cord	This is rare. Accumulation of fluid is limited to vas deferens only.

Q: What treatment options are available for a hydrocoele?

Infants with a hydrocoele may be managed conservatively until the age of 1 year when surgery is indicated. Secondary hydrocoeles resolve with treatment of the underlying cause. Treatment options for primary hydrocoeles may therefore be classified as follows:

Conservative	Surgical
Reassurance	**Aspirate:** This is both therapeutic & diagnostic.
Scrotal Support	**Phenol Injection:** Phenol is a sclerosing agent that may prevent recurrence.
	Lord's Plication: The hydrocoele sac is incised & plicated behind the testis.
	Jaboulay's Procedure: The hydrocoele sac is incised, partially excised & the remaining tissue is plicated behind the testis.

Q: What are epididymitis & orchitis?

Epididymitis is inflammation of the epididymis. Orchitis is inflammation of the testicle. Clinical features include acute pain, erythema & oedema. Clinical features of a urinary tract & systemic infection may also be present. Acute cases may progress to chronic, especially when TB is the cause.

Q: What are the causes of epididymitis & orchitis?

Cause	Examples
Viral	Mumps, Infectious Mononucleosis & Coxsackie B
Bacterial	Ascending UTI e.g. *E. coli*, STD e.g. *Chlamydia*, TB

Q: What is important about an acute presentation of epididymitis & orchitis?

It is important to differentiate this from torsion. Thorough history & clinical examination should point towards an infective cause rather than torsion. **If in any doubt, explore the scrotum**. The following investigations assist in diagnosis:

Investigation	Examples
Haematology & Biochemistry	FBC, U&E & CRP.
Serology	VDRL.
Microbiology	• **Swabs** for MC+S. • **MSU** for MC+S. • **3 x Early Morning Urine Samples for ZN Staining & Microscopy:** The presence of acid-fast bacilli indicates TB.
Radiology	USS.

Q: What are the treatment options for epididymitis & orchitis?

Treatment	Acute	Chronic
CONSERVATIVE	Bed Rest & Scrotal Support	Bed Rest & Scrotal Support
MEDICAL	Analgesia	Analgesia
	Antibiotics e.g. Ciprofloxacin	Antibiotics e.g. anti-TB regimen
SURGICAL	Abscess Drainage	Orchidectomy if severe

Q: What are epididymal cysts?

Fluid filled swellings of the epididymis which are palpated separately from the testes. They are often multiple, fluctuant & transilluminate. Large persistent cysts may be excised.

Q: What is a spermatocoele?

A cystic swelling that contains spermatozoa. It is most commonly found at the epididymis & spermatic cord. Clinical features & treatment are similar to epididymal cysts.

Q: What is a varicocoele?

A collection of dilated tortuous veins of the pampiniform plexus. Clinically, the scrotum appears as a 'bag of worms' when the patient is standing. This appearance disappears when the patient is lying. 98% are left sided as the left testicular vein (longer than the right) drains directly into the left renal vein (may be compressed where it is crossed by the colon). Varicocoeles appearing in late adulthood should be investigated further for possible invasion of the left renal vein by carcinoma. If symptomatic, surgical treatment options include radiological embolisation & ligation of the testicular vein proximal to the deep inguinal ring, either open or laparoscopically.

Testicular Torsion

Q: What is testicular torsion & why does it occur?

This is an acute condition where the testicle twists around the axis of the spermatic cord. It often affects teenagers & young adults, with a recent history of trauma, who may have an underlying abnormality. The **bell clapper** testicular abnormality describes a tunica vaginalis that doesn't anchor to the testicle, hence allowing free movement of the testicle like the clapper inside a bell.

Q: What are the clinical features of testicular torsion & how would you manage it?

Clinical features include an acutely hot, painful & tender scrotal swelling, abdominal pain, nausea & vomiting. The cord may be shorter & thicker than the contralateral side on palpation, due to twisting along its axis. This is a surgical emergency & there is only a 4–6 hour window in which to salvage the testicle. Management strategies include:

- Appropriate Resuscitation
- NBM
- FBC, U&E, G&S
- (IV) Fluids
- Analgesia
- Consent Patient for Scrotal Exploration +/- Bilateral Orchidopexy +/- Orchidectomy
- Place Patient on Emergency List
- Inform Anaesthetist

Q: What are the differential diagnoses for testicular torsion?

- Epididymitis & Orchitis
- Hydatid of Morgagni Torsion
- Strangulated Inguinal Hernia

Testicular Tumours & Cancer

Q: What testicular tumours do you know of?

Classification	Examples	Notes
BENIGN	**Leydig Cell Tumour**	Benign neoplasm of interstitial Leydig cells. May cause precocious puberty due to secretion of testosterone.
	Sertoli Cell Tumour	Benign neoplasm of Sertoli cells. May cause gynaecomastia due to release of oestrogens.
MALIGNANT	**Seminoma**	Malignant neoplasm of seminiferous tubule cells with a peak age of 30-40 years. Represents approximately 40% of testicular malignancy. Teratomas may secrete βhCG (never αFP).
	Teratoma	Malignant neoplasm containing elements from all 3 germ layers, derived from multipotent cells that display a wide range of differentiation. Represents approximately 30% of testicular malignancy. Teratomas may secrete αFP & βhCG.
	Mixed	Malignant neoplasm composed of both seminoma & teratoma. Represents approximately 20% of testicular malignancy.
	Lymphoma Choriocarcinoma Gonadoblastoma	Together represent approximately 10% of testicular malignancies.

Q: What are the clinical features of testicular malignancy?

- Painless, Hard Testicular Lump
- Sensation of Dragging
- Secondary Hydrocoele
- Back Pain (para-aortic lymphadenopathy)
- Respiratory Features (lung metastases)

Q: What staging systems do you know of for testicular malignancy?

Royal Marsden Staging:

Stage	Definition
I	Tumour confined to testis.
II	Para-aortic lymphadenopathy.
III	Supra-diaphragmatic lymphadenopathy.
IV	Extra-nodal matastases.
L	**L1:** <3 lung metastases.
	L2: >3 lung metastases all <2cm in diameter.
	L3: >3 lung metastases with ≥1 lesions >2cm in diameter.
H	Liver metastases.

TNM Classification:

Tumour Spread (T)		Regional Lymphadenopathy (N)	
Tx:	Tumour can't be assessed.	**N0:**	No regional lymphadenopathy.
T0:	No tumour present.	**N1:**	Regional lymphadenopathy <2cm in diameter.
Tis:	Carcinoma *in situ*.	**N2:**	Regional lymphadenopathy 2-5 cm in diameter.
T1:	Tumour confined to testicle or epididymis.	**N3:**	Regional lymphadenopathy >5cm in diameter.
T2:	Tumour confined to testicle or epididymis but either with local invasion of the tunica albuginea, vessels or lymph nodes.	**Distant Metastasis or Lymphadenopathy (M)**	
		M0:	No regional lymphadenopathy.
		M1a:	Lung metastases or distant lymphadenopathy.
T3: Tumour invades the spermatic cord.		**M1b:**	Any other organ metastases.
T4: Tumour invades the scrotum.			

Q: What investigations would you consider for a patient with a suspected testicular malignancy?

Investigations	Notes
Blood Tests	αFP, βhCG & LDH
Radiology	• **Scrotal USS:** Tumour assessment • **CXR:** Lung metastases • **CT:** Staging of disease

Q: What happens to αFP & βhCG levels in testicular tumours?

Tumour	Biochemistry
Seminoma	Raised βhCG
Non Seminoma	Raised αFP
• Teratoma	Raised βhCG
• Yolk Sac Tumours	

Q: What treatment options are there for testicular malignancy?

Treatment depends on underlying pathology & includes:

Treatment	Notes
Surgery	Orchidectomy via an inguinal approach, after clamping the cord. A scrotal incision is avoided to prevent seeding to scrotal skin that is drained by inguinal lymph nodes (not para-aortic).
Chemotherapy	Seminoma & Teratoma.
Radiotherapy	Seminoma.

CHAPTER 8
STOMA

BH Miranda
MJ Portou
MC Winslet

CHAPTER CONTENTS

STOMA EXAMINATION

START: Patient exposure is to underwear ideally. This also allows for further examination of the abdominal system.

The stoma may initially be examined with the patient standing, followed by lying flat.

The stoma bag should be taken off to allow for a thorough examination of the operation site & bag constituents.

Use sheet covers appropriately, to maintain patient dignity.

Memory: 'Small Bags Should Lay More Snugly On Committed Patients'

INSPECTION	Interpretation	
Site	Ideally should be sited away from bony prominences, scars & skin folds. Common stoma sites include:	
	• **Epigastric**	= PEG & Transverse Loop Colostomy.
	• **Right Iliac Fossa**	= Iliostomy (Fig 8.1).
	• **Left Iliac Fossa**	= Colostomy.
Bag & Contents	• **Fluid**	= Small Bowel Contents (Iliostomy) / Urine (Urostomy).
	• **Solid**	= Large Bowel Contents (Colostomy).
Spout?	• **Spout Present**	= Iliostomy (Fig 8.1).
	• **Flush to Skin**	= Colostomy.
Lumen	• **1 Lumen**	= End Iliostomy (Fig 8.1).
	• **2 Lumens**	= Loop Iliostomy.
Mucosa	Comment on whether the mucosa is healthy or unhealthy e.g. inflamed or ulcerated.	
Scar	Comment on associated scars that may indicate the underlying procedure.	
Old Sites	Comment on scars that may indicate previous stoma formation e.g. Crohn's Disease.	
Complications	Comment on presence of complications as follows:	
	• **Anatomical**	= Prolapse, Retraction, Stenosis & Parastomal Hernia (ask the patient to cough).
	• **Dermatological**	= Skin Discomfort & Excoriations Present (primarily due to leakage of iliostomy contents).
	• **Metabolic**	= Electrolyte Imbalance.
	• **Vascular**	= Haemorrhage, Ischaemia & Gangrene.
	• **Psychological**	= Psychosexual Disturbance.
	• **Other**	= Associated Gallstone Disease.
Perineum	The anus will be absent in an AP resection.	

Ask about pain.

Look at the patient's face throughout the examination.

Warm your hands by rubbing them together & warn the patient that they may be cold.

Feel for any temperature changes with the back of your hand.

PALPATION	Interpretation
Lumen	Place a finger into the lumen to ensure adequate patency.
Parastomal Hernia	This must be specifically palpated & may have a cough impulse.
Stoma Bag	Comment on the stoma bag as follows: • **1 x Piece** = The whole bag must be changed as 1 unit. • **2 x Piece** = There is a base plate on the skin & only the bag must be changed.

AUSCULTATION	Interpretation
Bowel Sounds	• Comment on presence or absence of bowel sounds e.g. Ileus (absent). • Comment on character of bowel sounds e.g. Bowel Obstruction (tinkling).

COMPLETION	Interpretation
Abdominal Examination	A full abdominal examination is vital *(see abdomen chapter)*.

FINISH:

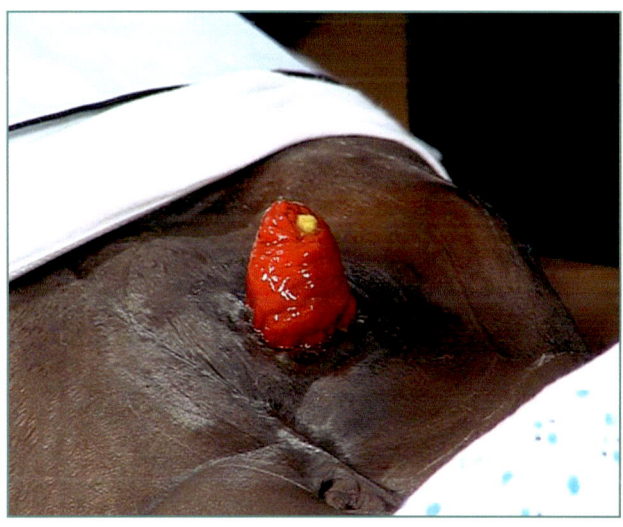

Fig 8.1: Active end ileostomy. Note the laparotomy scar & transverse scar from previous stoma formation.

OSCE QUESTIONS

Q: What is an enteric surgical stoma?

This is an iatrogenic opening that connects part of the bowel to the outside world. In the case of enteric stomas, a bag is required to collect the resulting discharge.

Q: How would you classify enteric surgical stomas?

These may be classified as end / loop & ileostomy / colostomy as follows:

Classification	Ileostomy	Colostomy
End	Panproctocolectomy	**Hartmann's Procedure** (rectosigmoid emergencies)
		AP Resection
Loop	Diversion	Palliative
	Protect Distal Anastomosis	Diversion (pre-chemo / radiotherapy)

Q: What are the clinical indications for an enteric surgical stoma?

Indications	Notes
Feeding	Enteral feeding is preferred to TPN e.g. PEG & PEJ.
Diversion	Temporarily protects distal bowel with view to later reversal e.g. defunctioning loop ileostomy. In these cases, primary bowel anastomosis may be contraindicated or a distal abscess / fistula may be present.
Lavage	Temporary stomas for on-table lavage prior to bowel resection.
Operation	**Hartmann's Procedure** fashions a temporary colostomy that may be later reversed e.g. rectosigmoid emergencies. Other examples include AP Resection & Panproctocolectomy, when permanent stomas are required.

SECTION A3: LIMBS, SPINE & VASCULAR

GALS & RHEUMATOLOGY

Dr Christopher Lutterodt
Dr Katherine Lindsay
Ms Prita Daliya

CHAPTER CONTENTS

GALS SCREEN EXAMINATION

The GALS Screen is a systematic 'screening examination' that assists identification of rheumatological & orthopaedic disease / conditions. It consists of brief targeted questioning, followed by a focused clinical assessment according to the framework:

Gait
Arms
Legs
Spine

Should the examining doctor identify positive findings, further targeted musculoskeletal / neurological examination(s) should be performed as appropriate *(see orthopaedics & neurosciences chapters).*

Note: Like all examination protocols, practice is key here. There are many variable components to the GALS screen. The trick is to ensure development of a comprehensive system that flows well both in an examination situation & during clinical practice.

START:

Begin the GALS screen by asking the following questions:

Q1.   Do you have pain or stiffness in any of your muscles, joints or back?
Q2.   Can you dress yourself completely without difficulty?
Q3.   Can you walk up & down stairs without difficulty?

Start with the patient exposed to their underwear.
Remember to ask about pain.

GAIT

Ask the patient to walk away a few steps, turn around & come back, whilst assessing:

- The Phases of Gait (stance, swing) *(see orthopaedics chapter)*
- Gait Fluidity
- Stride Length
- Ability to Quickly Turn

ARMS

Position the patient on the side of the bed, hands palmar surface down on a supporting pillow. Ensure that both upper limbs are systematically inspected throughout all joints & surfaces (e.g. neck, shoulder, upper arm, elbow, forearm, wrist hand & fingers).

LOOK	Interpretation
Scars	Post-operative, post-infective, traumatic.
Swelling	Soft tissue (RA, effusions, nodules), bony (dislocation, old fractures).
Symmetry	Symmetrical alignment of the shoulders, elbows & wrists.
Deformity	Nails (onycholysis in psoriasis), hands (OA, RA) (Figs 9.1, 10.7, 11.1–11.3), elbow (cubitus valgus, varus, hyperextension).
Erythema	Inflammation, infection.
	Note: signs of pallor / hyperaemia may indicate vasculitis or Raynaud's disease.
Sinus	Post-operative, post-infective.
Muscle Wasting	Thenar & hypothenar eminences, dorsal interossei, forearm, upper arm, shoulders.

Note: In particular, features of neurological involvement, RA & OA should be noted.

Fig 9.1: Rheumatoid hands.

Bilateral rheumatoid arthritis is seen, with ulnar deviation of the MCPJs, multiple swan neck deformities & rheumatoid nodules over the MCPJs including the right index & little fingers & left middle & little fingers.

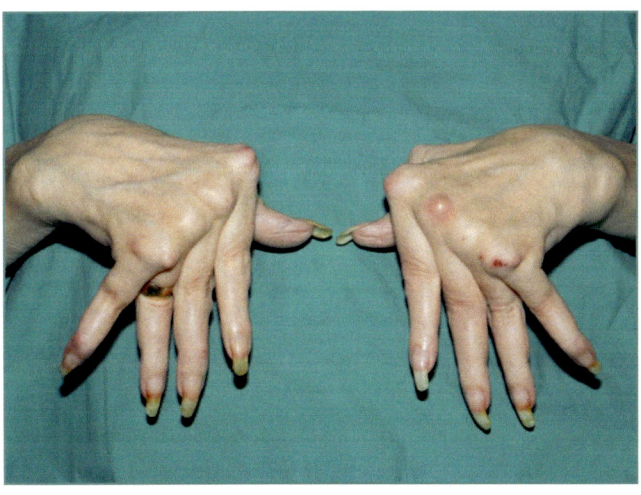

FEEL	Interpretation
MCPJ Tenderness	MCPJ squeeze may be tender in RA / other inflammatory joint disease causing metacarpophalangeal joint pain (Fig 9.2).

MCPJ squeeze may be tender in RA / other inflammatory joint disease causing metacarpophalangeal joint pain.

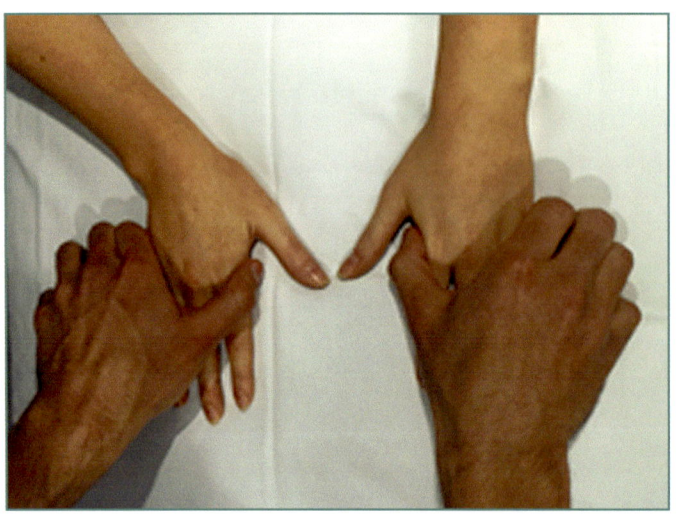

MOVE	Interpretation
Shoulder Abduction & External Rotation	Ask the patient to put their hands behind their head, pushing their elbows back. This is a good screening test for global active shoulder movement. These are the first movements affected in glenohumeral joint arthritis.
Shoulder Adduction & Internal Rotation	Ask the patient to put their hands behind their back, thumbs pointing to the ceiling. The thumbs should normally reach T6. This is a good screening test for global active shoulder movement.
Elbow Flexion / Extension	Ask the patient to bend their elbows, then stretch their arms straight out in front of them, palms facing upwards. Observe for any movement limitation, deformity or additional clinical features.
Wrist Supination / Pronation	Ask the patient to bend their elbows to 90° & tuck them into their sides. Now ask the patient to turn both of their hands over from palms up (supination) to palms down (pronation). Assesses the proximal & distal radioulnar joints.
Fingers	Ask the patient to make a fist, then fan out their fingers to assess the MCPJs & IPJs (Fig 9.3).
Opposition	Ask the patient to touch the tip of each finger to the tip of their thumb in turn.
Power Grip	Indicator of strength.
Fine Motor Function	Ask the patient to pick up a coin / paper clip, or un-button their shirt.

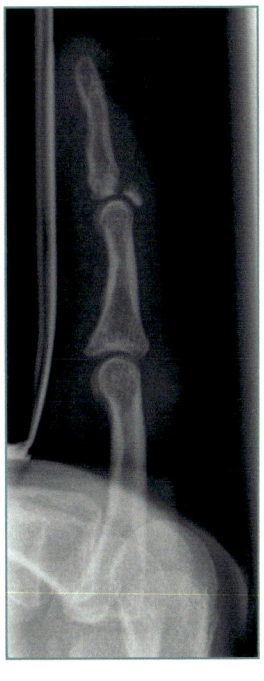

Lateral radiograph indicating a bony mallet deformity of the right index finger distal interphalangeal joint (DIPJ).

LEGS

Position the patient supine on the couch.
Note that areas not visualised with the patient lying, should be examined when the patient stands during assessment of the spine.

LOOK	Interpretation	
Scars	Post-operative, post-infective, traumatic.	
Swelling	Soft tissue (effusion, popliteal cyst), bony (OA).	
Symmetry	Assess symmetrical alignment of the iliac crests, knees & ankles.	
Deformity	Knee:	Flexion / extension, varus / valgus (Fig 9.4).
	Foot:	Systematically inspect the fore- / mid- / hind-foot.
		Look for callosities on the soles of the feet.
		Look at the foot arches.
		Examine the patient's shoes for unequal wear.
Erythema	Inflammation, infection.	
Sinus	Post-operative, post-infective.	
Muscle Wasting	Gluteals, quadriceps, hamstrings, calves.	
Note: In particular, features of neurological involvement, RA & OA should be noted.		

Fig 9.4: Genu valgum.

A valgus deformity of the knees is noted as the joint distal to the knee joint (ankle joint) is deviating away from the midline (arrowed).

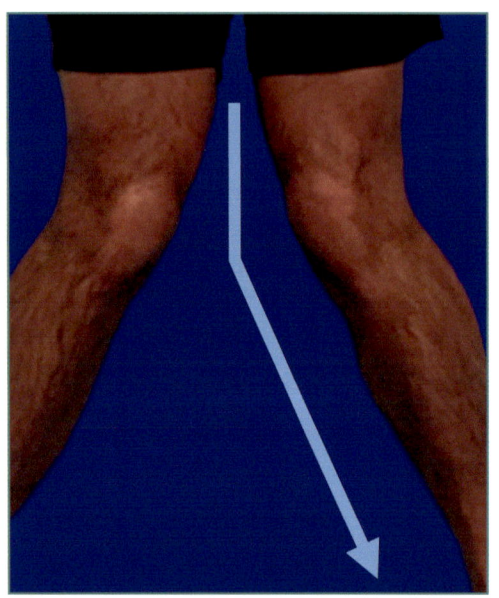

FEEL	Interpretation
Knee Effusions	The patellar tap, bulge & cross-fluctuation tests should be performed *(see knee examination)*.
Friction Test	Move the patella superiorly & inferiorly, pressing it down against the femur. Painful grating is experienced if the central portion of articular cartilage is damaged.
MTPJ Tenderness	MTPJ squeeze may be tender in RA / other inflammatory joint disease causing metatarsophalangeal joint pain.

MOVE	Interpretation
Knee Flexion & Crepitus	Passively bend the knee, pushing the patient's heel towards their bottom with one hand & supporting the knee with your other hand over the joint to feel for crepitus as you do.
Hip Flexion	Passively flex both the hip & knee to 90°, also feeling for joint crepitus over the knee again.
Hip Internal Rotation	With the hip flexed, fix the knee with your left hand & secure the heel with your right hand. Keeping the patient's thigh steady rotate the hip by moving the foot & ankle laterally & keeping the knee pointed medially. Internal rotation is the first affected movement in hip OA. External rotation may also be assessed here.

SPINE

Note: Some pathology from previous sections of the GALS examination may be more obvious with the patient standing e.g. pes planus. It is important to remember to re-consider these here.

Ask the patient to stand & inspect from the FRONT, BACK & SIDES as follows:

LOOK	Interpretation
Scars	Post-operative e.g. spinal fusion, discectomy.
Swelling	Bony e.g. gibbus (a bony prominence due to vertebral body collapse in skeletal tuberculosis)
Symmetry	Any signs of deviation / torticollis.
	Check the alignment of the iliac crests.
Deformity	Ensure a normal cervical lordosis, thoracic kyphosis, & lumbar lordosis. Comment on the presence / absence of an abnormal scoliosis (corrects on sitting if due to a leg length discrepancy).
	Observe for vertebral collapse.
Erythema	Inflammation, infection.
Sinus	Post-operative, post-infective.
Muscle Wasting	Paraspinal muscle bulk.

FEEL	Interpretation
Tenderness	Palpate the vertebral column & paraspinal muscles. Also palpate the temporomandibular joints (TMJs) bilaterally.
Fibromyalgia Pressure Points	Press over the mid-point of the supraspinatus muscle assessing for hyperalgesia in fibromyalgia.

MOVE	Interpretation
TMJ	Active side to side movement of the patients jaw will elicit pain in fibromyalgia & RA.
Cervical Spine Lateral Flexion	Ask the patient to touch their right ear to their right shoulder, & then repeat for the contralateral side. ROM is commonly decreased in cervical spondylosis. Normal = 45°.
Lumbar Spine Forward Flexion	Ask the patient to touch their toes, keeping their legs straight (also assesses hip flexion). Normal = finger to floor distance of <15cm.

SPECIAL TESTS	Interpretation
Schober's Test (Fig 9.5)	Draw a line through both posterior superior iliac spines (Dimples of Venus). Mark the spine 5cm below & 10cm above this line. Keeping the tape measure in place, ask the patient to touch their toes & record the new distance between the outermost marks. Normal flexion = 5cm. This is reduced in lumbar spine pathology e.g. ankylosing spondylitis.

Fig 9.5 Schober's test.

Draw a line through both posterior superior iliac spines (Dimples of Venus). Mark the spine 5cm below & 10cm above this line. Keeping the tape measure in place, ask the patient to touch their toes & record the new distance between the outermost marks. Normal flexion = 5cm. This is reduced in lumbar spine pathology e.g. ankylosing spondylitis.

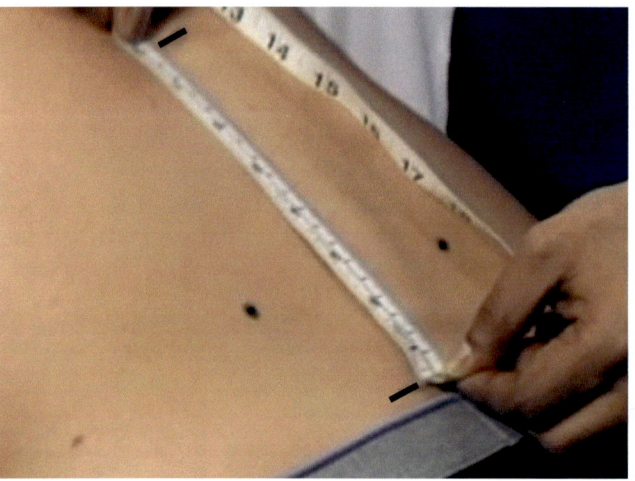

FINISH:

DOCUMENTATION

GALS screen findings may be easily documented using the following format. If an abnormality is detected it may be listed specifically, otherwise record NAD (no abnormality detected).

	Look	Feel	Move
Gait	NAD	NAD	NAD
Arms	NAD	NAD	NAD
Legs	NAD	NAD	NAD
Spine	Reduced cervical & lumbar lordosis	Lumbar paraspinal muscle tenderness	Limited by pain

OSCE QUESTIONS

Note: Further rheumatological topics are covered in the orthopaedics & hands chapters e.g. OA, RA, ankylosing spondylitis, Paget's disease of bone & gout.

Fibromyalgia

Q: What is fibromyalgia?

- Fibromyalgia is a chronic condition characterised by widespread pain, allodynia, joint stiffness, fatigue, & sleep disturbance.
- Psychological features are often present e.g. anxiety & depression.
- Commonly presents between 20-50 years of age.
- M : F = 1 : 9.

Q: How would you make a diagnosis of fibromyalgia?

The 2010 diagnostic criteria are based on the identification of pain in 19 potential areas (Fig 9.6) described as the Widespread Pain Index (WPI) & a calculation of a Symptoms Severity (SS) scale score. The SS scale score is calculated by asking patients to rate 4 areas (Fatigue, Waking feeling refreshed, Cognitive symptoms, Somatic symptoms) on a scale of 0 to 3 (where 0= no symptoms, 1= mild symptoms, 2= moderate symptoms, 3= severe symptoms).

Diagnosis	Criteria
American College of Rheumatology Criteria (2010)	1. WPI ≥7 & SS scale score ≥5 **or** WPI 3-6 & SS scale score ≥9
	2. Symptoms for ≥3 months
	3. Other differential diagnoses for pain excluded

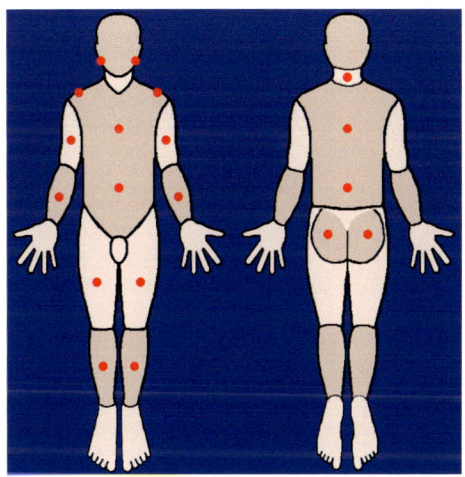

Fig 9.6: Widespread pain index (WPI).

There are 19 potential body areas in which the patient may have had pain during the last 7 days. These include; jaw (L/R), shoulder (L/R), upper arm (L/R), lower arm (L/R), upper leg (L/R), lower leg (L/R), chest, abdomen, neck, upper back, lower back, hip/buttock (L/R).

Q: What are the treatment options for fibromyalgia?

Treatment is symptomatic:

Conservative	Psychological	Medical
Patient Education: • Recognition of exacerbating features	**Counselling**	**Anti-Depressants:** • Tricyclics • Selective serotonin reuptake inhibitors (SSRIs) • Serotonin-norepinephrine reuptake inhibitors (SNRIs)
Stress Reduction: • Relaxation tapes • Support networks • Encourage optimal sleep	**Cognitive Behavioural Therapy**	**Analgesia:** • Tramadol • Pregabalin • Gabapentin
Low-Impact Aerobic Exercise: • Yoga • Tai-chi	**Support Groups / Networks:** • Fibromyalgia Society • Family	
Alternative Therapies: • Acupuncture • Massage	• Friends • Doctor	

Psoriatic Arthritis

Q: What is psoriatic arthropathy?

- Seronegative spondyloarthropathy.
- Presentation can include characteristic swelling of both the joints & soft tissue of the fingers & toes resulting in a 'sausage-like' appearance (**dactylitis**).
- It may also affect the spine, knees, ankles, shoulders, elbows & wrists.
- Strongly associated with nail changes such as pitting, onycholysis, subungual hyperkeratosis, & Beau's lines
- Up to 40% of patients with severe dermatological psoriasis also develop psoriatic arthritis. In a small proportion of patients the arthritis predates the skin changes.

Q: What are the different types of psoriatic arthritis?

Type	Features
Asymmetrical	• 70% of cases. • Dactylitis (swelling of the digits) is common. • Least severe, affecting <5 joints on one side of the body.
Symmetrical	• 15% of cases. • Can be difficult to distinguish from RA as has a similar joint pattern. • Milder disease course than RA with no extra-articular RA features.
Distal Interphalangeal Predominant	• 5% of cases. • Affects the distal interphalangeal joints of the hands. • Strongly associated with nail changes.
Spondylitis	• 5% of cases. • Similar pattern to Ankylosing Spondylitis (AS) • Inflammation mainly in the neck & spine, can also involve other joints
Arthritis Mutilans	• 5% of cases. • May cause severe joint destruction & deformity of the small joints of the hands, resulting in 'telescoping' of the digits.

Q: What radiological features may be seen in the different types of psoriatic arthritis?

Type	Features
Asymmetrical	• No changes **or** • Soft tissue swelling in the digits (dactylitis).
Symmetrical	• Proliferative marginal erosions (as opposed to non-proliferative erosions in RA).
Distal Interphalangeal Predominant	• Resorption of the distal interphalangeal tufts.
Spondylitis	• Similar appearances to ankylosing spondylitis, including spinal syndesmophytes.
Arthritis Mutilans	• Periarticular bone resorption causing erosions & a 'pencil-in-cup' appearance of the bones of the digits.

Q: How is psoriatic arthritis managed?

Conservative	Medical	Surgical
Hot & Cold Therapy	NSAIDs	Joint Replacement / Fusion (rare)
Physiotherapy	Intra-Articular Corticosteroid Injection	
Occupational Therapy	Disease Modifying Anti-Rheumatic Drugs (DMARDs):	
	- Methotrexate	
	- Leflunomide	
	- Sulfasalazine	
	Anti-TNF:	
	- Infliximab	
	- Etanercept	
	- Adalimumab	
	- Golimumab	

Scleroderma / Systemic Sclerosis

Q: What is scleroderma / systemic sclerosis?

- Systemic autoimmune disease of the connective tissue.
- Characterised by collagen deposition in the skin, organs & blood vessels.
- M: F = 1 : 4.

Q: How is scleroderma / systemic sclerosis classified?

Type		Characteristics	Features
LOCALISED	**Morphoea**	• Affects skin.	• Thick patches of skin with a waxy appearance. • Absence of auto-antibodies & systemic features.
	Linear	• Affects skin & occasionally deeper structures.	• Thickened linear streaks affecting the skin & occasionally joint stiffness & contractures.
SYSTEMIC	**Limited**	• Characterised by calcinosis. • Also known as **CREST** syndrome. • Better prognosis than diffuse but can have visceral involvement.	• **C**alcinosis (calcium deposits found in the skin & other tissues) (Fig 9.7). • **R**aynauds's phenomenon. • o**E**sophageal involvement. • **S**clerodactyly (thickened, tight skin overlying the digits giving an elongated appearance). • **T**elangiectasia (dilated small capillaries that blanche on pressure & refill from the centre outwards. Often on the face, hands & oral mucosa).
	Diffuse	• Characterised by skin & visceral involvement. • Calcinosis (Fig 9.7) only occurs on occasion.	**Skin & Joints:** • Thick & tight with occasional contractures. • Raynaud's phenomenon. • Telangiectasia. • *Musculoskeletal* (Fig 9.7)*:* Polyarthritis, Myositis. **Visceral:** • *Cardiac:* Restrictive cardiomyopathy. • *Respiratory:* Pulmonary fibrosis. • *Renal:* Renal failure. • *Gastrointestinal:* Dysphagia, Diarrhoea, Malabsorption, Weight loss.

Q: How would you diagnose scleroderma / systemic sclerosis?

There is no specific diagnostic test. History & clinical findings should guide further investigation.

Investigations	Interpretation

Blood Tests	• FBC (anaemia of chronic disease), ESR.
	
	• Presence of Anti-Nuclear Antibodies (ANA):
	
	   - Anti-Centromere Antibody present in limited type.
	
	   - Anti-Scl 70 Antibody present in diffuse type.

Organ Specific	Look for specific visceral complications of scleroderma to guide investigation: • *Pulmonary fibrosis:* CXR, pulmonary function tests, high resolution CT. • *Renal failure:* U&Es, BP, urine dip. • *Gastrointestinal problems:* endoscopy, transit studies. • *Pericarditis, cardiomyopathy:* ECG, echocardiogram.

Q: What treatment options are available for scleroderma / systemic sclerosis?

Treatment is variable dependent on the degree & range of organ involvement:

Symptom	Treatment
Raynaud's Phenomenon	• Avoid the cold • Use of gloves & hand-warmers • Smoking cessation • Calcium channel blockers
Cutaneous	• Topical steroids (ointment/injection) • Skin camouflage
Muscle Pain & Stiffness	• Exercise • Physiotherapy • Simple analgesia including NSAIDs
Respiratory	• Vaccination against influenza & pneumonia • Immunosuppressants (cyclophosphamide, azathioprine, steroids)
Renal	• ACE inhibitors • Renal replacement therapy if needed
Gastrointestinal	• Good fibre intake, bulking laxatives • PPIs, pro-motility drugs

Bilateral hand radiograph with features of scleroderma. Generalised **bone demineralisation** is noted with **erosive joint destruction** just visible at the PIPJs, **decreased joint space** visible at the MCPJs & terminal phalangeal **tuft resorption** most notable at the distal phalanges of the thumbs. **Calcinosis** is also noted with the largest foci at the ulnar side of the right wrist & left little finger metacarpal.

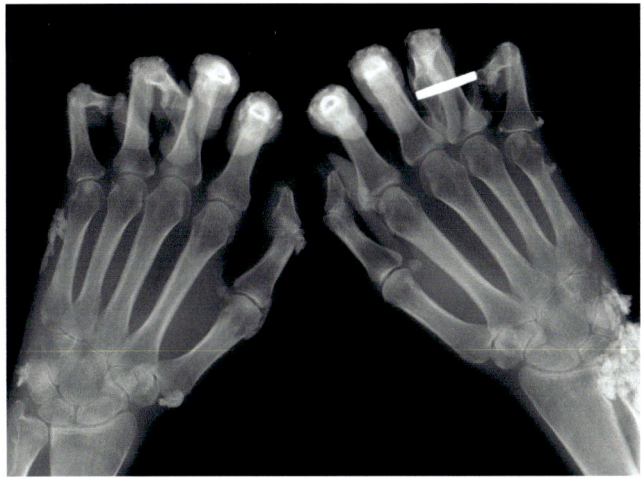

Polymyalgia Rheumatica

Q: What is polymyalgia rheumatica?

- Inflammatory disorder affecting muscles & joints.
- Characterised by pain & stiffness affecting the proximal muscles (predominantly the shoulders & hips, but also the neck).
- Systemic features are present on occasion e.g. fatigue, lethargy, fever, weight loss.
- 15% of patients with polymyalgia rheumatica develop temporal arteritis & 40-50% of patients with temporal arteritis at diagnosis also have polymyalgia rheumatica; these may therefore be considered as extremes of the same disease spectrum.

Q: How is polymyalgia rheumatica diagnosed?

Diagnosis is achieved by taking a **full history** & performing a **thorough clinical examination**, however the following investigations may be useful:

Investigation	Interpretation
Blood Tests	• FBC, U&Es, CRP, ESR.
Other Tests	• Radiology & muscle biopsy are usually normal. • Temporal artery biopsy may be necessary if clinical assessment suggests temporal arteritis.

Q: How is polymyalgia rheumatica treated?

Conservative	Medical
Physiotherapy: • Strengthen proximal muscle weakness	**Oral Prednisolone:** • Often for 1-2 years • Dose is slowly reduced from 15mg, guided by clinical improvement & falling ESR & CRP
Occupational Therapy	**Osteoporosis Protection** (from long-term steroids): • Calcium • Vitamin D • Bisphosphonates

Q: What is temporal arteritis?

- An inflammatory vasculitis affecting predominantly the temporal arteries.
- M:F = 1:2.
- Presentation is with headache, scalp tenderness, jaw claudication & visual disturbance in the presence of a visibly thickened, tender temporal artery.
- Involvement of the ophthalmic artery may result in blindness.
- Urgent high dose prednisolone is required to treat temporal arteritis (1mg/kg) or IV methylprednisolone.
- 15% of patients with polymyalgia rheumatica develop temporal arteritis & 40-50% of patients with temporal arteritis at diagnosis also have polymyalgia rheumatica; these may therefore be considered as extremes of the same disease spectrum.

Cervical Spondylosis

Q: What is cervical spondylosis?

- Degenerative condition of the lower cervical vertebrae & associated intervertebral discs.
- Intervertebral disc degeneration of the annulus fibrosus & osteophyte formation cause cervical nerve root compression.
- Advanced cases may involve spinal cord compression.
- Patients commonly present with neck pain & stiffness that may be associated with features of nerve root compression (radiculopathy).

Q: What is radiculopathy?

- Compression of a nerve root, resulting in sensory &/or motor symptoms in the distribution of that nerve root.
- Most commonly, due to a prolapsed lumbar intervertebral disc causing 'sciatica'.

Q: What are the clinical features of a cervical radiculopathy?

- Cervical nerve root compression causes predictable sensory (dermatomal) & motor (myotomal) clinical features relating to the level of compression.
- The most commonly affected root is C5/C6 which results in sensory features affecting the thumb & motor features affecting elbow flexion.

Q: What are the clinical features of a cervical myelopathy?

- May occur when cervical spinal cord compression results as a consequence of cervical spondylosis.
- Lower motor neuron signs are present at the cord compression level.
- Upper motor neuron signs are present below the cord compression level.

Area Affected	Clinical Features
Upper Limb (lower motor neuron features)	• Tendency to drop items. • Hand & forearm muscle weakness & wasting. • Paraesthesia affecting the hands. • Reduced sensation in the hands. • Areflexia.
Lower Limb (upper motor neuron features)	• Difficulty walking & unsteadiness. • Spasticity. • Reduced proprioception & vibration. • Brisk reflexes ± positive Babinski test. • Cauda equina syndrome *(see neurosciences chapter)*.

Q: What are the clinical features of an upper & lower motor neuron lesion?

	Upper Motor Neuron (↑)	Lower Motor Neuron (↓)
Power	↓ (reduced)	↓ (reduced ± fasciculations)
Tone	↑ (hypertonia/spasticity)	↓ (hypotonic/flaccidity)
Reflexes	↑ (hyperreflexia ± clonus)	↓ (hyporeflexia)
Plantar Response/ Babinski Reflex	↑ (up-going plantars/positive Babinski)	↓ (down-going plantars/negative Babinski)

Q: How is cervical spondylosis diagnosed?

After taking a **full history** & performing a **thorough clinical examination**, I would consider the following investigations:

Investigations	Interpretation
X-Ray	• Osteophytes • Reduced intervertebral joint space
MRI	• Nerve root / cord compression
CT Myelography	• If MRI contraindicated / not tolerated

Q: How is cervical spondylosis treated?

Conservative	Medical	Surgical
Lifestyle Modification	NSAIDs	Laminectomy
Physiotherapy	Muscle Relaxants (e.g. benzodiazepines)	Foraminotomy
Occupational Therapy	Local Steroid Injection	Spinal Fusion
	Adjuvant Medication (analgesic effect for neurological pain) • Amitriptyline • Carbamazepine • Tricyclic antidepressants	

Systemic Lupus Erythematosus (SLE)

Q: What is SLE?

- Autoimmune connective tissue disease.
- M : F = 1 : 9.
- Commonly presents at 15-35 years of age.
- May affect any part of the body including the joints, skin, heart, lungs & kidneys.

Q: How would you diagnose SLE?

Take a **full history**, perform a **thorough clinical examination** & **order appropriate investigations** to identify a minimum of 4 out of 11 of the diagnostic criteria described by the American College of Rheumatology.

Clinical Criteria	Investigation Criteria
• **Malar Rash:** Butterfly shaped rash across the cheeks & nasal bridge.	• **Anti-Nuclear Antibody (ANA):** Positive in 95% of patients with SLE.
• **Discoid Rash:** Large circular red rash, which can result in scarring.	• **Renal Disorder:** Proteinuria or cellular casts. May require renal biopsy for diagnosis.
• **Arthritis:** Painful, swollen joints.	• **Haematological Disorder:** Either anaemia, leucopenia, lymphopenia, or thrombocytopenia.
• **Serositis:** Pericarditis or pleuritis.	
• **Photosensitivity:** Aggravating rashes.	• **Neurological Disorder:** Seizures or psychosis.
• **Oral Ulcers:** Painful, aphthous ulceration.	• **Immunologic Disorder:** Anti-dsDNA antibodies, antiphospholipid antibodies as well as ANA may be present.

Q: What treatment options are available for SLE?

Conservative	Medical	
	Mild disease	**Severe disease**
Patient Education:	**NSAIDs:**	**High Dose Corticosteroids:**
• Recognising triggers	• Useful for symptom relief in arthritis & serositis	• Useful in renal inflammation, haematological problems & serositis
• Reduce fatigue		
• Exercise		
• Smoking cessation		
Support Groups	**Corticosteroid Creams:**	**Immunosuppressants:**
	• For topical use on rashes	• Azathioprine
		• Methotrexate
Sunlight Protection: (which may aggravate rashes)	**Hydroxychloroquine:**	**Cytotoxic drugs**
• Protective clothing	• Antimalarial agent useful for fatigue, rashes & musculoskeletal symptoms when NSAIDs have failed	
• Sunglasses		
• Sunscreen		

CHAPTER 10
ORTHOPAEDICS

S Kamalasekaran
AD Ebinesan
BH Miranda
J Saksena

CHAPTER CONTENTS

MUSCULOSKELETAL EXAMINATION TIPS

Scars, Swellings, Symmetry, Deformity, Erythema, Sinus, Muscle Wasting

As with all examination protocols, the key to success is to look slick & efficient! It is useful to have a standard introduction strategy when you 'look' at the patient. The above 7 clinical signs should be rehearsed in succession by the candidate, until they literally 'trip off the tongue'.

When examining a joint from all sides, the candidate will therefore be able to examine (e.g. the front, back & sides of the joint) for all of these signs in 1 movement around the patient. Examining for each of these 7 signs from the front, then each of these 7 signs from the sides, then each of these 7 signs from the back, takes longer & looks less slick!

This is particularly noticeable when the candidate is asked to comment as they go through the examination process. Rather than repeating each of the 7 signs (e.g. from the front, then sides, then back), the candidate can move around the patient with 1 movement, using a line as follows:

"I am examining the joint from the front, back & sides, for any scars, swellings, symmetry, deformity, erythema, sinuses & muscle wasting."

As with all examinations, if an obvious lump is seen, it should be inspected according to the *6 x S's (see lumps 'n' bumps chapter)*, prior to looking at the rest of the joint. Furthermore it should be palpated, prior to feeling the rest of the joint.

Like-for-Like

When testing power in any clinical examination, it is important (as far as possible) to test like-for-like, such that the same limbs & muscles are being used by the patient & examiner. This is to ensure that as much bias is removed as possible, due to discrepancies in patient–examiner muscle strength. For example, when testing elbow flexion of the right arm, the examiner should use flexion of their right elbow also.

Compare Each Side

Comparing each side assists in diagnosis of pathology that is either unilateral / worse on 1 side. This is always important. Furthermore, as it is not always possible to compare like-for-like, sometimes the only indication of pathology may be an imbalance between clinical signs on both sides e.g. left vs. right leg.

Valgus vs. Varus Deformity

Remember that these joint deformities are defined by the relationship of the distal joint.

- Valgus deformity implies that the distal joint is deviated away from the midline.
- Varus deformity implies that the distal joint is deviated towards the midline.

ORTHOPAEDIC NECK EXAMINATION

START: Patient sitting on chair, shirt off / exposed to level below the clavicles.

                Inspect from FRONT, BACK & SIDES as follows:

LOOK	Interpretation
Scars	Post-operative, post-infective.
Swelling	Soft tissue / bony mass. Remember to check the thyroid region separately. Also look in the supraclavicular fossae for fullness e.g. Pancoast tumour.
Symmetry	Torticollis (involuntary neck contractions result in head tilting towards the side of the precipitating lesion / underlying pathology).
Deformity	Kyphosis / loss of normal lordosis. Vertebral collapse due to e.g. fracture, TB or tumour. Klippel-Feil Syndrome (patients have a low hairline, shortened webbed neck & decreased cervical spine ROM due to variable vertebral fusion).
Erythema	Inflammation.
Sinus	Post-operative, infective.
Muscle Wasting	Previous trauma, neurological or infection e.g. TB.

Ask about pain.

To prevent causing distress, explain to the patient that you will be standing behind them.

Remember to feel the vertebrae, sides & front of the neck including the supraclavicular fossae.

Feel for temperature changes with the back of your hand.

FEEL	Interpretation
Tenderness	Feel midline structures, then paraspinal muscles, from occiput to C7/T1. **Note: The most prominent spinous process is that of T1 not C7 (vertebra prominens).** Tenderness in an isolated intervertebral space may be associated with cervical spondylosis.
Stepping	Run fingers down the midline of the spine from occiput to C7/T1. Feel for an abnormal 'step' that may be due to previous trauma, tumour or infection.
Mass	Soft tissue / bony mass. Remember to check the thyroid region separately.
Cervical Rib	Feel in the supraclavicular fossae for a cervical rib.
Lymph Nodes	Infection e.g. TB *(see head & neck chapter)*.

Listen / feel for crepitations during movement.

Repeat movements with downward pressure on head. Intervertebral foramen stenosis may be amplified, hence reproducing associated neurological symptoms.

MOVE	Interpretation
Flexion	Ask patient to touch chin to chest & record chin–chest distance. Normal = 80°.
Extension	Ask patient to look up at the ceiling. The plane of the nose & forehead should be horizontal. Normal = 50°.
Lateral Flexion	Ask patient to touch ear to shoulder on both sides. ROM commonly decreased in cervical spondylosis. Normal = 45°.
Rotation	Ask patient to look over shoulder on both sides, whilst standing behind patient & stabilising the contralateral shoulder. Normal = 80°.

SPECIAL TEST	Interpretation
Thoracic Outlet Syndrome *(also see thoracic outlet syndrome in vascular chapter)*	1. **Hand Ischemia:** Look for signs e.g. cold, discolouration & trophic changes. 2. **Roo's Test (Fig 10.1):** With the patient sitting in a chair, position the patient's arms in 90° shoulder abduction & full external rotation, with the elbow flexed to 90°. Ask the patient to open & close their hands for 3 minutes. A positive test is indicated by reproduction of the patient's neurological / vascular symptoms. This is indicative of thoracic outlet syndrome. 3. **Adson's Test (Fig 10.2):** Palpate the patient's radial artery while they are sitting in a chair. Position their shoulder in approximately 45° of abduction & full external rotation, with full elbow extension. Ask the patient to look over the shoulder of the side being tested, extend their neck & hold their breath. Gently extend the arm from this position, in a continuous movement. A positive test is recorded as the radial pulse disappears. This is indicative of thoracic outlet syndrome.

COMPLETION	Interpretation
Lymphadenopathy	Check associated lymph nodes.
Distal Neurovascular Status	Full examinations required *(see relevant chapters)*. Particularly focus on pulses, dermatomes & myotomes, look for cervical myelopathy & auscultate for a subclavian artery murmur suggestive of mechanical obstruction.
QoL Impingement & Sleep	Asking patient about these helps to assess impact on life & therefore necessity for intervention.
Help Patient Dress	Good practice if patient has functional limitation.
Radiographs	Soft tissue / bony abnormalities.

FINISH:

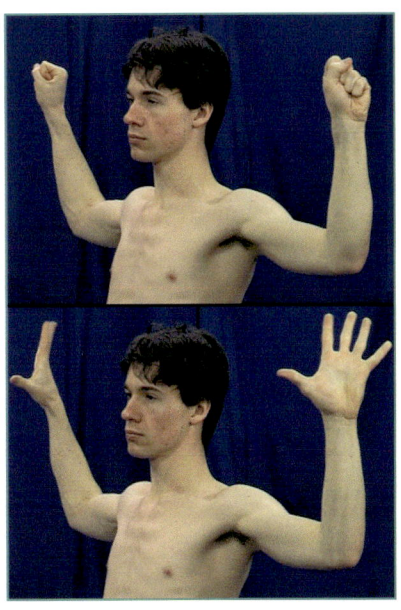

Fig 10.1: Roo's Test

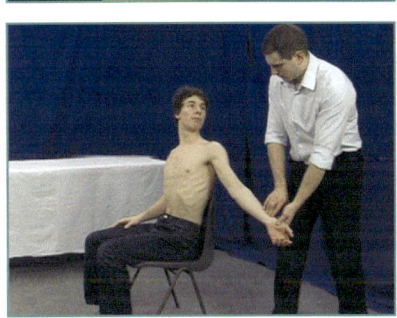

Fig 10.2: Adson's Test

SPINE EXAMINATION

START: Patient exposed to underwear.

First ask the patient to walk away a few steps, turn around & come back.

With the patient standing, inspect from FRONT, BACK & SIDES as follows:

LOOK	Interpretation
Scars	Post-operative e.g. discectomy (posterior midline), post-infective.
Swelling	Soft tissue / bony mass e.g. gibbus (fused vertebra causing abnormal protuberance at the thoracolumbar junction in TB / fracture).
Symmetry	Torticollis (involuntary neck contractions result in head tilting towards the side of the precipitating lesion / underlying pathology).
Deformity	• **Scoliosis:** May disappear with the patient sitting (secondary to leg length discrepancy) or persist (indicating a fixed / structural scoliosis). • **Kyphosis:** May disappear when the patient's shoulders are braced back (postural) or persist (fixed / structural). • **Lordosis:** May be obliterated e.g. OA, prolapsed IVD, ankylosing spondylitis. May be exaggerated e.g. spondylolisthesis, hip flexion deformity, exaggerated thoracic kyphosis.
Erythema	Inflammation.
Sinus	Post-operative, infective.
Muscle Wasting	Paraspinal muscles e.g. previous trauma, neurological or infection e.g. TB.

Ask about pain.

Feel for temperature changes with the back of your hand along the entire length of the spine.

FEEL	Interpretation
Pain	Systematically feel the bones, then soft tissues, starting from the top of the cervical spine, running down to the sacroiliac joints. Bony tenderness may indicate tumour / infection. Sacroiliac joint tenderness may indicate sacroiliitis e.g. ankylosing spondylitis. Paraspinal muscle tenderness may indicate mechanical back pain / spasm e.g. prolapsed IVD.
Stepping	Run fingers down midline of bony spine. An abnormal spinous process 'step' may indicate spondylolisthesis, fracture, tumour or infection.
Chest expansion	Ask the patient to breathe in, then out fully. Quickly place your thumbs (facing up) on the patient parasternally, then place your index fingers in the line of the 5th intercostal spaces. Ask the patient to take a deep breath in. Normal expansion = 5–7cm. This is grossly reduced in ankylosing spondylitis.

MOVE	Interpretation
Cervical Spine	• **Flexion** (80°) / **Extension** (50°) • **Lateral Flexion** (45°) • **Rotation** (80°) Repeat movements with downward pressure on head *(see orthopaedic neck examination)*.
Thoracic Spine	• **Lateral Rotation:** With the patient sitting on the edge of a chair, arms on each ipsilateral hip, ask the patient to twist to each side. Normal = 40°.
Lumbar Spine	• **Forward Flexion:** Ask the patient to touch their toes with their legs straight & measure the distance from their fingertips to the floor. Normal = 7cm. This should also be tested using Schober's Test *(see special tests)*. • **Extension:** Ask the patient to bend backwards. Normal = 30°. • **Lateral Flexion:** Ask the patient to slide their hand down the side of their leg. Normal = 30°.

SPECIAL TESTS	Interpretation
Schober's Test (Fig 9.5)	Draw a line through both PSIS (Dimples of Venus). Mark the spine 5cm below & 10cm above this line. Keeping the tape measure in place, ask the patient to touch their toes & record the new distance between the outermost marks. Normal flexion = 5cm. This is reduced in lumbar spine pathology e.g. ankylosing spondylitis.
Lumbar Disc / Sciatic Nerve Pathology	The following tests assess nerve root compression (L4–S1). • **Bragard's Test:** Perform a straight leg raise on the patient, with the patient lying supine. Stop when back / leg pain or paraesthesia is precipitated. Now dorsiflex the foot, which will worsen symptoms (positive test). • **Lasègue's Test:** Following straight on from Bragard's Test, maintaining the angle of foot dorsiflexion. Flex the knee until pain is relieved, then further flex the hip, which will worsen symptoms (positive test). **Note: A free straight leg raise without restriction rules out disc / sciatic nerve pathology.**
Reverse Lasègue / Femoral Stretch Test	With the patient lying prone, flex the knee to 90° & lift the ankle superiorly, perpendicular to the couch. Back / thigh pain suggests femoral nerve root (L1–L4) compression.
Pelvic Compression	Push down gently on both ASIS, with the patient lying supine. Pain in the sacroiliac region suggests sacroiliitis e.g. ankylosing spondylitis.
Lhermitte's Sign	With the patient sitting in a chair, flex the cervical spine. Radicular pain indicates cervical nerve root compression e.g. spondylosis, prolapsed IVD.
Beevor's Sign	Place the patient's arms behind their head, whilst they are lying supine on the couch. Ask the patient to lift their head off the couch & observe the umbilicus. If the umbilicus moves 'cranial', there is weakness of the inferior rectus, indicating T10-T12 spinal cord injury / nerve involvement.
Abdominal Reflex	Gently swipe your finger around the umbilicus, imagining 4 quadrants. Failure of the umbilicus to twitch towards the stimulated quadrant indicates thoracic cord compression on that side. The nerve supply for the upper quadrant = T6–T10 & lower quadrant = T11–T12.

COMPLETION	Interpretation
Lymphadenopathy	Check associated lymph nodes.
Full Neurological Examination	This is required to fine tune the diagnostic level of pathology including: • **Cauda Equina:** Check for saddle anaesthesia, perianal sensation & anal tone (via a per rectum examination), which are decreased in cauda equine syndrome. • **Reflexes:** *See peripheral neurology.* • **Extensor Hallucis Longus:** Weakness suggests L5 nerve root pathology.
Full Vascular Examination	Rule out AAA as a cause of back pain. Assess vascular status of upper & lower limbs.
Waddell's Tests	5 categories of test help to rule out non-organic causes of back pain i.e. tenderness, simulation, distraction, regional disturbances & overreaction tests.
QoL Impingement & Sleep	Asking patient about these helps to assess impact on life & therefore necessity for intervention.
Help Patient Dress	Good practice if patient has functional limitation.
Radiographs	Soft tissue / bony abnormalities.

FINISH:

SHOULDER EXAMINATION

START:　　　Patient exposure is ideally with blouse / shirt off. This is to assist the examination of the joint above (cervical spine) & below (elbow).

First ask the patient to walk away a few steps, turn around & come back, whilst checking for normal arm swing.

Remember to compare both sides throughout the examination.

Practice the elbow examination as a 'dance' in front of the mirror.

LOOK	Interpretation
Scapula Winging	Ask the patient to push their hands against a wall, with their elbows extended. Winging may be seen with a prominent medial scapula border. Lesions of the long thoracic nerve of Bell (C5–C7, innervates serratus anterior), may lead to winging.
With the patient sitting in a chair, examine the FRONT, SIDES, BACK, SUPERIOR joints & AXILLAE for:	
Scars	Traumatic or iatrogenic e.g. arthroscopy ports & post-operative scars.
Swelling	Look for soft tissue & bony swellings. Joint effusions present with swelling in the axilla. Apparent bony 'swellings' may indicate dislocation of the SCJ / ACJ. A swelling at the anterior-distal upper arm may represent a ruptured biceps tendon.
Symmetry	Check the alignment of the shoulder joint & associated muscle contour. This should be symmetrical. Significant asymmetry implies unilateral disease (or 1 shoulder is worse than the other). Symmetrical disease is associated with RA.
Deformity	Check for bony deformity, paying particular attention to the SCJ, clavicle & ACJ. SCJ & ACJ subluxation / dislocation may be more obvious from above. Shoulder dislocation may be present if the patient holds their arm in internal rotation (posterior dislocation) / external rotation (anterior dislocation).
Erythema	Inflammation e.g. RA.
Sinus	Post-operative, infective.
Muscle Wasting	Pectoral muscles (pectoral nerves), deltoid (shoulder contour is lost / square e.g. C5, axillary nerve lesion), trapezius (XI, accessory nerve), Supraspinatus (rotator cuff tear) & infraspinatus (C5–C6, suprascapular nerve lesion).

Ask about pain.

Feel for temperature changes with the back of your hand.

Systematically feel the shoulder joint, associated bony prominences & soft tissues.

FEEL	Interpretation
Pain	Start at the SCJ; feel along the line of the clavicle & around the ACJ. Feel around the glenohumeral joint & scapula. Feel trapezius, deltoid & infraspinatus. Extend the shoulder, feel supraspinatus & then the bicipital groove. The biceps tendon may be felt in this position by internally & externally rotating the humerus.
Axilla	The head of the humerus may be felt via the axilla. Also assess for lumps & lymphadenopathy.

Movements should ideally be tested actively & passively, with the patient standing.

Movements should be repeated with the scapula stabilised (pushing down on the shoulder).

Remember that shoulder ROM is particularly dependent on shoulder position.

MOVE	Interpretation
Abduction & External Rotation	Ask the patient to put their hands behind their head, pushing their elbows back. This is a good screening test for global active shoulder movement.
Adduction & Internal Rotation	Ask the patient to put their hands behind their back, thumbs pointing to the ceiling. The thumbs should normally reach T6. This is a good screening test for global active shoulder movement.
Abduction (coronal plane)	With the patient's arms by their sides, thumbs facing forward & elbows extended fully, ask the patient to fully abduct their arms. Supraspinatus initiates & is responsible for the first 0°–30° of abduction, deltoid is responsible for 30°–90° & the scapula-thoracic apparatus is responsible for the last 60° of abduction. Failure of abduction initiation may be due to supraspinatus tendinitis / rotator cuff tear. **Painful arc syndrome** represents pathology of the rotator cuff (this is usually due to compression of a chronically inflamed supraspinatus tendon, compressing against the acromion process resulting in pain between 60°–120° of abduction). Pain at the end of abduction (140°–180°) represents ACJ OA. Normal ROM = 0°–180°.
Flexion	Ask the patient to forward flex their shoulders, with their forearms fully pronated & elbows extended. Normal = 165° of flexion.
Extension	Ask the patient to extend their shoulders, with their forearms fully pronated & elbows extended. Normal = 60° of extension.
Adduction	Ask the patient to touch their opposite shoulder with each hand.
Internal Rotation	Ask the patient to internally rotate their shoulders, keeping their arms tucked into their sides (subscapularis). Normal = 60°–70° internal rotation (as the trunk prevents further movement). With the shoulder abducted to 90°, normal = 90° internal rotation. *Internal rotation may also be tested with the shoulder abducted & elbow flexed.*
External Rotation	Ask the patient to externally rotate their shoulders, keeping their arms tucked into their sides (infraspinatus & teres minor). Normal = 90° external rotation. *External rotation may also be tested with the shoulder abducted & elbow flexed.*

Muscle power is tested against resistance.

Remember to test muscle power 'like-for-like' where possible, comparing each side.

MUSCLE POWER	Interpretation
Supraspinatus	Resisted abduction 0°–30°. Position the patient's shoulder in 30° of forward flexion & 30° abduction, with the patient's forearm in full pronation (thumbs down). Test supraspinatus by asking the patient to 'push out' (abduct) against resistance.
Deltoid	Resisted abduction 30°–90°. Position the patient's shoulders in 90° of abduction, elbows fully flexed. Test deltoid by asking the patient to maintain this position against resistance.
Infraspinatus & Teres Minor	Resisted external rotation with elbows tucked into sides & flexed to 90°.
Gerber's Test	Position the patient's hand behind their back, with the dorsum of their hand touching their back & elbow flexed to 90°. Ask the patient to lift the dorsum of their hand off their back against mild resistance. If the patient is unable to do this or *'lift off'* even without resistance, this indicates **subscapularis** pathology.

SPECIAL TESTS	Interpretation
Multidirectional Instability	Ask the patient to lie supine at the edge of the couch, shoulder joint at the edge of the bed. Stabilise the scapula with one hand & test abnormal posterior / anterior movement of the humerus at the glenohumeral joint with your other hand. Instability implies capsule / ligament damage.
Apprehension-Relocation Test (Jobe's Test)	Ask the patient to lie supine on the examination couch, shoulder joint at the edge of the bed. Abduct the patient's shoulder to 90° & flex the elbow to 90°. Stabilise & feel the glenohumeral joint with one hand & externally rotate the joint with the other hand. Anterior instability is confirmed as the patient's face becomes 'apprehensive' due to pain (Apprehension Test). This pain may be relieved with the application of posterior (pushing down towards the couch) pressure to the shoulder (Relocation Test). This is positive for **anterior joint instability**. *It is best to avoid performing this test in the OSCE as it precipitates pain, so simply mention it instead.*
Neer's Test	Ask the patient to sit on the edge of the couch / in a chair. Internally rotate the patient's shoulder & pronate their forearm, keeping arms tucked by their sides. Stabilise the scapula & passively forward flex the shoulder in a continuous movement. If pain is reproduced, this is a positive test for rotator cuff impingement.

COMPLETION	Interpretation
Lymphadenopathy	Check associated lymph nodes.
Joint Above & Below	Full neck & elbow examination.
Distal Neurovascular Status	Full examinations required *(see relevant chapters)*. Particularly focus on pulses, dermatomes & myotomes. Axillary nerve (C5) sensation should be tested specifically over the lateral aspect of deltoid.
QoL Impingement & Sleep	Asking the patient about these helps to assess impact on life & therefore necessity for intervention.
Help Patient Dress	Good practice if the patient has functional limitation.
Radiographs	Soft tissue / bony abnormalities.

FINISH:

ELBOW EXAMINATION

START: Patient exposure is ideally with blouse / shirt off. This is to assist the examination of the joint above (shoulder) & below (wrist).

First look at the joint with the patient's arms alongside their body, in supination (palms forward). Comment on the carrying angle (normal 0°–15°).

Look at the joint with the patient's arms abducted to 90°, in supination (palms up).

Continue the examination, comparing both elbows, with the patient standing.

LOOK	Interpretation
Scars & Skin	Traumatic or iatrogenic e.g. arthroscopy ports & post-operative scars. Psoriasis patches on extensor aspects. Gouty tophi of joints (also check the pinna as tophi may occur here).
Swelling	Soft tissue e.g. RA, bone e.g. OA, bursa e.g. olecranon bursitis (student's elbow) (Fig 10.3)..
Symmetry	Check the alignment of the elbows & arms. This should be symmetrical. Significant asymmetry implies unilateral disease (or one elbow is worse than the other). Symmetrical disease is associated with RA.
Deformity	**Cubitus valgus** e.g. non-union of previous lateral condyle fracture, **cubitus varus** e.g. mal-union of previous supracondylar fracture in children, **ankylosis, flexion deformity.**
Erythema	Inflammation e.g. RA.
Sinus	Post-operative, infective.
Muscle Wasting	Wasting of arm & forearm muscles. Causes include previous trauma, neurological lesions or infection e.g. TB.

Ask about pain.

Feel for temperature changes with the back of your hand.

Systematically feel the elbow joint, associated bony prominences & soft tissues.

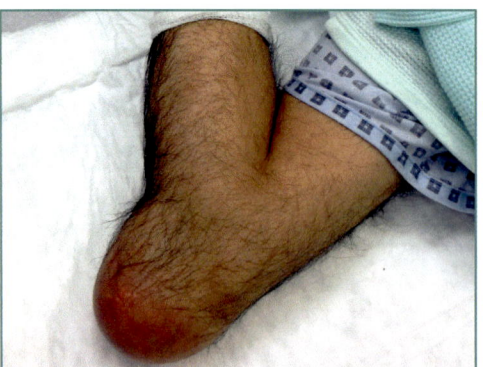

Fig 10.3 Olecranon bursitis (student's elbow) affecting the right elbow

FEEL	Interpretation
Pain	This may be bony or soft tissue in origin, depending on anatomical location. Comment on the following common pathologies: • **Lateral Epicondylitis:** Tennis elbow. • **Medial Epicondylitis:** Golfer's elbow. • **Olecranon Bursitis:** Student's elbow.
Relation of Bony Prominences	The olecranon, medial & lateral epicondyles together form an inverted triangle that is best seen from behind. This triangle is altered in dislocation.
Joint Line	In particular, palpate the head of the radius, whilst pronating & supinating the patient's forearm. Feel for clicking if loose bodies are present within the joint.
Rheumatoid Nodules	Often present on the extensor surfaces of the arms / elbow joint.
Ulnar Nerve	Lies superficially, posterior to the medial epicondyle. May be 'rolled' under the fingers. Hypersensitivity may be due to e.g. ulnar neuritis / tardy ulnar palsy. Thickening may be due to e.g. leprosy.
Antecubital Fossa	Brachial artery, median nerve & biceps tendon.

Movements should ideally be tested actively, passively & against resistance.

Remember to test muscle power 'like-for-like' where possible, comparing each side.

MOVE	Interpretation
Ulnar-Humeral Joint	Ask the patient to extend & flex their elbow. Normal ROM = 0°– 140°.
Radio-Ulnar Joint	Ask the patient to flex their elbows to 90°, tucking them into their sides. Ask the patient to point their palms to the ceiling (supination) & then the floor (pronation). Normal ROM = 90° of pronation through to 90° of supination.
Locking	May occur with loose bodies in e.g. trauma, OA, osteochondritis dissecans.

COMPLETION	Interpretation
Lymphadenopathy	Check associated lymph nodes.
Joint Above & Below	Full shoulder & wrist examination.
Distal Neurovascular Status	Full examinations required (see relevant chapters). Particularly focus on pulses, dermatomes & myotomes.
QoL Impingement & Sleep	Asking patient about these helps to assess impact on life & therefore necessity for intervention.
Help Patient Dress	Good practice if patient has functional limitation.
Radiographs	Soft tissue / bony abnormalities.

FINISH:

HIP EXAMINATION

START: Patient exposure to underwear. This is to assist examination of the joint above (spine) & below (knee).

First ask the patient to walk away a few steps, turn around & come back, to assess gait.

Comment on use of aids e.g. stick, frame, brace, shoes etc.

Perform Trendelenberg's Test *(see special tests)* **first.**

With the patient standing, inspect from the FRONT, BACK & SIDES of the joint.

LOOK	Interpretation
Scars	Traumatic or iatrogenic e.g. post-operative (anterior / posterior approach etc).
Swelling	Look for soft tissue & bony swelling e.g. lymphadenopathy, effusion (rare), tumour.
Symmetry	ASIS & greater trochanter levels should lie on a horizontal plane.
Deformity	Adduction / abduction (both may result in scoliosis), fixed flexion (may result in lordosis), leg length discrepancy (may result in scoliosis), rotational etc.
Erythema	Inflammation e.g. RA.
Sinus	Post-operative, infective e.g. TB.
Muscle Wasting	Gluteus, quadriceps etc.

Lay the patient on the couch supine.

Remember to examine the good side first.

Ask about pain.

Feel for temperature changes with the back of your hand.

FEEL	Interpretation
Pain	Systematically examine the hip: • **Greater Trochanter:** Palpated laterally (pain may suggest trochanteric bursitis). Also palpate the soft tissues around the greater trochanter. • **Femoral Head:** Lies deep to the femoral artery, at the mid-inguinal point. • **Adductor Longus:** Palpate medially along the entire length (adductor strain occurs in sports injury, adductor contracture occurs in OA). • **Ischial Tuberosity:** Palpated posteriorly (trauma). **Note: Turn the patient on their side to palpate the ischial tuberosities.**
Crepitus	Palpate for crepitus by rotating the hip medially & laterally. Crepitus suggests OA.
Lymphadenopathy	Assess inguinal lymph nodes.
Apparent Leg Length	Measure the distance from the xiphisternum to medial malleolus. Discrepancy indicates compensatory pelvic tilt, due to adduction / abduction deformity. **Note: Apparent length is longer for an abduction deformity & shorter for an adduction deformity.**
True Leg Length	Square the pelvis, aligning each ASIS in a horizontal plane. Demonstrate this by placing your elbow & hand (using the same upper limb) on each ASIS. Measure the distance from each ASIS to corresponding medial malleolus. Discrepancy indicates shortening of the affected limb. Isolate this to one of the following levels, first flexing the hips & knees to 90°, aligning the medial malleoli: • **Femoral Neck:** Place a thumb on each ASIS & middle finger on each greater trochanter. Imagine a line dropped vertically down from the ASIS & a 2nd line extended horizontally from the greater trochanter. Place your index finger at the point where these lines cross to form *Bryant's Triangle*. When the distance between the index & middle finger is shorter than the contralateral side, this indicates supratrochanteric shortening e.g. fracture, SCFE, Perthe's Disease, OA, DDH. • **Femoral Shaft:** Shortening is demonstrated as the knee of the affected limb lies proximal-inferior to the knee of the good limb e.g. fracture, infection. • **Tibia:** Shortening is demonstrated as the knee of the affected limb lies distal-inferior to the knee of the good limb e.g. fracture, infection.

Movements should ideally be tested actively, passively & against resistance, with the pelvis square.

Remember to compare each side, starting with the good side first.

Start with Thomas's Test *(see special tests)* to unmask fixed flexion deformity.

MOVE	Interpretation
Extension	Patient lies prone or on their side. Passively lifting the patient's leg may reveal 10° of normal hyperextension. In most hip pathologies, this is the first movement to be lost. Normal = 0°–10°. **Note: If Thomas's Test is positive, do not test extension.**
Flexion	Keeping the contralateral lower limb extended (back of thigh, calf & heel touching the couch = neutral position), flex the hip until the thigh touches the abdomen with the knee fully flexed, or until the pelvis starts moving. Normal = 150°.
Abduction	With the pelvis square, the angle of abduction is measured by drawing a vertical line distally from the ASIS. The angle subtended between this line & the long axis of the thigh is the angle of abduction. Normal = 45°. **Note: If there is an initial abduction deformity, measure true leg length by abducting the unaffected limb symmetrically to the affected limb.**
Adduction	With the pelvis square, the angle of adduction is measured by drawing a vertical line distally from the ASIS. The angle subtended between this line & the long axis of the thigh is the angle of adduction. Normal = 45°. **Note: If there is an initial adduction deformity, place the unaffected limb abducted off the side of the couch & adduct the affected limb in the horizontal plane, until the thumb appreciates movement of the ASIS.**
External & Internal Rotation	The hip & knee are flexed to 90°. Fix the knee with your left hand & secure the heel with your right hand. With the hip as a fulcrum, move the lower leg medially (normal external hip rotation = 30°) & laterally (normal internal hip rotation = 45°).

SPECIAL TESTS	Interpretation
Trendelenberg's Test (Fig 10.4)	*Perform at the start of the hip examination.* This assesses stability. Stand opposite the patient & hold out your supinated hands. Ask the patient to place their hands (pronated) on yours. Perform the test on the good leg first, asking the patient to bend the knee of their affected leg. Normally, the weight bearing hip is held stable by the abductors & the pelvis rises on the unsupported side. If the weight-bearing hip is painful / unstable, the pelvis drops on the unsupported side (positive test) e.g. OA, abductor weakness, hip pain (all causes). **Note: You must anticipate that the patient may fall when standing on their affected hip & support them with your corresponding outstretched hand.**
Thomas's Test (Fig 10.5)	*Perform before testing movements.* This unmasks a fixed flexion deformity. The patient should be lying flat on the couch. It may be easier to manipulate the patient kneeling down to the side of the couch. Place your left hand under the patient's lumbar spine. Ask the patient to flex both hips & knees fully (this will obliterate the normal lumbar lordosis). Perform the test on the good side first, asking the patient to hold their affected limb with both hands. With your other hand holding the lower leg / ankle, control full extension of the limb to be tested. Full extension is normally achieved with the lumbar lordosis still obliterated. If there is a fixed flexion deformity, the patient will arch their lumbar spine & the lumbar lordosis will reappear (pressure is relieved on your left hand). At the point where this occurs, bend the patient's knee such that their heel touches the couch & measure the angle between the couch & thigh = angle of flexion deformity.

COMPLETION	Interpretation
Lymphadenopathy	Check associated lymph nodes.
Joint Above & Below	Full spine & knee examination.
Distal Neurovascular Status	Full examinations required *(see relevant chapters)*. Particularly focus on pulses, dermatomes & myotomes.
QoL Impingement & Sleep	Asking patient about these helps to assess impact on life & therefore necessity for intervention.
Help Patient Dress	Good practice if patient has functional limitation.
Radiographs	Soft tissue / bony abnormalities.

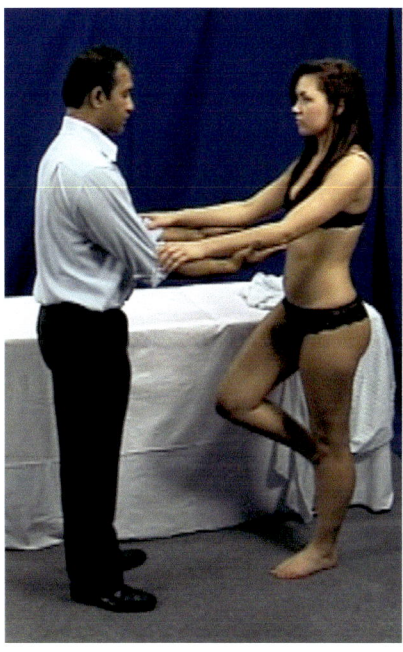

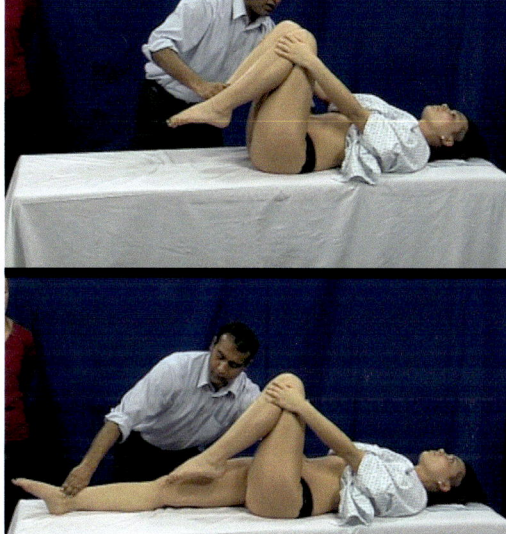

Fig 10.4: Trendelenberg's Test   Fig 10.5: Thomas's Test

FINISH:

KNEE EXAMINATION

START: Adequate patient exposure is ideally to underwear. This is to assist examination of gait, the spine, the joint above (hip) & below (ankle).

Comment on use of aids e.g. stick, frame, brace, shoes etc.

Ensure inspection from the FRONT, SIDES & BACK of the joint, comparing both knees with the patient standing.

LOOK	Interpretation
Scars	Traumatic or iatrogenic e.g. arthroscopy ports & post-operative scars.
	• **Anterior Midline Scar:** Total knee replacement.
	• **Suprapatellar Scar:** Quadriceps repair.
	• **Tibial Tubercle Scar:** Tubercle transfer for high riding patella / ACL surgery.
Swelling	• **Anterior:** Effusion, synovitis, prepatellar bursa, infrapatellar bursa.
	• **Lateral:** Meniscal cyst.
	• **Posterior:** Bakers cyst, popliteal aneurysm.
Symmetry	Check the alignment of the knees & legs. This should be symmetrical. Significant asymmetry implies unilateral disease (or one side is worse than the other). Symmetrical disease is associated with RA.
Deformity	Varus e.g. OA (measure interepicondylar distance, which will be increased). Valgus e.g. RA (measure intermalleolar distance which will be increased).
Erythema	Inflammation e.g. RA.
Sinus	Post-operative, infective.
Muscle Wasting	Check quadriceps VMO & calf muscles. Causes of muscle wasting include previous trauma, neurological lesions or infection e.g. TB.
With the patient on the examination couch, lying flat:	
Patella Tracking	Ask the patient to flex their knee to 90°. Tracking is confirmed as the patella moves in a J-shaped fashion (laterally in most cases) = tight vastus lateralis / patellofemoral ligament (PFL).

The remainder of the examination is also undertaken with the patient lying flat on the couch.

Ask about pain.

Feel for temperature changes with the back of your hand.

FEEL	Interpretation
Pain	Systematically examine the quadriceps, patella tendon, patella margins, knee joint margins & collateral ligaments. Pathology depends on site of pain & structural involvement e.g. lateral knee joint margin (meniscus), tibial tuberosity (Osgood Schlatter's Disease), patella tendon (tendinitis).
Continuity	Check continuity of the extensor apparatus.
Quadriceps	Measure the circumference of quadriceps bilaterally. Choose a fixed point e.g. 10cm above the superior border of the patella.
Effusion	• **Cross-Fluctuation Test:** Empty the medial compartment superiorly, then empty the suprapatellar pouch inferiorly, then compress the lateral compartment. Look for fluid transmission across the joint, appearing medially. • **Patellar Tap Test:** Empty the suprapatellar pouch inferiorly & then with the index finger of your other hand, push the patella downward, onto the femur. A spring back is positive. This is for moderate effusions. • **Bulge Test:** Empty the medial compartment superiorly & then compress the lateral compartment. Look for a bulge in the medial compartment. This is for minimal effusions.
Synovial Thickening	Try lifting the patella between your thumb & index finger. It will not be possible with a thickened synovium e.g. RA / TB synovitis.
Flexion Deformity	Place your hand under the patient's knee & ask them to push the back of their knee down to the couch. If your hand is compressed, there is no flexion deformity. If there is a gap under the patient's knee when they perform this manoeuvre, without hand compression, there is a flexion deformity. Flexion deformities may be classified as follows: • **Correctable:** Passive downward pressure corrects the deformity e.g. extensor lag. • **Fixed:** Passive downward pressure does not correct the deformity.

Movements should ideally be tested actively, passively & against resistance.

Remember to compare each side.

MOVE	Interpretation
Extension	Normal = 0°. Passively lifting the patient's leg may reveal 10° of normal hyperextension. >10° hyperextension = genu recurvatum.
Flexion	Normal = 150°.
Crepitus	Feel for crepitus with your hand over the patella-femoral junction at the same time as flexing & extending the knee e.g. trauma, OA.
Straight Leg Raise	Ask the patient to lift their leg off the bed, keeping their knee extended. If this is not possible, there may be extensor apparatus damage or a flexion deformity.

It may be more efficient to perform special tests in the following order:

SPECIAL TESTS	Interpretation
Posterior Sag Sign	Square the patient's legs with 90° knee flexion. Maintaining this position, flex the hips to 90°, supporting the lower legs from below, placing an arm underneath & in line with the ankles. The test is positive when the tibia of the affected knee sags towards the examination couch, indicating **posterior cruciate ligament rupture**. This is clearly seen as the prominence of the tibial tuberosity, usually visible in the lower leg, becomes obliterated. It is important to assess posterior sag prior to performing Lachman's test, as if it is missed, a false positive Lachman's Test may be elicited.
Posterior Drawer Test	Square the patient's legs with their knees flexed to 90°. Explain to the patient that you are going to sit on their foot, check that they have no pain, gain permission & sit on the patient's feet. Grasp the upper tibia firmly, thumbs placed on the anterior joint line & apply posterior pressure. Significant posterior glide is positive for a **posterior cruciate ligament rupture**.
Lachman's Test	Performed with 20–30° knee flexion, with the patient's heel on the couch. Stabilise the patient's thigh with one hand & pull the tibia anteriorly with your other hand (thumb on joint line, hand behind calf). The test is positive if there is anterior tibial translation. This indicates an **anterior cruciate ligament rupture**. **Continue straight on to testing the collateral ligaments as you are in a position that facilitates easier assessment already.**
Collateral Ligaments	Test the collateral ligaments with 30° knee flexion. Tuck the patient's foot under your arm & stabilise their knee on either side of the joint with both hands. Use a combination of body movement & pressure on the knee to apply valgus (testing the medial collateral ligament) & varus stress (testing the lateral collateral ligament). Springiness with a firm endpoint is normally felt. Absence of an endpoint is positive for a collateral ligament rupture. Repeat collateral ligament tests with 0° knee extension. Valgus / varus deviation in 0° knee extension is always abnormal.
McMurray's Test	Place the thumb & index finger of one hand along the joint line to detect any 'clicks' & pain that is positive for a meniscus tear. Fully FLEX the leg, then in one smooth motion EXTEND the knee joint (by moving the patient's lower leg with your other hand). To test each meniscus, the following leg orientations are required throughout extension to open up the joint line: • **Medial Meniscus:** Foot external rotation & lower leg abduction (valgus) (throughout extension). • **Lateral Meniscus:** Foot internal rotation & lower leg adduction (varus) (throughout extension).
Patella Tests	• **Friction Test:** Move the patella superiorly & inferiorly, pressing it down against the femur. Painful grating is experienced if the central portion of articular cartilage is damaged. • **Zolen's / Clark's Test:** Press the patella down against the femur & ask the patient to contract their quadriceps. Pain is suggestive of patellofemoral OA. • **Apprehension Test:** Displacing the patella laterally with the thumb, whilst gently flexing the knee may induce pain & anxiety. This is a positive test & the patient will resist further movement. Diagnostic of recurrent patella subluxation / dislocation.

COMPLETION	Interpretation
Lymphadenopathy	Check associated lymph nodes.
Joint Above & Below	Full examination of the ankle & hip required *(see relevant sections)*.
Distal Neurovascular Status	Full examinations required *(see relevant chapters)*. Particularly focus on pulses, dermatomes & myotomes.
QoL Impingement & Sleep	Asking patient about these helps to assess impact on life & therefore necessity for intervention.
Help Patient Dress	Good practice if patient has functional limitation.
Radiographs	Soft tissue / bony abnormalities.

FINISH:

ANKLE & FOOT EXAMINATION

START: Patient exposure is ideally with trousers / skirt off.

Check the patient's shoes for pattern of wear.

First ask the patient to walk away a few steps, turn around & come back.

MUSCLES & TENDONS	Interpretation
Plantarflexors	Ask the patient to walk on their tip-toes.
Dorsiflexors	Ask the patient to walk on their heels.
Inverters	Ask the patient to stand on the outside edges of their feet.
Everters	Ask the patient to stand on the inside edges of their feet.

Remember to compare both sides throughout the examination.

Look at the ankle & foot with the patient standing, then sitting in a chair.

With the patient standing, look at the 3 x foot arches (medial / lateral / transverse).

With the patient sitting, look between the toes for ulcers, corns or callosities.

Do not forget to look at the plantar surface of the foot.

LOOK	Interpretation
Scars	Traumatic or iatrogenic e.g. post-operative.
Swelling	Look for soft tissue & bony swelling that may be traumatic, inflammatory or systemic. Suspect systemic cause with bilateral ankle oedema.
Symmetry	Asymmetrical callosities imply uneven distribution of load.
Deformity	Previous fracture, short / ruptured Achilles tendon, talipes (club foot), pes planus (flat foot), hallux valgus, mallet toe (DIPJ flexion deformity), hammer toe (PIPJ deformity), claw toes (DIPJ & PIPJ deformity), overriding toes. Most deformities are exaggerated on weight bearing.
Erythema	Inflammation e.g. RA.
Sinus	Post-operative, infective.
Muscle Wasting	Check the anterior, posterior & lateral compartments of the lower leg.

The patient should already be sitting in a chair.

Ask about pain.

Feel for temperature changes with the back of your hand.

FEEL	Interpretation
Pain	**Soft Tissues:** Achilles tendon (may palpate defect in rupture), peroneal tendons (behind lateral malleolus), dorsiflexion tendons, medial foot ligaments e.g. deltoid, lateral foot ligaments e.g. bifurcate, plantar fascia (plantar fasciitis). **Bones:** Palpate each joint individually. Check for malleolar tenderness. Squeeze the metatarsophalangeal joints (RA). Individually assess the remaining small bones of the feet.
Capillary Refill	Normal = 2–3 seconds.

MOVE	Interpretation
Ankle Joint	Grasp the lower leg with your left hand & hold the heel with your right hand. Assess dorsiflexion (normal = 15°) & plantar flexion (normal = 55°). Movements may be painful & restricted in arthritis or absent with arthrodesis.
Subtalar Joint	Grasp the lower leg with your left hand & hold the heel with your right hand. Assess inversion & eversion (normal = 15°). Movements may be painful & restricted in arthritis.
Midtarsal Joint	Grasp the heel with your left hand & hold the mid-foot with your right hand. Assess inversion & eversion (normal =15°).
Toes	Ask the patient to curl & extend their toes. Test the hallux individually & against resistance.

SPECIAL TESTS	Interpretation
Tenosynovitis	**Flexors / Inverters:** Palpate along the tendons behind the medial malleolus. Milk out synovial fluid from the tendons by running fingers proximally along them. **Tibialis Posterior:** Plantarflexion & eversion of the foot will precipitate pain just posterior to the medial malleolus. Check for gaps that indicate rupture e.g. RA & pes planus. **Peroneal:** Plantarflexion & inversion of the foot will precipitate pain behind the lateral malleolus. Now ask the patient to evert against resistance & feel for 'snapping' of a thickened, inflamed peroneal tendon.
Thompson's Test	Position the patient prone with their feet off the edge of the couch. Squeezing the calf should cause plantar flexion of the ankle. If not, this is pathognomonic of a ruptured Achilles tendon.
Tinel's Tarsal Tunnel Test	Percuss the posterior tibial nerve as it runs through the tarsal tunnel. This is located posterior to the medial malleolus. Reproduction of symptoms suggests tarsal tunnel syndrome.

COMPLETION	Interpretation
Lymphadenopathy	Check associated lymph nodes.
Joint Above & Below	Full knee examination. There is no joint below!
Distal Neurovascular Status	Full examinations required *(see relevant chapters)*. Particularly focus on pulses, dermatomes & myotomes. Glove in stocking distribution of paraesthesia / anaesthesia is suggestive of DM.
QoL Impingement & Sleep	Asking patient about these helps to assess impact on life & therefore necessity for intervention.
Help Patient Dress	Good practice if patient has functional limitation.
Radiographs	Soft tissue / bony abnormalities.

FINISH:

OSCE QUESTIONS

Gait

Q: What are the different phases of a normal gait?

Phase	Notes

Stance	• The foot is in contact with the ground during the stance phase.
	• The stance phase represents 60% of the gait cycle when walking.
	• The stance phase may be further classified as follows:
	  • **Heel Strike**: The heel hits the floor.
	  • **Foot Flat:** The whole of the foot makes contact with the floor.
	  • **Mid Stance:** Weight is transferred from the heel to the front of the foot.
	  • **Toe-Off**: Pushing off with the toes for forward propulsion.

Swing	• The swing phase represents 40% of the gait cycle when walking. • The foot swings forward (to become the leading foot again) & the contralateral leg supports the body.

Note: During walking there is a **'double stance'** period when both feet are in contact with the ground. When running, the stance phase becomes progressively shorter until a point is reached when neither foot is in contact with the ground, the so-called **'flight phase'**.

Q: What different types of gait do you know of?

Gait	Notes
Antalgic	Decreased stance & increased swing phase on the affected leg (due to pain).
Cerebellar	Broad based 'drunkard' gait (cerebellar ataxia).
High Stepping	Due to foot drop (common peroneal nerve damage).
Parkinsonian	Shuffling 'festinant' gait.
Short Leg	The affected hip appears to dip (congenital, iatrogenic, previous fracture).
Spastic	Jerky & scissoring (upper motor neuron lesion).
Trendelenberg	The patient lurches over the side of the bad hip to compensate for 'abductor weakness'. Causes of abductor weakness include OA, DDH, neuromuscular disorders & trauma.

Bone Structure

Q: What types of bone do you know of?

Type	Notes
Woven	Haphazardly organised collagen fibres = mechanically weak. Seen in foetal bones (replaced by lamellar bone from the 3rd trimester) & fracture healing.
Lamellar	Regular parallel alignment of collagen fibres = mechanically strong. Replaces woven bone in the foetus from the 3rd trimester & during fracture healing.
Compact / Cortical	The hard outer layer of bone, composed of tightly packed osteons. Osteons consist of lamellae, surrounding a central Haversian canal. Turnover is slow.
Cancellous / Trabecular	The porous central layer of bone, composed of a network of irregular bony rods & plates. Cancellous bone is less dense than compact bone, although turnover is much faster.

Q: What is the composition of bone?

Composition	Notes
Cellular	Osteoprogenitor Cells, Osteoblasts, Osteoclasts, Osteocytes, Lining Cells
Matrix	• **Inorganic (60%):** Calcium Hydroxyapatite, Osteocalcium Phosphate • **Organic (40%):** Collagen (type I), Proteoglycans, Proteins, Cytokines, Growth Factors

Osteoarthritis (OA)

Q: What is osteoarthritis?

This is a disease of synovial joints, characterised by cartilaginous loss & bony response, resulting in joint degeneration & destruction. OA is the most common joint disease worldwide.

Q: What are the causes of osteoarthritis?

Cause	Explanation / Examples
Primary	No underlying cause is attributable to joint degeneration. Chronic degeneration of joints occurs with age.
Secondary	An underlying cause is attributable to joint degeneration. These may be classified as follows:
	• **Congenital:** Perthe's Disease / SUFE
	• **Endocrine:** Acromegaly
	• **Infective:** Osteomyelitis
	• **Inflammatory:** RA
	• **Metabolic:** Diabetes / Gout
	• **Nutritional:** Obesity
	• **Traumatic:** Iatrogenic / Accidental
	• **Other:** Paget's Disease of Bone / SLE

Q: What are the clinical features of osteoarthritis?

Features	Explanation
Pain	• Sharp ache / burning sensation.
	• Worse with movement.
	• Worse at the end of the day.
Stiffness	• Worse at the end of the day.
	• Decreased range of motion due to pain / joint destruction.
Loss of Function	• Due to bony response e.g. osteophytes, Heberden's (DIPJ) & Bouchard's (PIPJ) Nodes.
	• Due to deformity e.g. valgus / varus.

Q: How would you make a diagnosis of osteoarthritis?

Diagnosis involves taking a **full history** & performing a **thorough clinical examination**. No laboratory or pathological tests are useful. Diagnosis is confirmed by radiological features as follows (Fig 10.6):

Memory: 'LOSS' for the radiological features of OA.

Loss of Joint Space (or narrowing)

Osteophyte Formation

Subchondral Sclerosis

Subchondral Cysts

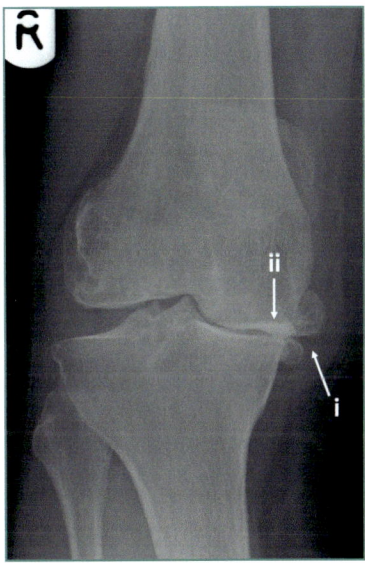

Fig 10.6: AP radiograph illustrating osteoarthritis of the right knee.

Most pathology is seen at the medial joint line with loss of joint space, osteophytes (i) & subchondral sclerosis (ii) present.

Q: What are the treatment options for osteoarthritis?

These may be classified as follows:

Conservative	Medical	Surgical
Aids e.g. Walking Stick	Analgesic Ladder	Osteotomy (realign)
Lifestyle Modification	Intra-Articular Corticosteroids (if there is a superadded inflammatory component)	Arthroplasty (replace)
OT / PT		Arthrodesis (fuse)
Patient Education		

Rheumatoid Arthritis (RA)

Q: What is rheumatoid arthritis?

A chronic, systemic inflammatory disorder, with an autoimmune component, that primarily affects joints (polyarthritis) in a symmetrical pattern. The characteristic pathology includes chronic synovitis, polyarthritis, joint deformity & ankylosis. RA affects <1% of the population & is 4 times more common in women.

Q: What are the clinical features of rheumatoid arthritis?

The hallmark feature of RA is a symmetrical polyarthritis & joint deformity. Clinical features may be classified as intra- / extra-articular as follows:

Intra-Articular	Interpretation
Pain	Due to synovitis & worse with movement. The joint may be warm & tender.
Swelling	Due to localised inflammation & joint effusions.
Stiffness	Characteristic early morning stiffness (>1 hour) or after prolonged inactivity.
Loss of Function	Due to joint swelling & destruction.
Deformity	Many deformities exist e.g. valgus, varus, subluxation, ulnar deviation of the MCPJs, radial deviation of the wrist (Figs 9.1, 10.7), Z-thumb, swan neck, boutonniere (Figs 11.1–11.3), CMCJ subluxation, atlanto-axial joint subluxation.
Extra-Articular	**Interpretation**
Skin	Rheumatoid nodules, erythema nodosum, pyoderma gangrenosum, palmar erythema.
Cardiovascular	Myocarditis, pericardial effusion, pericarditis, vasculitis.
Eyes	Keratoconjunctivitis sicca, episcleritis, uveitis.
Kidneys	Chronic inflammation causing amyloidosis, damage due to treatment (Gold, NSAIDs).
Lungs	Fibrosis due to disease or treatment, effusions, nodules (Caplan Syndrome).
Neurological	Carpal tunnel syndrome.
Felty's Syndrome	RA associated with splenomegaly, anaemia, neutropaenia, thrombocytopaenia & lymphadenopathy.

Q: How would you make a diagnosis of rheumatoid arthritis?

After taking a **full history** (including family history & association with EBV) & performing a **thorough clinical examination**, I would consider the following:

Diagnosis	Interpretation
Blood Tests	• FBC, U&Es, CRP, ESR. • Rheumatoid Factor (positive in 80%). • HLA–DR4.
X-Ray	Changes may be: • **Early:** No change or soft tissue swelling & loss of joint space. • **Late:** Bony erosions, severe joint destruction & subluxation.
American College of Rheumatology Criteria (1987)	4 criteria must be met to diagnose RA: • Morning stiffness >1 hour on most mornings for ≥6 weeks. • Arthritis & soft-tissue swelling of ≥3 joint groups, for ≥6 weeks. • Arthritis of hand joints, present for ≥6 weeks. • Symmetrical arthritis, present for ≥6 weeks. • Subcutaneous nodules in specific places. • Rheumatoid factor at a level >95th percentile. • Radiological changes suggestive of joint erosion **Note: Treatment should be started prior to meeting criteria, as early treatment is associated with decreased joint erosion.**

Q: What is this radiograph & what are points A & B?

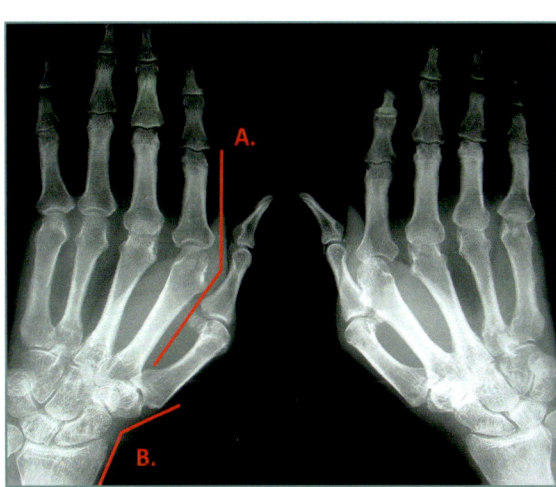

Fig 10.7: Radiograph of the hands, with characteristic features of rheumatoid arthritis.

A: Ulnar deviation of the metacarpophalangeal joints (MCPJ).

B: Radial deviation of the wrist.

Q: What is the management of rheumatoid arthritis?

Conservative	Medical	Surgical
Aids e.g. Walking Stick	Analgesic Ladder	Osteotomy (realign)
Lifestyle Modification	Corticosteroids	Arthroplasty (replace)
OT / PT	Disease Modifying Anti-Rheumatic Drugs (DMARDS) e.g. Gold, Penicillamine	Arthrodesis (fuse)
Patient Education		Tendon Transfer
	TNFα Inhibitors	Synovectomy

Gout

Q: What is the urate reference range?

- Urate / uric acid, is a product of purine metabolism i.e. adenine & guanine.
- Normal reference range = 3.5 –7 mg/dl.

Q: What are the consequences of hyperuricaemia?

Acute	Chronic
Gout: *Classically a hot, painful & swollen 1st metatarsophalangeal joint, although other joints may be affected e.g. ankle, knee, hands, wrist & spine.*	Destructive Joint Disease
Low Grade Fever	Polyarthritis
Painful Skin Tophi (Fig 10.8)	Urate Renal Calculi
	Renal Failure
	Skin Tophi Ulceration & Chalky Discharge

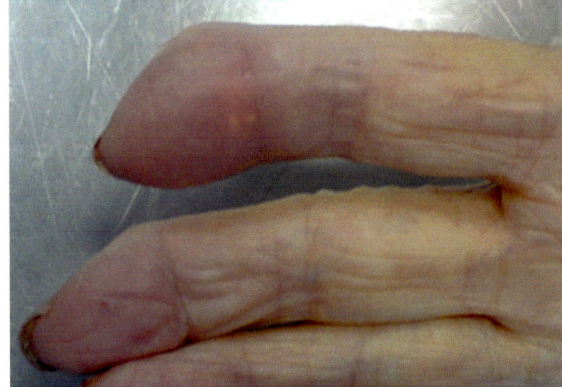

Fig 10.8: Gouty Tophi.

Gouty tophi affecting the right index finger tip (palmar surface).

Q: What are the causes of hyperuricaemia?

Primary	Secondary
Idiopathic	Alcohol
Inborn Errors of Metabolism	Diuretics
	Protein Rich Foods

Q: What are the pathological features of gout?

10% of patients with hyperuricaemia develop gout. There is rapid uric acid crystal deposition in cartilage, synovium & tendons of the affected joint. Larger deposits, known as **tophi**, may also ulcerate through skin.

Q: What are the specific investigations for gout?

Investigations	Notes	
Blood Tests	• **Urate**	Indicates hyperuricaemia.
	• **FBC**	Excludes infective cause.
	• **CRP**	Indicates presence of inflammation.
Joint Aspiration	• **MC+S**	Negatively birefingent crystals, which appear yellow under polarised light is pathognomonic. Also excludes infective cause.
Radiology	• **X-Ray**	May show joint destruction.

Q: What is the treatment of gout?

Conservative	Medical Treatment	Medical Prophylaxis
Rest & Elevated Acutely Affected Joint	Non-Steroidal Anti-Inflammatory Drugs	Allopurinol (not to be given during an acute attack)
Reduce Alcohol	Colchicine	Febuxostat (if allopurinol contraindicated or not tolerated)
Reduce Purine Rich Foods	Joint Aspiration +/- Intra Articular Corticosteroid Injection	Uricosuric Agents e.g. Sulfinpyrazone (used less commonly)
Weight Loss		

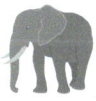

Memory: Colchicine whilst it's seen   &   Allopurinol once it's been!

(Medical Treatment)   (Medical Prophylaxis)

Septic Arthritis

Q: What is septic arthritis?

- An acute infective arthritis caused by bacteria (also fungi, mycobacteria or viruses).
- Presentation is usually with a red, hot, swollen, painful joint with a restricted range of movement.
- Associated systemic features can include fever, rigors, nausea, vomiting & shock.

Q: How can a septic arthritis develop?

Route	Features
Haematogenous Spread	• Organisms present in the blood.
	• Patients with a prosthetic joint & bacteraemia from another source (e.g. infective endocarditis) are at higher risk.
Bone to Joint	• Local spread from osteomyelitis affecting the epiphysis or metaphysis.
Soft Tissue to Joint	• Local spread from an overlying cellulitis or infected bursitis.
Direct Inoculation	• Local spread following a penetrating wound.
Iatrogenic	• Direct inoculation following joint injection / aspiration.
	• Direct inoculation following arthrodesis / arthroplasty.

Q: What are the common bacterial causes of septic arthritis?

Bacterial Species	Notes
Staphylococcus spp.	*Staphylococcus aureus* is the most common pathogen in all age groups.
Streptococcus spp.	Including *Streptococcus pyogenes* & *pneumoniae*.
Pseudomonas aeruginosa	Particularly in IV drug users, at the extremes of age & the acutely unwell.
Escherichia coli	Particularly in IV drug users, at the extremes of age & the acutely unwell.
Neisseria gonorrhoea	A cause of adolescent septic arthritis.
Salmonella spp.	Rare. Can occur in the very young or in patients with sickle cell disease.
Mycobacterium tuberculosis	Rare, except in the immunocompromised.
Haemophilus influenzae	Now uncommon in western Europe due to widespread immunisation

Q: How is septic arthritis diagnosed?

The diagnosis of septic arthritis is following clinical assessment & prompt joint aspiration, however after taking a **full history** & performing a **thorough clinical examination**, I would consider the following:

Investigations	Interpretation
Blood Tests	• FBC, U&Es, CRP, ESR.
	• Blood Cultures.
Plain Radiographs	• Predominantly to exclude other differential diagnoses of arthritis.
	• Radiological changes of an **acutely** septic joint will be limited to soft tissue swelling.
	• If underlying bone is also infected (usually a more chronic clinical picture) then evidence of osteomyelitis may be seen (osteopaenia ± periosteal reaction ± joint destruction).
Joint Aspiration	Aspiration of a joint must **always** be performed under *full aseptic technique & full sterile technique (i.e. theatre)* in those patients with a prosthetic joint.
	• Macroscopic: turbid, non-viscous fluid or pus.
	• Microscopic: neutrophilia, positive gram stain or culture.

Q: How is septic arthritis managed?

Septic arthritis is a rheumatological & orthopaedic emergency & should be managed following a resuscitative approach as patients may present in septic shock. I would consider the following steps to **simultaneously assess & treat** the patient:

Initial Management	
Airway	• Consider giving high flow oxygen (15L/minute via a non-rebreathe mask).
Breathing	• Assess for tachypnoea.
	• Measure oxygen saturation.
	• Consider performing an ABG (to measure the degree of hypoxia & lactic acidosis).
Circulation	• Assess for a tachycardia & hypotension.
	• Obtain intravenous access & take blood tests for FBC, U&Es, CRP, ESR & blood cultures.
	• Consider intravenous fluid replacement.
	• Consider urinary catheterisation & fluid balance measurement.
Disability	• Assess for neurological impairment using either GCS or AVPU.
Exposure	• Perform a top to-toe examination to identify source of sepsis.
	• Measure core body temperature.
	• Send cultures for MC+S (e.g. blood, sputum, urine, wound swabs as relevant).

Osteomyelitis

Q: What is osteomyelitis?

An inflammatory lesion due to infection of bone or bone marrow. It may be classified as acute or chronic, by route of infection or causative organism.

Q: What are the most common causative organisms of osteomyelitis, relating to age group?

Age	Organism
<4 Months	*Staphylococcus aureus, Streptococcus* Groups A & B, *Enterobacter, Escherichia coli.*
4 Months–Late Teenager	*Staphylococcus aureus, Streptococcus* Group A, *Haemophilus influenzae, Enterobacter.*
Adult	*Staphylococcus aureus, Enterobacter,* Streptococcus Group B, *Pseudomonas, Escherichia coli.*

Q: Are any causative organisms of osteomyelitis related to specific diseases?

There are many important causes e.g. MRSA. The remainder may be classified according to disease:

Disease	Organism
Diabetes Mellitus	Anaerobes
Immunocompromise	*Aspergillus fumigatus, Candida albicans, Mycobacterium Avium-Intracellulare Complex*
HIV	*Mycobacterium tuberculosis*
Sickle Cell Anaemia	*Salmonella*

Q: What is the pathogenesis of osteomyelitis?

- A focus of acute inflammation develops around capillaries in the bone metaphysis.
- As this progresses, capillaries & other vessels become compressed, blood supply to bone trabeculae is compromised & osteonecrosis ensues.
- Dead bone fragments separate from healthy bone, forming a **sequestrum**.
- If the lesion persists, a new surrounding bone layer may form beneath the periosteum. This is the **involucrum**.
- Pus & debris may drain to the skin's surface via sinus formation.

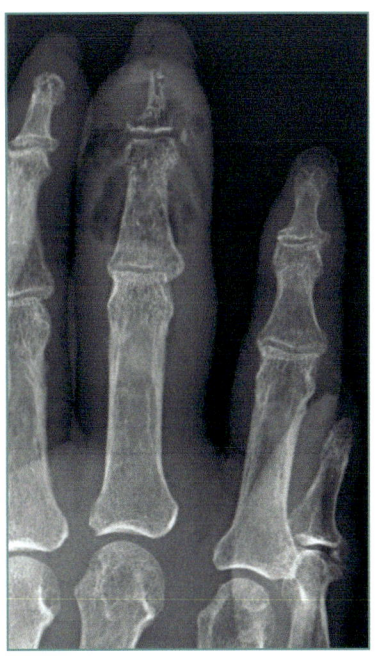

Fig 10.9: Radiograph illustrating an acute abscess of the left hand middle finger tip, with associated osteomyelitis & distal phalanx destruction.

Q: What are the complications of osteomyelitis?

- Sinus Formation
- Overlying Soft Tissue Infection
- Metastatic Infection e.g. Brain (abscess), Joints (septic arthritis), Lungs (abscess)
- Septicaemia
- Limb Length Discrepancy
- Pathological Fractures
- Chronic Osteomyelitis

Q: What would your management of a patient with osteomyelitis be?

- **Full History**
- **Thorough Clinical Examination**
- **Appropriate Investigations:**

Investigation	Examples
Blood Tests	FBC, U&E, LFT, CRP.
Microbiology	Blood cultures & wound swabs.
Radiographs	AP & true lateral long bone radiograph.
Other	More complex scans as appropriate.

- **Treatment:**

Treatment	Examples	Interpretation
MEDICAL	**Dressings**	These may be biological or synthetic, adherent or non-adherent.
	Analgesia	According to analgesic ladder.
	High Dose (IV) Antibiotics	This may be for weeks, with continued oral treatment in the community after hospital discharge.
SURGICAL	**Debridement**	Of necrotic & infected tissue.
	Reconstruction	After infection cleared.
	Amputation	May be required.

Ankylosing Spondylitis (AS)

Q: What is ankylosing spondylitis?

An inflammatory disorder from the group of seronegative spondylarthropathies. Progressive inflammation typically affects the vertebral column & sacroiliac joints, leading to bony ankylosis (fusion). Ankylosing spondylitis is 3 times more common in males & presents around the age of 25 years. The annual incidence is 7/100,000 & it is associated with HLA-B27.

Q: What are the clinical features of ankylosing spondylitis?

Intra-Articular	Interpretation
Back Pain	Low back pain that is worse in the morning. Other joints may be affected e.g. hips & knees. Sacroiliitis may also be present & painful.
Stiffness	Back & joint stiffness, characteristically worse early in the morning. Early morning stiffness may gradually ease with activity.
Loss of Function	Limitation of spinal movement due to bony ankylosis. Lateral flexion is commonly 1st to be affected.
Enthesitis	Inflammation of a tendon, ligament or joint capsule insertion point into bone.
Fractures	More common in patients with ankylosing spondylitis.
Osteoporosis	More common in patients with ankylosing spondylitis.
Other	Increased thoracic kyphosis, loss of lumbar lordosis, chest expansion <5cm.
Extra-Articular	Interpretation
Cardiovascular	Aortitis, conduction defects, myocarditis.
Eyes	Anterior uveitis (most common & affects 20%), iritis.
Lungs	Apical pulmonary fibrosis.
Neurological	Cauda equina syndrome.

Q: How would you make a diagnosis of ankylosing spondylitis?

Diagnosis depends on taking a **full history** & performing a **thorough clinical examination**. There are no laboratory or pathological tests available to diagnose ankylosing spondylitis, however the following investigations should be considered:

Investigations	Interpretation
Blood Tests	• FBC, CRP, ESR.
	• Rheumatoid factor (negative).
	• HLA-B27 (positive in 90% of patients).
Spine X-Ray	• Intervertebral disc ossification.
	• Bamboo spine (syndesmophytes are bony bridges that span the intervertebral joints, giving it the appearance of bamboo) (Fig 10.10).
	• Sacroiliac joint fusion (Fig 10.11).
CT / MRI	• May show early signs of sacroiliitis.

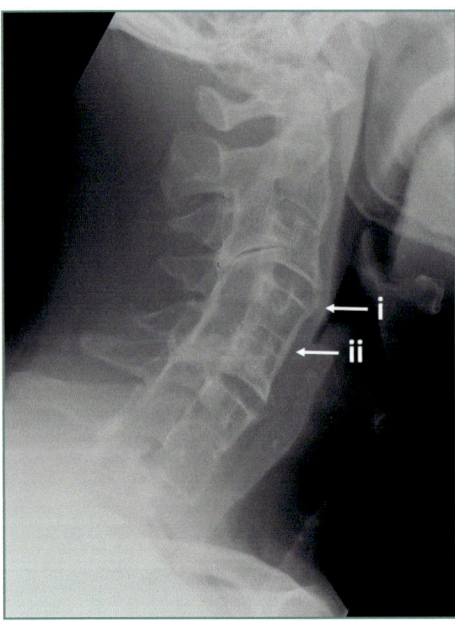

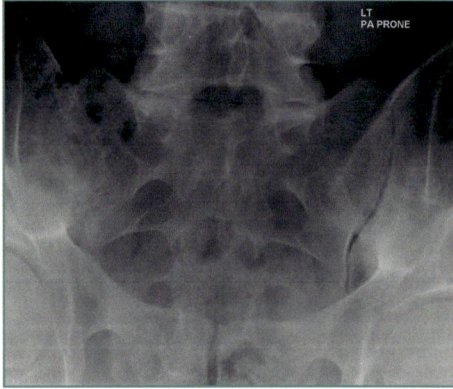

Fig 10.11: PA radiograph of the pelvis in a patient with ankylosing spondylitis.

Sacroiliac joint fusion is visible on the right side when compared with the left, where the joint line is clearly visible.

Fig 10.10: Lateral cervical spine radiograph of a patient with ankylosing spondylitis.

Bamboo spine, with syndesmophytes (i) & vertebral fusion (ankylosis) (ii) present.

Q: What are the treatment options for ankylosing spondylitis?

Conservative	Medical	Surgical
Aids e.g. Walking Stick	Analgesic Ladder	Osteotomy (realign)
Lifestyle Modification	Corticosteroid Injections	Arthroplasty (replace)
OT / PT	TNFα Antagonists	Arthrodesis (fuse)
Patient Education		

Paget's Disease of Bone

Q: What is Paget's Disease?

Paget's Disease (also known as osteitis deformans) is a chronic condition of bone involving mixed osteoclast & osteoblast activity. It is the 2nd most prevalent metabolic bone disease, commonly affecting middle-aged / elderly populations. The aetiology is largely unknown, however environmental, genetic & viral factors have been suggested. There are 3 distinct phases:

Phase	Notes
Osteolytic	Characterised by enhanced bone resorption due to osteoclast activity. This results in discrete lytic lesions of affected bone (Fig 10.12)
Mixed	Osteoblasts also become active & lay woven bone. The result is disorganised bone formation.
Osteosclerotic	Osteoclast & osteoblast activity decline. Resulting in abnormal, eroded & sclerotic bone.

Note: Paget also described Paget's Disease of the nipple.

Q: What does the following radiograph show?

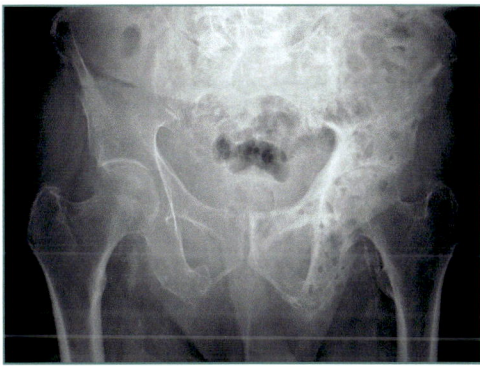

Fig 10.12: Paget's Disease of the left hip.

This is a radiograph of the pelvis. There is a mixed lytic & sclerotic picture, with:

- **Lytic lesions** affecting the left hemi-pelvis & femoral head.
- **Bony sclerosis** of the left acetabulum region.

The most likely diagnosis is Paget's Disease of the left hip.

Q: What are the clinical features of Paget's Disease?

Paget's Disease is usually asymptomatic. Clinical features are related to the extent & phase of disease, including the presence or absence of complications. They include:

Features	Examples
Symptoms	• **Bone Pain** (due to microfractures). • **Muscle Weakness** (due to disuse / pain). • **Neurological Symptoms** e.g. deafness (due to cranial nerve VIII compression) / trigeminal neuralgia (due to cranial nerve V compression).
Signs	• **Bony Deformity & Enlargement.** • **Localised Pain.** • **Skin Erythema & Warmth** (due to vascular response). • **Gait Abnormalities** (due to bony deformity / pain).
Complications	• **Bony:** Deformity, OA & pathological fractures. • **Cardiovascular:** High output cardiac failure (due to increased vascularity). • **Endocrine:** Secondary hyperparathyroidism may develop in 10% of patients. • **Metabolic:** Hypercalcaemia (due to prolonged immobility). • **Neurological:** Focal neurological deficits & neuropathic pain (due to spinal cord / cranial nerve / peripheral nerve compression). • **Neoplastic:** Osteosarcoma may develop in 1% of patients. • **Social:** Immobility.

Q: What specific investigations would assist your diagnosis of Paget's Disease?

After taking a **full history** & performing a **thorough clinical examination**, I would consider the following specific tests in addition to those ordered as part of a comprehensive work up:

Investigation	Interpretation
Blood Tests	• **Alkaline Phosphatase:** Raised with increased osteoblastic activity & reflects disease extent. • **Calcium:** Usually normal. May be raised with prolonged immobility. • **Phosphate:** Normal. • **TFT:** Thyroid function tests rule out secondary hyperparathyroidism.
Urine Tests	• **Urinary Hydroxyproline:** Raised with increased osteoblastic activity (it is a collagen breakdown product).
Radiology	• **X-ray:** Lytic lesions in early disease (Fig 10.12). Thickened, eroded & sclerotic bone in late disease. Bony enlargement, with increased radiodensity & trabeculations is pathognomonic. • **CT / MRI:** Helpful to assess complications including joint involvement, articular abnormalities & spinal cord involvement. • **Bone Scan:** Helpful to assess disease extent.

Q: What is the management of Paget's Disease?

Conservative	Medical	Surgical
Aids e.g. Walking Stick	Analgesic Ladder	Repair Fractures
OT / PT	Bisphosponates	Osteotomy (realign joint)
Hot / Cold Packs	(decrease bone turnover)	Arthroplasty (replace joint)
Massage	Calcitonin	Nerve / Spinal Cord Decompression
Patient Education		Tumour Resection / Amputation

Painful Shoulder

Q: What is the differential diagnosis of a painful shoulder?

Pathology	Example
Soft Tissues	Adhesive capsulitis (frozen shoulder), rotator cuff injury / rupture, supraspinatus tendinitis, subacromial bursitis, long head of biceps tendinitis, suprascapular nerve entrapment.
Joint	Acromioclavicular OA, glenohumeral OA, recurrent dislocation, subluxation.
Bone	Infection, neoplasm.
Referred Pain	Cervical spondylosis, cardiac ischaemia.

Q: What is adhesive capsulitis (frozen shoulder)?

An idiopathic condition characterised by decreased ROM & chronic pain. Active & passive ROM becomes limited in all directions, however external rotation is usually worst affected. Adhesions gradually form until the glenohumeral joint is stiff & only scapular-thoracic movement remains. Diagnosis is based on a full history & thorough clinical examination, although other causes of shoulder pathology must be ruled out e.g. infection / rotator cuff injury.

Q: What is the management of adhesive capsulitis?

Conservative	Medical	Surgical
Physiotherapy	Analgesic Ladder	Manipulation Under Anaesthetic
	NSAIDs	Arthroscopic Release
	Corticosteroid Injection	

Q: What is shoulder impingement syndrome?

Impingement of the supraspinatus tendon passing through the subacromial space causing inflammation of the tendon, eventually leading to its rupture. This condition also is known as the painful arc syndrome.

Features	Examples
Symptoms	• Painful shoulder (overhead activity). • The painful arc (60^0–120^0 abduction). • Limited range of movements. • Weakness.
Signs	• Impingement testing (Neer's Test, Hawkin's Test, Jobe's Test).
Causes	• Trauma (can cause complete rupture of tendon). • Idiopathic. • Bony spur (from OA of ACJ or under surface of acromium). • Subacromial bursal pathology.

Diagnosis	• **Clinical investigation:** Injection of local anaesthetic into the subachromial space, relieves pain during clinical examination, hence assisting in diagnosis.
	• **Radiological diagnosis:**
	  • **X-ray:** May show a calcified tendon or bony spur in the subacromial space.
	  • **MRI:** Delineates rotator cuff muscle pathology (including rupture).

Complications	• Inflammation can lead to tendon rupture. • Instability of shoulder. • Poor shoulder function.

Q: What is the treatment of shoulder impingement syndrome?

Conservative	Medical	Surgical
PT (strength)	Analgesic Ladder	Subacromial Decompression +/- ACJ Excision
Limit Impingement Position Activity	Steroid Injection	Rotator Cuff Repair (arthroscopic or open)

Ankle & Foot Pathology

Q: Can you briefly explain the following conditions: Achilles tendon rupture, claw toes, hallux rigidus & valgus, hammer toes & talipes equinovarus?

Condition	Explanation
Achilles Tendon Rupture	Inability to plantar flex foot due to rupture.
Claw Toes	Flexion deformity of PIPJ & DIPJ with compensatory hyperextension of MTPJ.
Hallux Rigidus	Degenerative joint disease of big toe MTPJ causing joint pain & stiffness.
Hallux Valgus	Prominence of 1st metatarsal head (the most common foot deformity). This may be associated with valgus deviation of the great toe.
Hammer Toes	Flexion deformity of PIPJ with compensatory DIPJ extension.
Talipes Equinovarus (club foot)	Plantar flexion, inversion, adduction deformity of the foot, with the heel in varus. The foot appears 'clubbed'.

Q: What is the pathophysiology of these conditions?

Condition	Explanation
Achilles Tendon Rupture	Spontaneous or traumatic (direct injury). Sudden plantar flexion (forced) causes tendon rupture. Spontaneous ruptures are associated with an increased risk of future contralateral rupture.
Claw Toes	Usually seen in neurological disorders e.g. poliomyelitis & peroneal muscle atrophy (Charcot-Marie-Tooth Disease). Also seen in RA.
Hallux Rigidus	Osteoarthritis of 1st MTPJ (either primary or secondary).
Hallux Valgus	Underlying deformity is forefoot splaying (metatarsus primus varus).
Hammer Toes	Caused by imbalance between extrinsic & intrinsic muscles causing fixed PIPJ flexion.
Talipes Equinovarus (club foot)	Most common congenital foot deformity.

Q: What operative treatment might you consider for these conditions?

All these conditions can be treated conservatively & medically e.g. appropriate footwear & analgesic ladder. Specific operative treatments for the various conditions are as follows:

Condition	Operative Treatment
Achilles Tendon Rupture	*Non-Operative:* Serial Casts (in equinus, semi-equinus & neutral positions). *Operative:* Open / Percutaneous Repair & Cast Immobilisation.
Claw Toes	Tendon Transfer (long toe flexor to extensors), Joint Excision, Arthrodesis.
Hallux Rigidus	Silastic Joint Replacement, Arthrodesis.
Hallux Valgus	Bunionectomy & Realignment Osteotomy (Scarf, Akin, Chevron, Wilson's, Mitchell's).
Hammer Toes	Tendon Transfer, Joint Excision, Arthrodesis.
Talipes Equinovarus (club foot)	Plaster / Wedging / Splinting (Ponseti), Surgical Correction e.g. Percutaneous Tibialis Anterior Lengthening.

Fractures - Overview

Q: How are fractures classified?

These may be classified according to cause, extent, pattern, displacement & structural involvement as follows (Fig 10.13):

Classification	Example	Interpretation
CAUSE	**Traumatic**	Due to strong deforming force.
	Stress	Occur in normal bone subjected to repeated trauma.
	Pathological	Occur when bone is weakened by pre-existing disease, such that minimal insult results in fracture e.g. metastasis, osteoporosis.
EXTENT	**Partial**	Only part of the cortex is involved.
	Complete	Both cortices are involved.
	Transverse	Fracture lies 90^0 to long axis of bone.
	Oblique	Fracture lies off the long axis of bone ($>30^0$).
	Spiral	Due to twisting around the long axis of bone.
	Comminuted	>2 bone fragments produced.
	Avulsion	Fractured segment is pulled off e.g. by inserting tendon.
	Butterfly	Force to 1 side of bone blows out a triangular wedge on the other side.
PATTERN	**Segmented**	Force to 1 side of bone blows out a complete bone segment.
	Crush	Compressive forces result in bone collapse e.g. vertebral column in patients with osteoporosis.
	Wedge	Flexion-extension injuries may produce a V-shaped bone defect, such that 1 cortex side appears wider than the other at radiography.
	Burst	Compressive forces may result in many fragments of bone bursting away from the area of greatest force.
	Greenstick	1 cortex side is broken & the other undergoes plastic deformation. Affects children.
	Subluxation	Partial loss of contact between 2 joint surfaces that usually articulate.
	Dislocation	Complete loss of contact between 2 joint surfaces that usually articulate.
DISPLACEMENT	**Translation**	Fracture displacement is in the same plane e.g. medial, lateral, superior, inferior.
	Angulation	May be anterior, posterior, varus, valgus etc.
	Rotation	May be external, internal etc.
STRUCTURAL INVOLVEMENT	**Simple**	Fracture does not communicate with the outside & no additional structural damage.
	Open / Compound	Fracture communicates with the outside e.g. open wounds, skull fractures communicating with air sinuses.
	Complicated	Additional structural damage present e.g. nerve, vascular, visceral.
	Intra-Articular	Fracture involves an articulating joint.

Memory: When describing fractures, consider the above classification system in order to structure your answer.

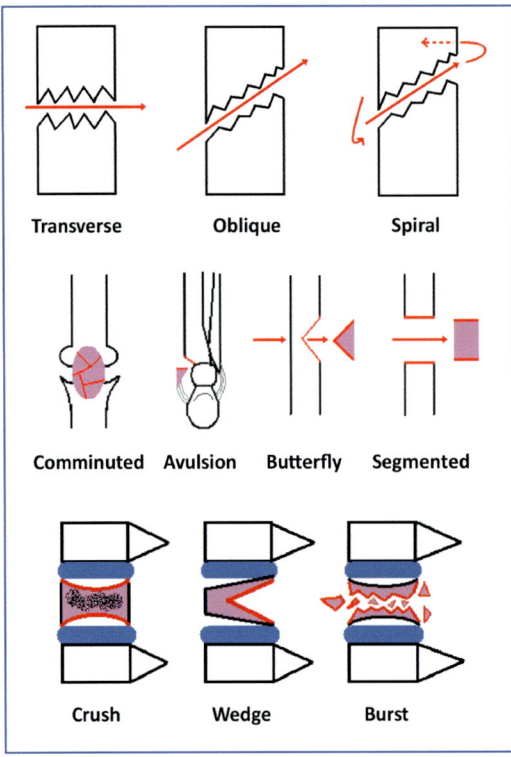

Fig 10.13 Diagrammatic representation of various fracture patterns.

Transverse   Oblique   Spiral

Comminuted   Avulsion   Butterfly   Segmented

Crush   Wedge   Burst

Q: What is the Salter-Harris fracture classification?

A classification system for fractures involving the epiphyseal growth plate in children (Fig 10.14). A higher class implies a more severe fracture.

Memory: **SALT CRUSH**

S	= **S**eparated from growth plate	(Class I)
A	= **A**bove growth plate	(Class II)
L	= **L**ower than growth plate	(Class III)
T	= **T**ogether both above & below growth plate	(Class IV)
CRUSH	= Impacted growth plate	(Class V)

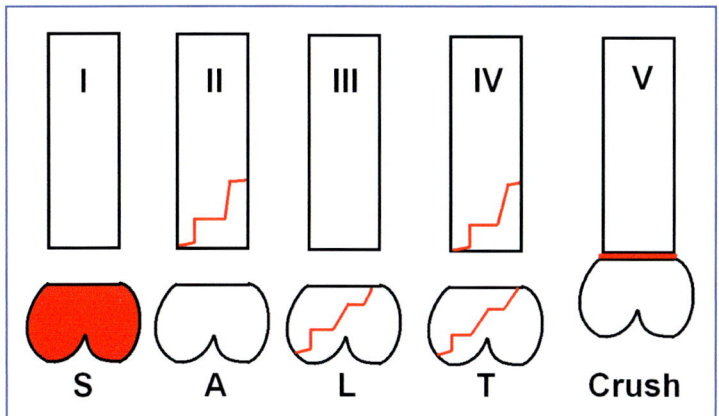

Fig 10.14: Salter-Harris classification. Note: This diagrammatic representation only works with the growth plate orientated inferiorly.

Q: What are the phases of fracture healing?

There are 3 major phases that may be further sub-classified as follows (Fig 10.15):

 Memory: 3 x **R**s of fracture healing.

Phase	Sub-Classification	Description
REACTIVE	**Inflammation**	Haemorrhage & tissue destruction with haematoma formation. Necrosis of osteocytes at the fracture ends.
	Granulation	Fibroblast proliferation & capillary growth at the site of haematoma. Granulation tissue is formed.
REPARATIVE	**Callus**	Periosteal cells transform into chondroblasts (forming hyaline cartilage) & osteoblasts (forming bone). These tissues grow & bridge the fracture.
	Lamellar Bone Formation	Lamellar bone replaces woven bone & cartilage. This bone is trabecular & has most of the original bone strength.
REMODELLING	**Remodelling**	Compact bone substitutes trabecular bone. Bone shape returns to normal as influenced by stress forces encountered during rehabilitation.

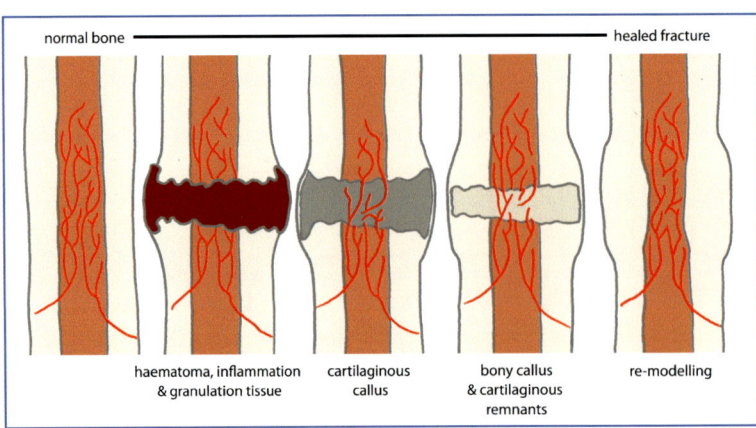

Fig 10.15:
Diagram of
fracture healing.

normal bone ——————————————————————— healed fracture

haematoma, inflammation & granulation tissue | cartilaginous callus | bony callus & cartilaginous remnants | re-modelling

Q: What are the principles of fracture treatment?

This requires **ATLS** resuscitation (with appropriate history & clinical examination) & includes:

Principle	Interpretation
Reduce	The fractured ends of bone need to be realigned. This may be done either in the acute setting or under general anaesthetic. Open reduction involves surgical exposure prior to fracture reduction.
Hold	Immobilisation times are governed by the fracture type, location & extent. This may be achieved by a number of fixation methods: • **Internal Fixation** Screw, Plate, Intramedullary Nail • **External Fixation** External Fixation Device, Pin-Traction • **Non-Invasive Stabilisation:** Cast, Splint, Strap **Note: K-wires may be used as internal / percutaneous fixation.**
Rehabilitate	Involves physiotherapy & occupational therapy. Rehabilitation protocols are governed by evidence-based research & must be adhered to in order to maximise recovery. Protocols are highly variable depending on fracture type, location & extent.

Q: What factors affect bone healing?

General Factors	Local Factors
Age	Blood Supply
Co-Morbidities	Infection
Nutrition	Injury Severity
Smoking	Stabilisation
Drugs (NSAIDs, Steroids)	Site
	Soft Tissue Interposition

Q: What are the complications of fractures?

Complication	Local	General
EARLY	Haemorrhage	Hypovolaemic Shock
	Structural Damage e.g. Nerve, Vessel, Viscera	Urinary Retention
	Loss of Function	DVT
	Tetanus	Pneumonia
	Wound Infection & Gangrene	Fat Embolism
	Compartment Syndrome	Crush Syndrome
LATE	Delayed Union	Pulmonary Embolism
	Non-Union	Pneumonia
	Mal-Union	Immobility
	CRPS	PTSD
	Myositis Ossificans	
	Avascular Necrosis	
	Joint Stiffness / Contracture	
	Osteomyelitis	

Fractured Neck of Femur

Q: What is the epidemiology in relation to a fractured neck of femur?

- 1.7 million worldwide per annum.
- Most prevalent in osteoporotic women.
- Increasing incidence with age.

Q: What are the clinical features?

Often sustained after a low-energy fall in an elderly patient who presents as follows:

- Non weight-bearing.
- Shortened leg on affected side.
- Externally rotated leg on affected side.

Q: What is the vascular supply to the femoral head:

- Ligamentem teres obturator artery branch (absent in 20% of the population).
- Retinacular (capsular) vessels arising from the medial & lateral circumflex femoral branches of the profunda femoris artery.
- Intramedullary vessels.

Q: What is the radiological diagnosis & classification of a fractured neck of femur?

- Intracapsular vs. extracapsular (Fig 10.16).
- Further subclassification according to anatomical position (Fig 10.17).

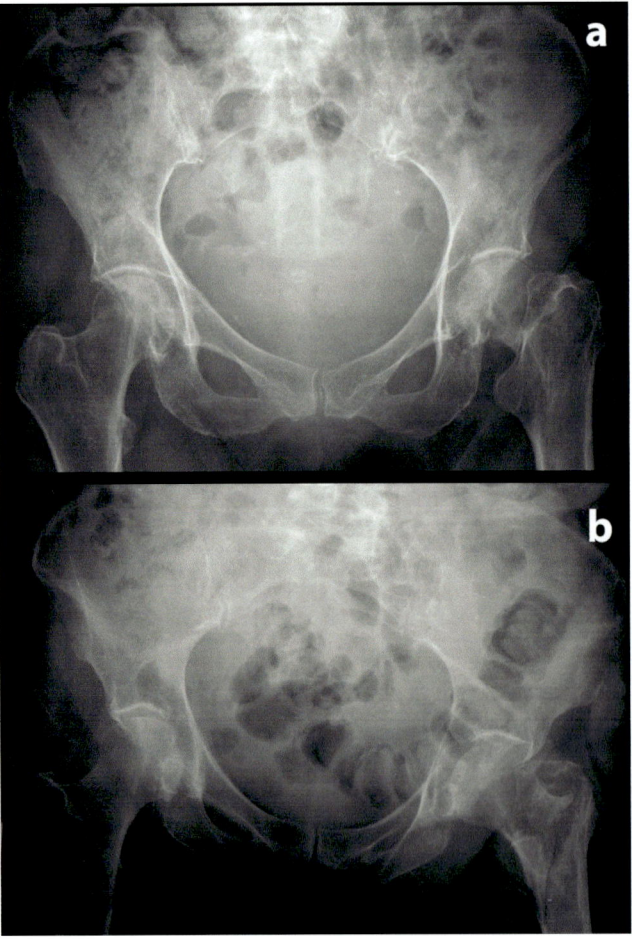

Fig 10.16: Femoral neck fracture radiographs.

Fractures of the left femoral neck are visualised

a = Intracapsular

b = Extracapsular

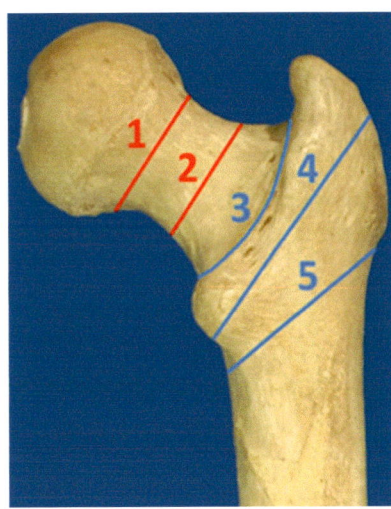

Fig 10.17: Anatomical classification of femoral neck fractures.

Intracapsular (red):
1 = Subcapital
2 = Transcervical

Extracapsular (blue):
3 = Basal
4 = Intertrochanteric
5 = Sub-Trochanteric

Q: What is the surgical treatment for femoral neck fractures?

- Initial management is according to **ATLS** guidelines, including adequate resuscitation, history, examination & appropriate investigations.
- In general, surgical fixation (Fig 10.18) is guided by radiological classification:
  - **Intracapsular fracture = hemiarthroplasty.**
  - **Extracapsular fracture = dynamic hip screw.**
- Hemiarthroplasty replaces the femoral head which is at higher risk of avascular necrosis with intracapsular fracture patterns due to disruption of the retinacular (capsular) vessels supplying the femoral head.
- Dynamic hip screws facilitate compression at the fracture site, assisting the fracture healing process.

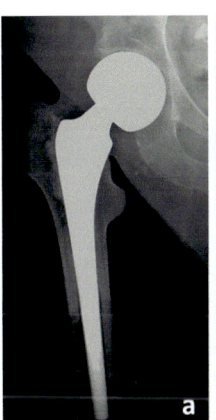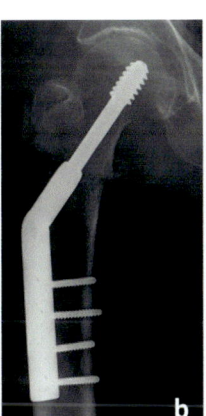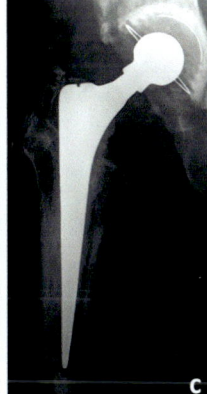

Fig 10.18: Hip prostheses radiographs.

(a) = Hemiarthroplasty

(b) = Dynamic hip screw

(c) = Total hip replacement

Q: What further important investigations should be considered in a patient who sustains a femoral neck fracture?

Investigation	Reasoning
FBC	Is there anaemia? Is there underlying infection?
U&E	Dehydration is a common cause of falls. Are there electrolyte Imbalances that may be associated with arrhythmias?
CRP	Acute phase reactant.
Blood Glucose	Hypoglycaemia is a common cause of falls.
CK	The patient may have been lying on the floor for hours. Rhabdomyolysis may have ensued, with a risk of renal failure.
Cross Match	2 units for hemiarthroplasty, otherwise group & save.
Urine Biochemistry	Myoglobinuria may be detected in association with rhabdomyolysis.
Urine Dipstick / MC+S	Urinary tract infection is a common cause of falls.
Chest X-Ray	Pneumonia is a common cause of falls. Are there rib fractures? For pre-anaesthetic purposes.
Electrocardiogram (ECG)	Is there a new arrhythmia?
Osteoporosis Screen	If underlying osteoporosis is present, treatment should be commenced in hospital. The GP should also be notified.

Q: What is the % mortality at 1 year following a femoral neck fracture?

25%.

Lower Limb Trauma

Q: What are the management strategies for open tibia fractures / lower limb trauma?

- Guidelines vary between countries, however principles of best-practice are similar.
- The following protocol is based on the British Orthopaedic Association & Association of Plastic Reconstructive & Aesthetic Surgeons Standard for Trauma Guidelines.

Management	Notes
ATLS	• Initial assessment, resuscitation & management according to ATLS principles.
	• Splint limb as appropriate.
Antibiotics	• (IV) co-amoxiclav (1.2g) / cefuroxime (1.5g) <3h post injury.
	• Continue 3 times daily until wound debridement.
	• (IV) clindamycin (600mg) if penicillin allergic.
Wound	• Only handle wound to remove gross contamination & allow photography.
	• Cover wound with saline soaked gauze & impermeable film to prevent desiccation.
	• Immediate wound handling may be indicated with gross contamination e.g. murine, agricultural or sewage.
Neurovascular Assessment	• Performed systematically & repeated at regular intervals.
	• Vascular injury requires immediate surgery within 6 hours of warm ischaemia time.
Compartment Syndrome	• Early clinical features include disproportionate pain at rest (resistant to opiates) & pain on passive stretch.
	• Diagnosis confirmed when there is an intra-compartmental pressure reading ≤30mmHg difference of the diastolic blood pressure reading.
	• This is a surgical emergency requiring immediate fasciotomy with 4 compartment decompression via 2 incisions.
Surgery	• Combined management plan for soft tissues & bone formulated by Orthopaedic & Plastic Surgeons.
	• Ideally undertaken in a specialist treatment centre unless there are no other options.
	• Surgery <24 hours post-injury unless heavily contaminated.
	• (IV) co-amoxiclav (1.2g) & gentamicin (1.5mg/kg) are administered at wound excision.
	• Antibiotics continued for 72 hours or until definitive wound closure has occurred.
	• Definitive skeletal stabilisation & wound cover achieved <72 hours post-injury ideally but not to exceed 7 days.
Negative Pressure Dressings	• These do not replace definitive wound management in open tibial fractures.
	• Indicated only if definitive skeletal & soft tissue reconstruction is not to be undertaken in a single stage.

Q: What is the Gustilo classification for open tibia fractures?

- Gustilo & Anderson (1976) classified 3 grades.
- Grade III was high energy, severe crush, comminuted/segmental fractures with extensive soft-tissue damage including neurovascular structures, bone loss, gunshot wounds or traumatic amputations.
- Gustilo & Mendoza (1984) further classified Grade III into a-c.

Grade	Bone	Skin / Wound / Soft Tissues	Surgery
I	Simple Fracture Without Comminution	• <1cm Skin Defect • Minimal Soft Tissue Damage	• Intramedullary Nail = 28 Weeks for Union
II	Simple Fracture Without Comminution	• >1cm Skin Defect • Minimal Soft Tissue Damage	• Intramedullary Nail = 28 Weeks for Union
IIIa	• High Energy Injury Regardless of Soft Tissue Cover • Comminuted or Segmental Fracture / Bone Loss	• Crush Injury • Extensive Soft Tissue Damage • Primary Wound Closure Sometimes Possible	• Intramedullary Nail = 35 Weeks for Union
IIIb	Exposed Bone & Periosteal Stripping	• Contaminated Wound • Extensive Soft Tissue Damage • Primary Wound Closure Not Possible	• Intramedullary Nail = 35 Weeks for Union • Flap Cover Required
IIIc	-	• Arterial Injury Requiring Repair • Extensive Soft Tissue Damage	• Arterial Repair to Salvage Limb • Consider BKA • Flap Cover Required

Q: How is a lower limb fasciotomy performed for compartment syndrome?

- 4 compartment decompression via 2 incisions (Fig 10.19).
- Posterior-medial incision 1cm posterior to the posterior-medial subcutaneous tibial border. Extended in a coronal plane to decompress the deep & superficial posterior compartments of the lower limb.
- Anterior-lateral incision 2cm lateral to the anterior subcutaneous tibial border. Extended circumferentially & posteriorly to decompress the anterior compartment, then continued through into the lateral compartment.

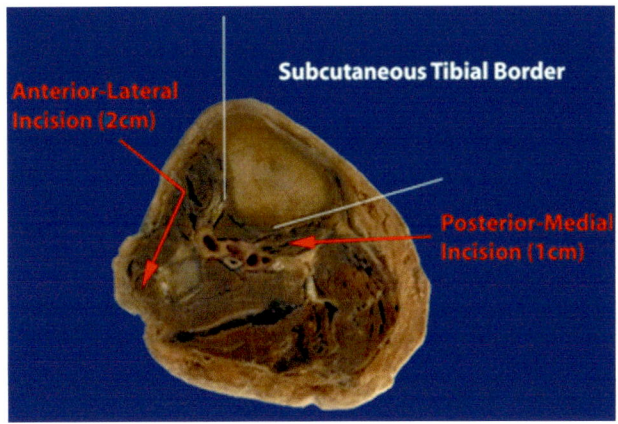

Subcutaneous Tibial Border

Anterior-Lateral
Incision (2cm)

Posterior-Medial
Incision (1cm)

Fig 10.19: Lower limb fasciotomy incisions.

Fasciotomy Incisions for Lower Limb Compartment Syndrome.

(right leg, mid-calf level, view from below).

Q: What is the Webber classification of ankle fractures?

- Webber (1972) re-classified Danis's (1949) classification of lateral malleolus ankle fractures relating to the level from the tibia-fibular syndesmosis:

Type	Level	Stability
A	Below the syndesmosis level	Usually Stable
B	At the syndesmosis level	May be Stable / Unstable
C	Above the syndesmosis level	Unstable Requiring Surgery

CHAPTER 11
HANDS

K Asaad
BH Miranda
M Nicolaou
SK Al-Ghazal

CHAPTER CONTENTS

HAND EXAMINATION

START: Patient sitting opposite you, with hands resting on a table / supported by a pillow.

Expose patient above the elbows bilaterally.

Look for any aids e.g. splints.

LOOK	Interpretation
Scars	Trauma, post-operative e.g. carpal tunnel release, tendon repair.
Swelling	Soft tissue or bony mass.
	Describe *6 x S's* as for any lump *(see lumps 'n' bumps chapter)*.
Symmetry	Symmetrical disease is associated with RA.
Deformity	Dupuytren's contracture, nerve lesions *(see upper limb nerves chapter)*, OA, RA.
Erythema	Inflammation, infection.
Sinus	Post-operative, infective.
Muscle Wasting	Thenar / hypothenar eminences, dorsal intermetacarpal wasting (Fig 11.4).
Other	• Raynaud's Phenomenon.
	• Onycholysis (nail separation from the nail bed e.g. psoriasis).
	• Gangrene.
	• Check elbows for psoriatic plaques.

Memory: Look for features of OA & RA specifically

OA	RA
Heberden's Nodes (bony DIPJ swelling)	**Rheumatoid Nodules** (Fig 11.1) (25% of patients with RA have rheumatoid nodules)
Bouchard's Nodes (bony PIPJ swelling)	**Boutonniere Deformity** (Fig 11.2) (PIPJ flexion & DIPJ hyperextension)
Thumb Squaring (1st CMCJ subluxation)	**Swan-Neck Deformity** (Fig 11.3) (PIPJ hyperextension & DIPJ flexion)
	Z-Thumb (MCPJ extension & IPJ flexion)
	Radial Deviation of the Wrist (Fig 10.7)
	Ulnar Deviation of the Digits (Fig 10.7) (capsular loosening & ligamentous laxity of the MCPJ)

Ask about pain.

Feel for temperature changes (dorsal & ventral) with the back of your hand.

FEEL	Interpretation
Capillary Refill	Gently press fingertip for 5 seconds then observe time for colour to change from white to pink. Normal = 2–3 seconds.
Dupuytren's Contracture	Feel for palmar fascia thickening & look for associated Garrod's Pads (Figs 11.4 & 11.5).
Rheumatoid Nodules	Subcutaneous lesions, usually on extensor surfaces.
Tenderness	Palpate each joint separately & systematically.
	Check the anatomical snuffbox for tenderness that may be associated with a scaphoid fracture, particularly in the acute setting.
Hand Nerves	Screen for the following nerve injuries, by assessing fine touch. If an injury is suspected, perform a thorough nerve examination *(see upper limb nerves)*:
	• **Radial Nerve:** (1st dorsal web space).
	• **Median Nerve:** (thenar eminence).
	• **Ulnar Nerve:** (palmar aspect of little finger).

Remember to test like-for-like.

MOVE	Interpretation
Global Functional Assessment	• Flex thumb.
	• Make a fist & fan out fingers.
	• Abduct & adduct fingers.
	• Demonstrate opposition.
	• Power grip.
Range of Motion	• Both active & passive range of motion should be recorded.
	• Prayer sign (normal = 70° wrist extension).
	• Reverse prayer sign (normal = 90° wrist flexion).
	• Radial deviation (normal = 20° wrist radial deviation).
	• Ulnar deviation (normal = 50° wrist ulnar deviation).
	• Pronation / supination (normal = 85° / 80°).

MOVE	Interpretation
Digital Tendons	*Thumb:*
	• **Abductor pollicis brevis** (against resistance).
	• **Flexor pollicis longus** (against resistance).
	• **Extensor pollicis longus** (patient keeps palmar surface of hand flat on a table & lifts thumb).
	Digital Flexors:
	• **Flexor digitorum profundus** (against resistance).
	• **Flexor digitorum superficialis** (against resistance).
	Digital Extensors:
	• **Extensor digitorum communis** (against resistance).
	• **Extensor indicis & extensor digiti minimi** (tested together by asking the patient to make a fist & extend their index & little fingers – 'Bullhorns').

SPECIAL TESTS	Interpretation
Tinnel's Test	Take the patient's hand, palmar surface up. Tap their forearm, proximal to distal, along the course of the median nerve (warn the patient that you are going to do this). Ensure that tapping is extended over the region of the carpal tunnel, which may reproduce carpal tunnel syndrome symptoms e.g. tingling.
Phalen's Test	Ask the patient to hold their wrists in complete & forced flexion (similar to the reverse prayer sign), pushing the dorsal surfaces of both hands together for 1 minute. This compresses the median nerve as it runs through the carpal tunnel, such that reproduction of carpal tunnel syndrome symptoms may occur.
Finkelstein's Test	Positive for De Quervain's Tenosynovitis. Pain & inflammation of the extensor pollicis brevis & abductor pollicis longus tendons, may be reproduced / exacerbated by asking the patient to flex their thumb, form a fist over it, then ulnar deviate their wrist.
Fine Functional Assessment	Pick up a key (pincer grip). Unbutton & button shirt. Pick up a pen & write a short sentence.
Two-Point Discrimination Test	Normal: <6mm.
	Fair: 6–10mm.
	Poor: 11–16mm.
	Protective: 1 point perceived.
	Anaesthetic: No points perceived.

FINISH	Interpretation
Lymphadenopathy	Check associated lymph nodes.
Joints	Full examination of the wrist & elbow is required (joints above).
Upper Limb Neurovascular Status	Full examinations required (see relevant sections). Particularly focus on pulses, dermatomes & myotomes.
QoL Impingement & Sleep	Asking patient about these helps to assess impact on life & therefore necessity for intervention.
Help Patient Dress	Good practice if patient has functional limitation.
Radiographs	Soft tissue / bony abnormalities.

FINISH:

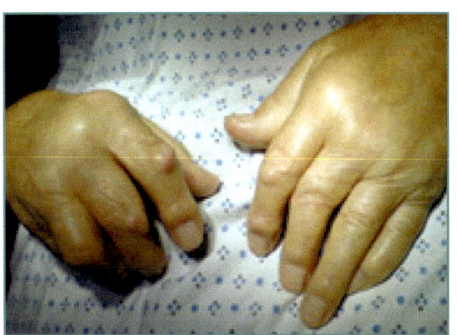

Fig 11.1: Rheumatoid Nodules.

Symmetrical polyarthropathy of the hands with rheumatoid nodules visible on the extensor surfaces of the digits.

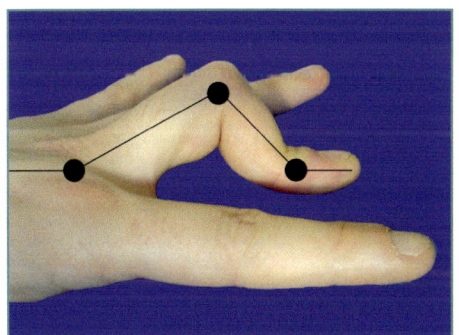

Fig 11.2: Boutonniere's Deformity of the left middle finger.

There is PIPJ flexion with DIPJ hyperextension.

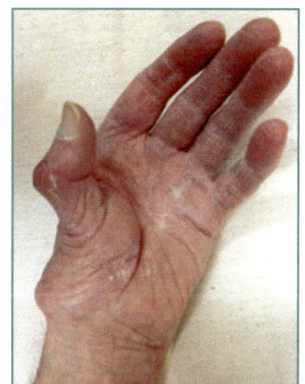

Fig 11.3: Z-Thumb Deformity.

Left Z-thumb deformity in a patient with rheumatoid arthritis.

OSCE QUESTIONS

Dupuytren's Disease

Q: What is Dupuytren's Disease?

This is a fibrotic disease of the palmar & digital fascia (superficial & deep) characterised by subcutaneous nodules, cords & flexion deformity (Fig 11.4). Persistent flexion deformity may result in formal joint contracture formation.

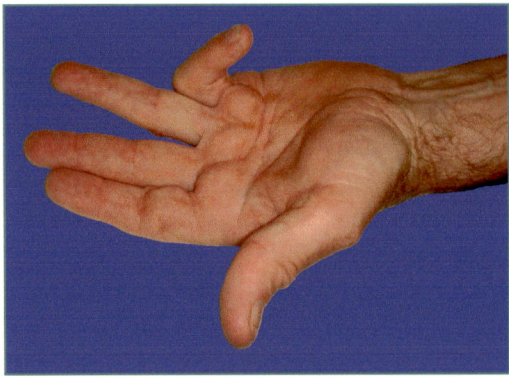

Fig 11.4: Dupuytren's Disease affecting left hand.

Note the flexion deformity of the little finger PIPJ, with palmar fascia thickening.

Q: What are the risk factors?

Congenital	Acquired
Genetic e.g. Caucasians of Celtic / Northern European Origin	Age >50
Male: Female = 10:1	Smoking
Diabetes	Epilepsy (possibly anti-epileptic medication)
	Infection
	Manual Labour (evidence is equivocal)

Q: Where else would you look for associated conditions?

Location	Description
Dorsal PIPJ	Garrod's Pads (Fig 11.5).
Plantar Surface of Foot	Ledderhose's Disease (fibrosis of the plantar fascia).
Penis	Peyronie's Disease (fibrotic plaques of the corpus cavernosa & tunica albuginea).

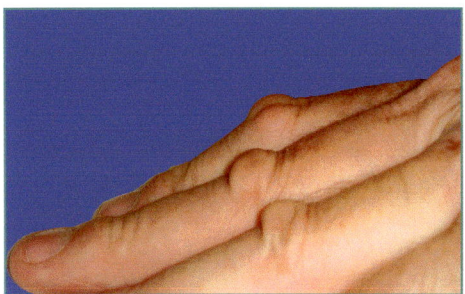

Fig 11.5: Garrod's Pads.

These present as thickenings of the dorsal surfaces of the PIPJs.

Q: What are the indications for release of the diseased cord?

- Positive Hueston table top test
- Pain & increasing disability
- MCPJ flexion deformity >30°
- Any PIPJ flexion deformity

Q: How is collagenase used to treat Dupuytren's disease?

Collagenase is an enzyme that breaks down collagen peptide bonds. It is secreted by *Clostridium histolyticum* bacteria & is used to perform a chemical fasciotomy (non-surgical division of the diseased cord). Collagenase is injected directly into the disease cord; 24-72 hours later, the digit is carefully manipulated into extension until the diseased cord 'snaps' apart.

Q: What are the options for surgery?

This depends on the patient's co-morbidities, wishes & functional demands on the hand. Options include:

Surgical Option	Notes
Fasciotomy	Division of the diseased cord.
Fasciectomy	Excision of diseased fascia.
Dermofasciectomy	Excision of diseased fascia & overlying skin (may require a skin graft).
Amputation	Considered in severe cases.

Q: What are the complications of surgery?

Immediate	Early	Late
Neurovascular Damage	Haematoma	Recurrence (50% at 10 years)
	Infection	Incomplete Joint Release
	Skin Flap Necrosis	Wound Breakdown
		CRPS
		Scar Contracture

Ganglion

Q: What is a ganglion?

- A mucinous filled cyst commonly located near a joint / tendon.
- It may communicate with the joint itself.
- It is the most common benign soft tissue tumour of the hand.

Q: What are the common sites for ganglia?

- **70% on the dorsal wrist.**
- **20% on the volar wrist.**
- **10% other sites:**   Dorsal DIPJ (known as mucous cysts).

  Flexor sheath.

  PIPJ.

Q: What investigations would assist your diagnosis of a ganglion?

Diagnosis centres primarily on taking a **full history** & performing a **thorough clinical examination**. Investigations to consider include:

Investigation	Notes
X-Ray	Rule out co-existing degenerative joint disease.
USS	Inexpensive & non-invasive method of visualisation.
	Differentiates solid from liquid lesions.
MRI	For more detailed visualisation of extent.

Q: What are the treatment options?

Conservative	Interventional	Surgical
Patient Education & Monitoring	Aspiration +/- Steroid Injection	Excision
	(high risk of recurrence)	(open or arthroscopic)

Trigger Finger

Q: What is a trigger finger?

Difficulty extending the finger from a flexed position. The finger may catch (or trigger) during motion or lock in the flexed position. It may be primary or congenital. It is associated with diabetes, carpal tunnel syndrome, De Quervain's Tenosynovitis, hypothyroidism, rheumatoid arthritis, renal disease & amyloidosis.

Q: Can you describe the arrangement of tendon sheath?

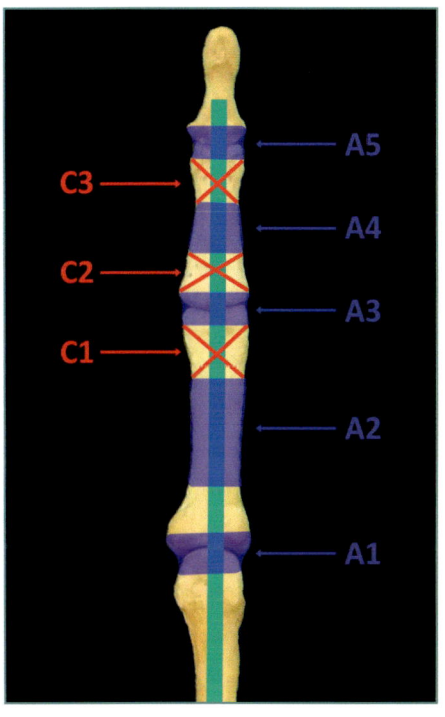

Fig 11.6: Diagrammatic representation of the flexor tendon sheath, illustrating:

Line of Flexor Tendons (FDP & FDS)

Annular Pulleys (A1–A5)

Cruciate Pulleys (C1–C3)

- The FDS & FDP tendons glide under a complex pulley system to enable the PIPJs & DIPJs to bend.
- There are 5 annular pulleys (A1–A5). A1 is the most proximal, located approximately at the level of the MCPJ. The A3 & A5 pulleys are located approximately at the level of the PIPJ & DIPJ respectively. The A2 & A4 pulleys are located at the shaft of the proximal & middle phalanges respectively.
- There are 3 cruciate pulleys (C1–C3). These alternate between the A2–A5 pulleys.

Q: What is the mechanism of triggering?

- Pathological narrowing of the tendon sheath tightens the gliding space for the tendons.
- Increased friction causes inflammation & further space reduction.
- The tendon may then catch or become stuck at the annular pulley (A1).

Q: What are the treatment options?

Conservative	Medical	Surgical
Patient Education & Monitoring.	Steroid Injection of Tendon Sheath.	Surgical Division of A1 Pulley.
Behaviour Modification e.g. Night Time Splinting (for adults).		

Scaphoid Fracture

Q: What are the clinical features of a scaphoid fracture?

- Anatomical snuffbox tenderness is associated with fractures of the scaphoid, one of the most commonly missed traumatic diagnoses.
- A high index of clinical suspicion, as indicated by history & examination is required for diagnosis.
- Furthermore radiographs may be normal at first presentation.

Q: How would you manage a patient with a suspected scaphoid fracture?

- **ATLS Resuscitation** (if acute trauma)
- **History**
- **Clinical Examination**
- **Appropriate Investigations:** X-Ray (Fig 11.7)
- **Treatment:** Analgesia
  Scaphoid Cast (2 weeks)
  Follow Up (2 weeks) & Further Radiographs

Q: What plain radiographs are indicated in a suspected scaphoid fracture?

Scaphoid views involve 4-view radiography of the scaphoid bone & are specifically requested when a scaphoid fracture is suspected.

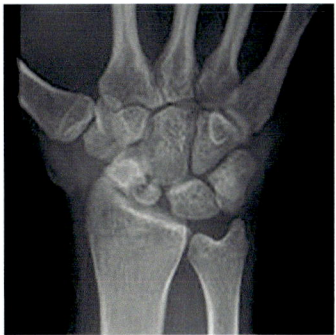

Fig 11.7: Scaphoid fracture radiograph.

Right wrist radiograph showing a fracture of the waist of the right scaphoid.

Note: Scaphoid views involve 4-view radiography of the scaphoid bone.

Q: Why can avascular necrosis occur as a complication of a scaphoid fracture?

- Avascular necrosis (AVN) of the proximal segment may occur as the blood supply to the scaphoid bone is from distal to proximal.
- The blood supply is from the palmar branch of the radial artery.
- The scaphoid bone spans both rows of the carpus, so if AVN ensues, there may be severe pain & limitation of mobility.

Q: What are the repair options for a scaphoid fracture?

Repair Option	Explanation
Scaphoid Cast (6-12 weeks)	For undisplaced & simple fractures.
Open Reduction & Internal Fixation	For displaced or non-healing fractures e.g. cannulated screws (Fig 11.8).
Bone Grafting	For severe displacement or non-union.

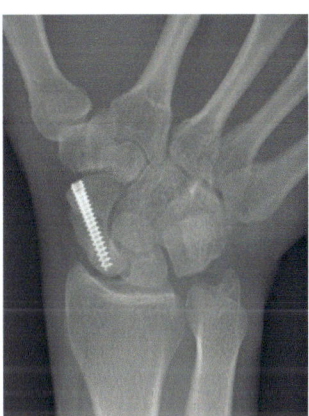

Fig 11.8: Right scaphoid fracture cannulated screw radiograph.

A cannulated compression screw has been used to fix a right scaphoid waist fracture. Example screw types include the Herbert & Acutrak screws.

CHAPTER 12
VASCULAR

M Singh
J Lorains
K Asaad
DJA Scott

CHAPTER CONTENTS

Peripheral Arterial Examination

Varicose Veins Examination

OSCE Questions

- Arterial Insufficiency
- Abdominal Aortic Aneurysm
- Thoracic Outlet Syndrome
- Raynaud's Syndrome
- Carotid Artery Stenosis
- Deep Vein Thrombosis
- Deep Venous Insufficiency & Venous Hypertension
- Varicose Veins
- Gangrene

PERIPHERAL ARTERIAL EXAMINATION

START: Patient lying on bed, with shirt unbuttoned / off & legs exposed.

INSPECTION	Interpretation
Memory: SNUGGS	
Skin	**Hands:** Tar staining, wasting of small muscles of the hand (a rare finding in thoracic outlet syndrome). **Face:** Xanthelasma, corneal arcus. **Abdomen:** Obvious pulsatile mass. **Legs:** Discolouration (due to haemosiderin deposition), shiny skin.
Nails	Tar staining, onycholysis, thick & brittle.
Ulcers	Malleoli & pressure areas. Check between toes. Lift the lower limbs to check the heels & underneath the legs. Remember to describe any ulcer BEDS *(see lumps 'n' bumps chapter).*
Guttering & Gangrene	Venous guttering, gangrene (Fig 12.1), tissue loss.
Scars	Amputations (Fig 12.2), scars from previous surgery (cephalic & basilic vein harvesting scars from bypass procedures may be present on the arms).

Ask about pain.

Examine each side comparing both upper & lower limbs.

Examine the good side first.

PALPATION	Interpretation
Memory: PC BOAT	
Pulses	Radial, brachial, carotid, feel for AAA, femoral, popliteal, DP & TP. Note presence of any aneurysms & describe as for any other lump *(see lumps 'n' bumps chapter).*
Capillary Refill	Test the capillary refill time in the upper & lower limbs until blanching occurs, then release. Normal reperfusion occurs over 2–3 seconds. **Note: Capillary refill time may be affected by conditions other than PAD.**
Buerger's Angle & Test	Gently raise each leg & note the angle at which pallor occurs. In a normal subject pallor should not develop, even with 90° of leg elevation. Pallor developing with ≤20° leg elevation indicates severe peripheral arterial disease. Also note any venous guttering. **Buerger's Test** is then performed by swinging the leg down over the side of the bed & looking for reactive hyperaemia indicative of peripheral arterial disease (positive test). This should be repeated on the contralateral limb. The **Pole test** can also be used, which involves the application of a Doppler probe to the toe, then elevating the leg & measuring the height at which the Doppler signal disappears by means of a calibrated pole.
Oedema	DVT, lymphoedema, post-surgical.
Allen's Test	This assesses ulnar & radial arterial supply to the hand. Occlude both arteries, then ask the patient to repeatedly open & close their hand until it becomes pale. Release the artery to be tested & note the time for reperfusion. Repeat for the other artery. The ulnar artery is usually dominant.
Temperature	Feel for temperature changes by running the back of your hand proximally to distally over limb.

AUSCULTATION	Interpretation
Memory: **CALF**	
Bruits	Listen for arterial bruits, indicative of turbulent flow:
	• **C**arotid
	• **A**orta
	• I**L**iac
	• **F**emoral

COMPLETION	Interpretation
ABPI	Measure BP at the brachial artery. Using a hand-held Doppler, measure the BP at the DP & TP, then divide the highest ankle BP by the highest brachial BP. If resting ABPI is normal, get the patient to do 10 heel toe raises & re-check the ABPI.
VV Examination	Can have mixed arterial & venous disease.
Cardiac Examination	Full cardiac examination & ECG.
Neurological Examination	Full neurological examination e.g. diabetic neuropathy may be present.
BP & HR	Hypertension & AF common.
Investigations	Order appropriate investigations including Duplex, MRA, CTA, IADSA.

FINISH:

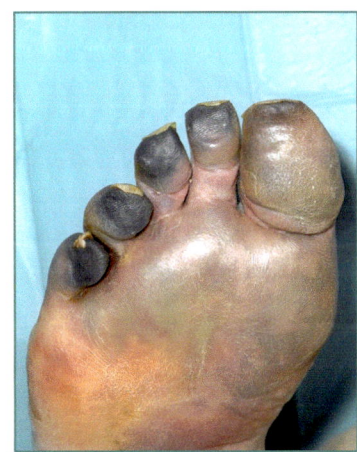

Fig 12.1: Right foot (plantar view) of a patient with peripheral arterial disease. The forefoot appears dusky & there are black, dry areas on the toes indicative of gangrene.

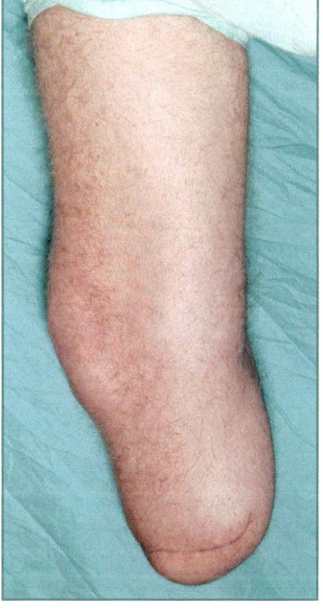

Fig 12.2: Right below knee amputation. Note the flap formed from the skin & muscles of the posterior compartment.

VARICOSE VEINS EXAMINATION

START: Patient initially standing, exposed to underwear.

INSPECTION	Interpretation
6 x S's	Describe dilated tortuous varicose veins as for any other lump (Fig 12.3) *(see lumps 'n' bumps chapter)*. **Note: Varicosities above the SPJ relate to the LSV, but those that are below the SPJ may relate to either the LSV or SSV.**
Skin	Venous eczema, haemosiderin deposition, lipodermatosclerosis. Note the gaiter area especially.
Oedema	Could be secondary to DVT or lymphoedema.
Ulcers	LSV distribution is usually over the medial malleolus. SSV distribution is usually over the lateral malleolus. Remember to describe any ulcer BEDS *(see lumps 'n' bumps chapter)*.
Scars	Groin crease scar e.g. high tie & LSV stripping. Popliteal fossa scar e.g. SPJ ligation surgery. Small scars along leg e.g. stab avulsions.

Ask about pain.

Examine each side comparing one limb to the other.

Examine the good side first.

PALPATION	Interpretation
SEC FFP TR	Assess compressible dilated tortuous varicose veins as for any other lump *(see lumps 'n' bumps chapter)*.
Saphena Varix	Palpate over the SFJ for a saphena varix. This lies 4cm below & lateral to the pubic tubercle & is a smooth, soft bluish swelling that disappears on lying down.
Cough / Tap Test*	Palpate VV distally & tap proximally or ask the patient to cough. A transmitted impulse distally suggests incompetent valves proximal to the point of palpation.
Trendelenberg Test*	Patient lying down. Empty veins by milking proximally. Place pressure over SFJ & ask patient to stand up. If control is achieved then possible SFJ incompetence exists.
Tourniquet Test*	Patient lying down. Empty veins by milking proximally. Place tourniquet proximally around thigh & ask patient to stand up. If control is achieved then the level of incompetence is at / above the tourniquet level. If not, then move the tourniquet down the thigh & repeat until control is achieved.
Perthe's Test*	Once control has been achieved by the tourniquet test, ensure the patient is standing & ask them to move up & down on tip toes. If veins distend or the patient experiences pain, this suggests an incompetent deep venous system & therefore a LSV strip may worsen symptoms.

*Note: These clinical tests have now been superseded by hand-held Doppler & portable Duplex scanning & have little place in current practice.

| Hand-Held Doppler | With patient standing, place Doppler over the SPJ. Squeeze the calf & listen for Doppler sound. One whoosh with abrupt cut-off suggests a competent valve. If followed by a second whoosh this suggests reflux. Repeat by listening over the SFJ. Currently most vascular surgeons will use a portable Duplex scanner to assess varicose veins. |

AUSCULTATION	Interpretation
Bruits	Listen over the femoral arteries for bruits, there may be an AVF e.g. post-femoral artery catheterisation / IVDUs.

COMPLETION	Interpretation
Full Abdominal Examination	Including PR examination for any masses that may cause venous obstruction.
ABPI	NICE guidelines 2022: ABPI >1.3 – Avoid compression stockings due to calcified vessels. ABPI between 0.8 & 1.3 – Safe to use compression. ABPI <0.8 – Compression stockings are contraindicated due to arterial insufficiency. The patient should be referred for specialist vascular assessment.
Investigations	Order appropriate investigations including Duplex scan, MRV.

FINISH:

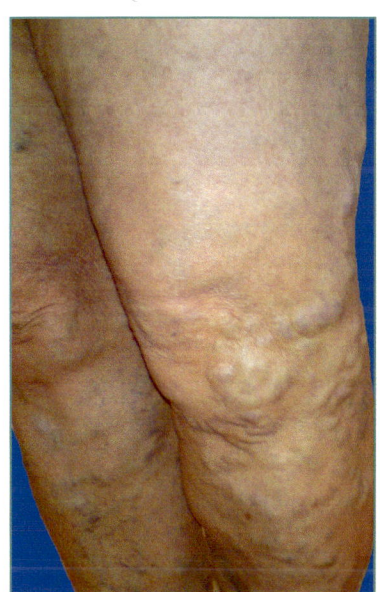

Fig 12.3: Bilateral varicose veins in a 54-year-old lady. There are multiple bluish, dilated & tortuous varicosties on the thigh & lower legs bilaterally. The limbs are oedematous & there are some venous telangicctasia present.

OSCE QUESTIONS

Arterial Insufficiency

Q: What are the symptoms & signs of acute arterial insufficiency?

 Memory: The 6 x P's of acute arterial insufficiency:

Symptom/Sign	Notes
Pain	Acute/sudden onset of pain in the affected limb.
Paraesthesia	Presence of a pins & needles sensation.
Pallor	Pale appearance.
Pulselessness	Loss of distal pulses in comparison to opposite limb.
Paresis	Motor weakness progressing to paralysis.
Perishingly Cold	Cold on palpation.

Q: What is the Fontaine Classification?

Grade	Description
I	Asymptomatic.
IIA	Intermittent claudication walking >200m & no rest pain.
IIB	Intermittent claudication walking <200m & no rest pain.
III	Rest / nocturnal pain.
IV	Gangrene / necrosis.

Q: What is the significance of the ABPI?

- An ABPI ≤0.9 may be used as a haemodynamic marker of PAD
- ABPI measurements relate to the severity of chronic ischaemia as follows:

ABPI	Notes
>1.3	Abnormal vessel hardening e.g. arterial calcification due to diabetes.
0.8-1.3	Normal range.
0.5-0.8	Arterial disease present.
<0.5	Severe arterial disease.

Q: What is critical limb ischaemia?

- Chronic ischaemic rest pain or the presence of ischaemic skin lesions (ulcers or gangrene).
- The term *'critical limb ischaemia'* only applies to chronic ischaemic disease (Fontaine Classification Grade III / IV), lasting >2 weeks.
- Some papers further classify this into:

i) **Subcritical Ischaemia:** Rest pain + ankle pressure >40mmHg.

ii) **Critical Ischaemia:** Rest pain + tissue loss/ankle pressure <40mmHg.

Abdominal Aortic Aneurysms (AAA)

Q: What is an abdominal aortic aneurysm?

Abnormal dilation of the abdominal aorta by >50% of its normal diameter (Fig 12.4).

Q: What are the clinical features of AAA?

Classification	Clinical Features
Asymptomatic	Most are asymptomatic & diagnosed incidentally on ultrasound.
Mass	Pulsatile abdominal mass.
Compression	Early satiety, nausea, vomiting, urinary tract symptoms & venous thrombosis.
Erosion	Back pain due to erosion into adjacent vertebrae.
Embolisation	Ischemic toes.
Rupture	Hypovolaemic shock & sudden death.

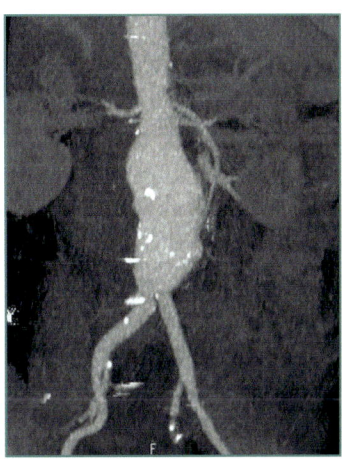

Fig 12.4: Aortic Aneurysm CT Reconstruction:

Sagittal CT reconstruction of a large abdominal aortic aneurysm.

Q: What is the risk of rupture of an AAA?

Risk of rupture is related to diameter as follows:

AAA Diameter	Rupture Risk (per annum)
<5.5cm	<1%
5–5.6 cm	10%
6–6.5 cm	20%
6.5–7 cm	25%
7–8 cm	33%
>8 cm	>50%

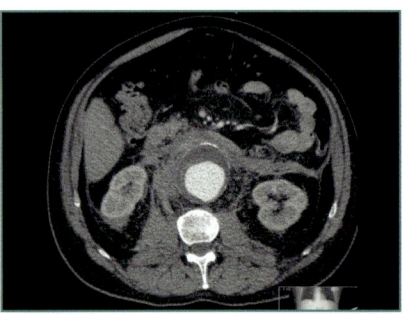

Fig 12.5: Ruptured AAA CT.

Contrast enhanced CT scan illustrating a ruptured abdominal aortic aneurysm. The contrast is high density in the aorta, which is surrounded by thrombus & a high density calcified wall. There is mixed density fluid surrounding the aorta consistent with rupture of the aneurysm.

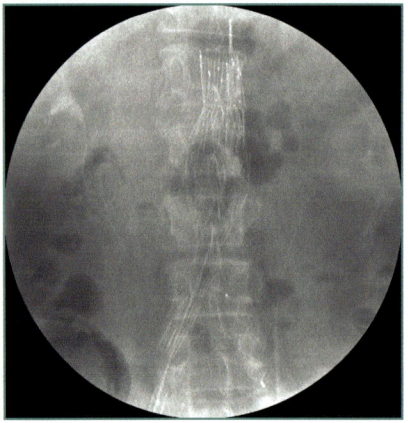

Fig 12.6: EVAR Radiograph.

Endovascular aneurysm repair (EVAR) of an abdominal aortic aneurysm.

Q: What is the elective management of a AAA?

Management depends on **AAA diameter** & should be discussed within the context of a **Vascular MDT referral**:

Diameter	Management
<3cm	No aneurysm.
3–4.4cm	Annual USS monitoring.
4.5–5.4cm	3-monthly monitoring offered.
>5.5cm	Referral to vascular surgeon.
	Patient offered elective repair (open repair or EVAR if possible). (Fig 12.6)

Q. What are the indications for AAA repair?

- Symptomatic patient
- Diameter >5.5cm
- Diameter increasing by 1cm per annum

Thoracic Outlet Syndrome

Q: What is thoracic outlet syndrome?

- A syndrome describing the symptoms & signs caused by arterial, venous or nerve compression as these major structures pass between the clavicle & 1st rib.

Q: What are the causes of thoracic outlet syndrome?

Cause	Example
Congenital	Cervical rib.
Acquired	Pathological enlargement of the 1st rib.
	Scalenus muscle hypertrophy.
	Fractured clavicle.

Q: What are the clinical features of thoracic outlet syndrome?

Clinical features are related to the compressed structure as follows:

Compression	Clinical Features
Artery	Arm / hand claudication (worse on raising arm above head).
	Acutely ischaemic hand (secondary to emboli).
	Subclavian aneurysm.
Vein	Venous hypertension.
	Arm swelling.
	Venous thrombosis.
Nerve	Motor or sensory deficit (commonly affects the lower 2 nerve roots, C8 & T1).

Special tests for thoracic outlet syndrome include Roo's Test (Fig 10.1) & Adson's Test (Fig 10.2) (*see orthopaedics chapter*).

Q: What are the differential diagnoses for thoracic outlet syndrome?

Classification	Examples
Arterial	Raynaud's Disease / Syndrome
	Thrombangiitis Obliterans
	Takayasu's Arteritis
Venous	Axillary Vein Thrombosis
	Damage to Axillary Drainage e.g. Post-Mastectomy
Neurological	Cervical Spondylosis
	Pancoast Tumour
	Cervical Intervertebral Disc Protrusion
	Ulnar Nerve Neuropathy

Raynaud's Syndrome

Q. What is Raynaud's Syndrome?

This is a syndrome characterised by digital vasospasm, resulting in 3 distinct phases, with visible colour changes noticed in the fingers as follows:

Colour	Cause
White	Arterial spasm causing blanching of the digits (may lead to gangrene).
Blue	Cyanosis & pain caused by insufficient oxygenation.
Red	Reactive hyperaemia once blood flow restored.

Q: How do you classify the causes of Raynaud's Syndrome?

Primary	Secondary
Idiopathic	**Arterial Disorders** e.g. Atherosclerosis
(Raynaud's Disease)	**Blood Disorders** e.g. Polycythaemia
	Connective Tissue Disorders e.g. RA, Scleroderma
	Drugs e.g. β-Blockers, Caffeine, OCP, Smoking
	Trauma e.g. Vibrating Tools (chronic usage)

Q: What is the management of Raynaud's Syndrome?

Conservative	Medical	Surgical
Heated Gloves	Nifedipine	Sympathectomy (commonly thoracoscopic T1-T3, rarely performed open)
Avoid Precipitants e.g. β-Blockers, Caffeine, Cold Weather, OCP, Smoking	α-Blockers	Digital Sympathectomy
	Iloprost Infusion	Amputation (if gangrene present)

Carotid Artery Stenosis

Q: How do you classify carotid artery stenosis?

- Carotid artery stenosis is classified as either **symptomatic** or **asymptomatic**. Symptomatic stenosis is associated with amaurosis fugax, TIA or CVA.

Q. What is the management of carotid artery stenosis?

Conservative	Medical	Surgical
Smoking Cessation	Statins	Carotid Stenting
Exercise	Antihypertensives	Carotid Endarterectomy
Healthy Diet	Aspirin	
	DM control	

Q: What are the indications for carotid endarterectomy?

- Controlled trials have shown that surgery reduces the risk of stroke in symptomatic patients with 50–99% carotid stenosis, more effectively than best medical therapy, if performed within 2 weeks of an event.
- In asymptomatic patients, <75 years, with a significant stenosis, surgery reduces the 5-year risk of stroke by 50%.

Symptomatic patients with >70% stenosis   (clear benefit from surgery)

Symptomatic patients with 50–69% stenosis   (less benefit from surgery)

Asymptomatic patients with >60% stenosis   (some benefit from surgery, especially if male)

Q: How can risk of stroke be estimated after a TIA?

Using the ABCD^2 scoring system:

Risk Factor		Points	2 Day Stroke Risk
Age:	≥60 years	1	Score 0–3 = Low Risk
Blood Pressure:	≥140/90mmHg	1	
Clinical Features:	Unilateral weakness	2	Score 4-5 = Moderate Risk
	Speech impairment (no weakness)	1	
Duration of Symptoms:	≥60mins	2	Score 6-7 = High Risk
	10–59mins	1	
Diabetes Mellitus:	Present	1	

Deep Vein Thrombosis (DVT)

Q: What is a deep vein thrombosis (DVT)?

Phlebothrombosis of deep veins.

Q: What are the causes of DVT?

Causal factors are related to **Virchow's triad**, which describes general causes of thrombosis anywhere in the body:

Endothelial Damage	Stasis / Turbulent Blood Flow	Hypercoagulable States
Atheroma	Immobility	Dehydration
Radiotherapy	Obesity	Malignancy
Trauma e.g. Cannulation	Pelvic Surgery	Oral Contraceptive Pill
	Lower Limb Surgery	Hormone Replacement Therapy
	Aneurysm	Smoking
	Cardiac / Vascular Stents	Protein C & S Deficiency
	Cardiac Valve Replacements	Factor V Leiden
	DVT History	Antithrombin Deficiency

Q: What are the clinical features of DVT?

- 75% clinically silent.
- Painful calf / leg swelling that is hot & erythematous.
- Homan's sign = pain on foot dorsiflexion.
- Distended superficial veins due to blockage within deep venous system.
- **Phlegmasia alba dolens** = painful white leg swelling (iliofemoral vein partial occlusion).
- **Phlegmasia cerulea dolens** = painful blue leg swelling resulting in gangrene (iliofemoral vein complete occlusion).

Q: What investigations might you consider?

A high index of suspicion is required. Diagnosis involves eliciting risk factors from the history e.g. recent long-haul travel / surgery, thorough examination & confirmation by Duplex scan.

Q: What are the management options?

- Management strategies should be primarily preventative.
- When indicated, treatment-dose low molecular weight heparin (on-ward) may be commenced, with concurrent warfarin treatment until a therapeutic INR is reached.
- The patient may then be discharged on warfarin as per protocol.
- Patients are often anticoagulated for 3 months in the 1st instance.
- With recurrence, anticoagulation may be lifelong.
- Specific treatment strategies include:

Conservative	Mechanical	Medical	Surgical
Maintain Good Hydration	Intermittent Pneumatic Compression Devices	Oral Contraceptive Pill – Stop 4 Weeks Prior to Elective Surgery	Avoid General Anaesthesia if Possible
Leg Exercises		Low Molecular Weight Heparin Prophylaxis	Early Mobilisation After Surgery
Thromboembolic Deterrent Stockings		(IV) Fluids	Vena Cava Filters – Prevent Pulmonary Embolism

Q: What are the complications of DVT?

- The most serious complication is pulmonary embolism & sudden death.
- DVT may also damage venous valves resulting in venous insufficiency & venous hypertensive disease.

Deep Venous Insufficiency & Venous Hypertension

Q: What is deep venous insufficiency?

- Also known as the post-thrombotic / post-phlebitic limb.
- Disruption of the venous return of the deep venous system, with associated valvular incompetence, results in high pressure reflux into superficial veins.

Q: What are the causes?

- Congenital absence of deep vein valves.
- DVT resulting in deep vein valve damage.
- Arterio-venous malformations.

Q: What are the clinical features?

Clinical Features	Notes
Varicose Veins	Tortuous dilated veins, often affecting the lower limbs (see below).
Varicose Eczema	Varicose pruritic rash results in scratching. Potential skin abrasion increases risk of venous ulceration & infection.
Haemosiderin Pigmentation	Venous leak into soft tissues
Lipodermatosclerosis	Silvery-grey patches of skin where fibrous tissue has replaced normal cutaneous tissue.
Peripheral Oedema	May be inflammatory or directly related to venous hypertension & increased intraluminal hydrostatic pressure.
Venous Ulceration	Due to venous hypertension. Scratching results in repeat excoriations. Skin affected by lipodermatosclerosis is less robust, nutrient exchange is decreased & it is therefore more prone to delayed healing. These precipitate a vicious cycle which delays healing.
Infection	Cellulitis most commonly.

Q: What specific investigations would you consider?

- Duplex Scan
- Venography

Q: What are the treatment options?

Treatment is of primarily of the underlying cause & subsequent complications e.g. varicose veins / venous ulceration. Conservative options include avoidance of long periods standing, leg-elevation & compression stockings.

Varicose Veins

Q: What are varicose veins?

- Tortuous dilated veins.
- Most often affecting the long (greater) & short (lesser) saphenous veins of the lower limbs.

Q. What are the causes of varicose veins (Fig 12.3)?

Primary	Secondary
Idiopathic	DVT
Familial	Pregnancy
	Tumour
	Klippel-Trenaunay Syndrome (varicose veins, port-wine stains, soft tissue limb hypertrophy)
	Parkes-Weber Syndrome (AVFs, limb hypertrophy)

Q: What investigations would you consider for varicose veins?

- Diagnosis begins with a full history & thorough clinical examination.
- Investigations must include a venous Duplex scan to assess:
  - i.   site of incompetence (superficial / deep).
  - ii.   deep venous system.

Q: What is the management of varicose veins?

After taking a **full history** & performing a **thorough clinical examination**, management should be considered in relation to the underlying cause:

- **Investigations:** Must include a venous Duplex scan to assess (i) the site of incompetence (superficial / deep) & (ii) the deep venous system.
- **Treatment:** May be conservative / surgical *(see below)*.

Conservative	Surgical
Support Stockings	Injection Foam Sclerotherapy
Weight Loss & Exercise	Ligation (SFJ / SPJ), Vein Stripping (LSV / SSV) & Stab Avulsions
	Endovenous Laser Therapy (EVLT)
	Radiofrequency Ablation (RFA)

Note: The CLASS (Comparison of Laser, Surgery & Foam Sclerotherapy) randomised controlled trial concludes that endovenous laser ablation (EVLA), performed under local anaesthetic, should be considered as the treatment of choice for suitable patients. These findings are driven by greater estimated QALY & utility gains at 6 months versus foam sclerotherapy & surgery, lower costs at 6 months versus surgery, & marginally lower estimated recurrence rates versus foam sclerotherapy & surgery.

Gangrene

Q: What is gangrene?

Gangrene is abnormal & irreversible tissue necrosis due to decreased vascular-nutrient supply (Fig 12.1).

Q: How would you classify gangrene?

Classification	Notes
Dry	Mummification of tissue without infection e.g. peripheral arterial disease.
Wet	Superadded infection, often anaerobic e.g. *Clostridium perfringens* / *Bacteroides*.
Gas	*Clostridium perfringens* is a gas forming, gram positive anaerobe that produces exotoxin which may cause tissue necrosis, disease spread & local crepitus (palpable crackling of skin due to gas formation).

Q: What are the treatment options for gangrene?

- Treatment strategies are primarily preventative or aimed at the underlying cause.
- Where infection is involved, appropriate antibiotics are used.
- Surgical options include debridement / amputation.

SECTION A4: NEUROSCIENCES

CHAPTER 13
NEUROSCIENCE

V Kakar
BH Miranda
J Nagaria

CHAPTER CONTENTS

ABBREVIATED MENTAL TEST SCORE (AMTS)

This is a screening test consisting of 10 questions.

A score <6/10 suggests dementia / delirium & should precipitate a mini mental state examination.

It is appropriate to perform an AMTS examination on all elderly patients.

Question	Score
How old are you?	1
What is the time (to the nearest hour)?	1
Ask the patient to remember an address e.g. 10 James Street. Explain that you will ask them to recall it at the end of the AMTS examination (do not forget to do this)!	1
What is the year?	1
What is the name of the hospital (or place where the patient is being examined)?	1
Can you identify 2 people (doctor, nurse, family member etc.)?	1
What is your date of birth?	1
What date did World War 2 begin (or another well known date)?	1
Who is the current prime minister (or monarch / president / dictator)?	1
Ask the patient to count backwards from 20 to 1.	1
Total	**10**

MINI MENTAL STATE EXAMINATION (MMS)

This test provides more information than the AMTS with respect to cognitive impairment.

It should be undertaken in all patients who achieve an AMTS score <6/10.

Score 24–30 implies no cognitive impairment.

Score 18–23 implies mild cognitive impairment.

Score 0–17 implies severe cognitive impairment.

Question	Max Score
ORIENTATION	
What is the year? What is the season? What is the date? What month is it? What is the day of the week?	5
What country is this? What region? What city? What hospital is this? What floor?	5
REGISTRATION	
Ask the patient to remember 3 items that you have clearly named e.g. pen, book, shoe. Ask the patient to repeat these items back & record the number of trials it takes for the patient to do this correctly.	3
ATTENTION & CALCULATION	
Ask the patient to count backwards from 100 in 7's until the patent has done this 5 times (93, 86, 79, 72, 65). Alternatively ask the patient to spell WORLD backwards.	5
RECALL	
Can you recall the 3 items that you remembered earlier? (Skip this if the patient was unable to remember the 3 items initially).	3
LANGUAGE & PRAXIS	
Show the patient 2 objects e.g. pen, watch. Ask the patient to name them.	2
Repeat the phrase: *'No ifs, ands or buts.'*	1
Instruct the patient to take a piece of paper in their right hand, fold it in half & put it on the table.	3
Write the following on a piece of paper: *Close your eyes*. Instruct the patient to follow the command that you have written.	1
Instruct the patient to make up any complete sentence & write it on a piece of paper. The sentence must be grammatically accurate.	1
Ask the patient to copy the following picture:	1
Total	**30**

GLASGOW COMA SCALE (GCS)

START: Patient sitting on a chair (unless scenario dictates otherwise).

Ask the patient if they are in pain.

Ask / check for prescription medications that may alter the patient's level of consciousness.

Best Eye Response	Interpretation
4	Open spontaneously
3	Open in response to speech
2	Open in response to pain
1	No response

Best Verbal Response	Interpretation Adults	Interpretation Pre Verbal Children
5	Orientated	Smiles, orientated to sounds, follows objects, interacts
4	Confused	Cries but is consolable, inappropriate interactions
3	Inappropriate speech	Inconsistently consolable, moaning
2	Incomprehensible sounds	Inconsolable, agitated
1	No response	No response

Best Motor Response	Interpretation
6	Obeys commands
5	Localises to pain
4	Flexion withdrawal
3	Abnormal flexion to pain (Decorticate)
2	Abnormal extension to pain (Decerebrate)
1	No response

FINISH:

REMEMBER

- The GCS is a reproducible, objective assessment of a patient's conscious level.
- Assessment in young children can be difficult & a modified verbal scoring system exists.
- GCS ≤8 defines coma & warrants intubation.
- Beware that language barriers may appear to inhibit the patient's response.
- Other trauma may prevent following commands (e.g. spinal injury).

CRANIAL NERVES EXAMINATION

START: Patient sitting on a chair.

              Ask the patient if they are in pain.

INSPECTION	Interpretation
Speech	Whilst interacting with the patient at the START of the CNS examination, note any of the following **3 x D's**:
	• **Dysarthria:** Disorder of articulation that may be due to alcohol, cerebellar disease, head injury & lesions to cranial nerves V, VII, IX, X, XII.
	• **Dysphonia:** Disorder of phonation due to vocal organ impairment e.g. vocal cords.
	• **Dysphasia:** Disorder of language that may be expressive, receptive or mixed
Facial Appearance	Look for ptosis, facial asymmetry & weakness.
Dyskinesia	Look for any movement disorders that may include:
	• **Fasciculation:** Small involuntary muscular contractions (LMN).
	• **Tremor:** Involuntary & **r**hythmical oscillatory muscle movements.
	• **Dystonia:** Sustained involuntary muscle contractions, resulting in twisting & repetitive movements or abnormal postures.
	• **Chorea:** Rapid involuntary jerky movements that may be highly variable in location.
	• **Tic:** Rapid involuntary sudden movements that are stereotypical in location.

CRANIAL NERVES	No.	Interpretation
Olfactory	I	Ask the patient if they have noticed any change in their sense of smell. Test each nostril individually with coffee or chocolate. **Note: Substances e.g. tobacco or ammonia are too noxious & result in trigeminal (V) nerve stimulation.**
Optic	II	Check the following 5 parameters:

Optic, II (continued):

1. **Visual Acuity:** Test each eye separately using a **Snellen Chart**. Do this without vision aids, then with best corrected vision e.g. contact lenses, glasses or pinhole camera. Vision is recorded as a fraction, such that normal vision is 6/6. The numerator is the distance that the patient is standing from the chart (metres) & the denominator is the line that the patient can read on the chart. The following should be done in succession until the patient is able to see something, or until no perception of light is detected (in which case NPL should be recorded):

   - Bring the patient closer to the chart.
   - Ask the patient how many fingers you are holding up.
   - Ask the patient to identify your hand movements.
   - Ask the patient if they can see light.

2. **Visual Fields:** Test each eye separately by confrontation. A red hat pin is best for testing scotomas, as colour vision fails early in optic nerve & retinal disorders.

3. **Colour Vision:** Test each eye separately using **Ishihara Plates**.

4. **Pupils:** Note **size & symmetry**. Test **direct & consensual light reflexes** in a dark room. Test **accommodation**, asking the patient to focus on an object behind you, then on an object close to their face. The normal accommodation reflex for close objects is bilateral pupil constriction. Test **swinging light reflex** for an afferent pathway defect by swinging a pen torch from one eye to the other. Both pupils constrict when the light shines on the normal eye, but when the light shines on the affected eye, that pupil continues to dilate slightly (Marcus Gunn Pupil), indicating optic nerve injury / MS.

5. **Fundoscopy:** Elicit the red reflex & look for any opacities, that will appear dark, outlined by the red glow. Check the optic disc for colour, contour & cupping. Excessive cupping is associated with glaucoma. Assess for indistinct disc margins & lack of retinal venous pulsations (papilloedema). Assess the macula by asking the patient to briefly look straight into the light.

Oculomotor	III	Stabilise the patient's head by gently placing your left hand under the patient's chin. Then, ask the patient to follow your right index finger. Perform the **'H-Manoeuvre'** on each eye separately (Fig 13.1). Remember that eye movements are controlled by III, except for **'SO$_{IV}$'** = superior oblique muscle, innervated by IV, adducts the eye with inferior gaze & **'LR$_{VI}$'** = lateral rectus, innervated by VI, abducts the eye.
Trochlear	IV	
Abducent	VI	

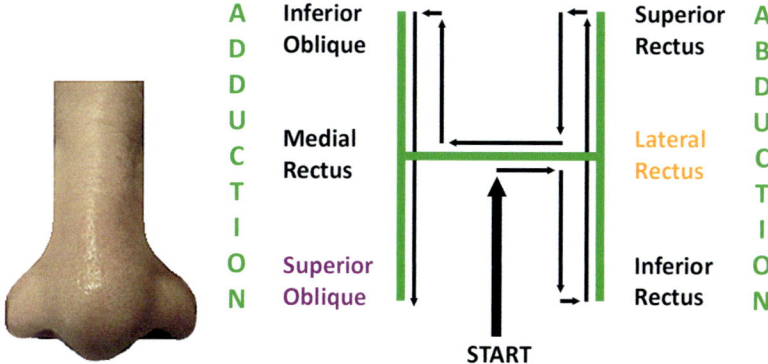

A	Inferior			Superior	A
D	Oblique			Rectus	B
D					D
U					U
C	Medial			Lateral	C
T	Rectus			Rectus	T
I					I
O	Superior			Inferior	O
N	Oblique			Rectus	N

START

Fig 13.1: The H-Manoeuvre (left eye).

'SO$_{IV}$' = superior oblique muscle, innervated by IV, adducts the eye with inferior gaze.

'LR$_{VI}$' = lateral rectus, innervated by VI, abducts the eye.

Note: Arrows represent movement of the pupil.

Trigeminal	V	**Sensory:** Assess fine touch, using cotton wool, of the ophthalmic (V1), maxillary (V2) & mandibular (V3) branches (Fig 13.2). Elicit the corneal reflex.
		Motor: Ask the patient to open their mouth. If there is a unilateral lesion affecting the pterygoid muscles, **the jaw will deviate towards the side of the lesion**.
		Jaw Jerk: Put a finger on the patient's mandible, in the midline & gently tap your finger with a tendon hammer. A positive reflex results in masseter activation & jaw closure. This reflex is usually slight or absent. If exaggerated, an UMN lesion is present.
Facial	VII	**Facial Asymmetry:** This may have been detected on inspection already.
		Sensory: The chorda tympani nerves may be tested by using a substance that is either salty, sweet, bitter or sour on the anterior $^2/_3$ of each side of the tongue.
		Motor: Test the branches of the facial nerve by asking the patient to raise their eyebrows, screw up their eyes (against resistance), blow out their cheeks, show their teeth, tense & flare their neck muscles.

Vestibulocochlear	VIII	**Hearing:** Ask the patient to reproduce a word that you whisper in their ear. Then perform Rinne's & Weber's Tests as follows: • **Rinne's Test:** Place a vibrating tuning fork (256Hz / 512Hz) on the mastoid process to test bone conduction. When the sound is no longer detected by the patient, place the vibrating arms immediately lateral to the ear. A patient with normal hearing should detect the sound again as air conduction is better than bone conduction. *Conductive hearing loss* may be suspected if the patient is unable to detect the sound again. • **Weber's Test:** Place a vibrating tuning fork on the forehead in the midline. Ask the patient where the sound is heard loudest. A patient with normal hearing should detect the sound equally in the midline. A patient with *conductive hearing loss* will detect the sound loudest in the affected ear. A patient with *sensorineural hearing loss* will detect the sound loudest in the good ear. **Vestibular Function:** Test the oculocephalic reflex in a comatose patient. Slightly flex the neck & quickly rotate the head from side to side. The eyes should move to the left when the patient's head is turned to the right & vice-versa (like doll's eyes).
Glossopharyngeal	IX	Test for a gag reflex that may indicate either IX or X pathology. Ask the patient to say 'ahh' & look at the uvula. If there is a unilateral X lesion, **the uvula will deviate away from the side of the lesion**.
Vagus	X	
Spinal Accessory	XI	Ask the patient to shrug their shoulders against resistance (trapezius). Ask the patient to turn their head to the side against resistance (sternocleidomastoid). *Remember that the sternocleidomastoid laterally rotates the head to the contralateral side.*
Hypoglossal	XII	Ask the patient to protrude their tongue. Assess for symmetry, wasting & fasciculations. If there is a unilateral lesion, **the tongue will deviate towards the side of the lesion**.

FINISH:

PERIPHERAL NERVOUS SYSTEM EXAMINATION (PNS)

START: Patient exposed to underwear.

Maintain their dignity.

Chaperone is recommended.

Ensure thorough inspection from the FRONT, BACK & SIDES of the patient.

INSPECTION	Interpretation
Gait	Ask the patient to walk away, turn around & walk back. Comment on any gait abnormalities.
Spine	Comment on abnormal kyphosis, lordosis & scoliosis.
Fasciculation	Look for involuntary muscle contractions.
Wasting	Look for muscle wasting, associated with weakness.
Romberg's Test	Ask the patient to stand with their feet together, arms by their sides & eyes closed. Loss of proprioception will result in loss of stability (positive Romberg's Test).
Cerebellar Signs	Performing a quick cerebellar screen is useful to help fine-tune the candidate's differential diagnosis early on in the examination. A helpful memory aid is **DANISH**: **D**ysdiadochokinesia *(see coordination)* **A**taxia **N**ystagmus **I**ntention Tremor & Past Pointing **S**lurred Speech **H**ypotonia.

Ask about pain.

Ideally, continue with the patient on a couch, lying at 45° (upper limbs) or flat (lower limbs).

Assess tone, power, coordination, sensation & reflexes, remembering to compare each side.

TONE	Interpretation	
UPPER LIMB	Hold the patient's hand as if you were going to greet them with a hand shake. Support the patient's upper arm, just proximal to the elbow joint, with your other hand. Tell the patient to relax & 'go floppy' & test tone by quickly moving each joint in succession as follows:	
	• **Shoulder:**	Abduction, adduction, flexion, extension, internal & external rotation.
	• **Ulnar-Humeral Joint:**	Flexion & extension of the elbow.
	• **Radial-Ulnar Joint:**	Pronation & supination of the hand / forearm.
	• **Wrist:**	Flexion & extension.

NEUROSCIENCE EXAMINATION

TONE	Interpretation
LOWER LIMB	• Facing the patient's feet, place 1 hand just proximal to each knee joint & quickly roll the knees externally & internally. Look for symmetrical movement of the toes.
	• Place both hands under the patient's leg, just proximal to the knee & quickly 'flick' each knee off the table. The patient's heel should remain on the examination couch unless there is hypertonia, in which case the heel will also lift off the couch.
	• Examine for **clonus**, supporting the patient's flexed knee with 1 hand. Quickly dorsiflex the foot & hold this position. Clonus is present if the foot continues to move in a rhythmical manner & is indicative of an UMN lesion.

Muscle movements are tested for power in both the upper & lower limbs.

Remember that the primary goal is to locate particular nerve root pathology.

Ensure that the movements being tested cover the appropriate myotomes.

Compare movements on each side & record the Medical Research Council (MRC) Power Grade *(see box below)*.

POWER	Root	Movement	Muscle	Nerve
UPPER LIMB	C5	Shoulder Abduction	Deltoid	Axillary
	C5/C6	Elbow Flexion	Biceps	Musculocutaneous
			Brachioradialis	Radial
	C7/C8	Elbow Extension	Triceps	Radial
	C7	MCPJ Extension	Extensor Digitorum Communis (EDC)	Posterior Interosseous (branch of radial nerve)
	C8	Thumb IPJ Flexion	Flexor Pollicis Longus (FPL)	Anterior Interosseous (branch of median nerve)
	T1	Finger Abduction	Dorsal Interossei	Ulnar
	T1	Thumb Abduction	Abductor Pollicis Brevis (APB)	Median
LOWER LIMB	L2/L3	Hip Adduction	Hip Adductors	Obturator
	L2/L3	Hip Flexion	Iliopsoas	Femoral
	L4/L5	Hip Extension	Gluteus Maximus	Sciatic
	L3/L4	Knee Extension	Quadriceps	Femoral
	L5/S1	Knee Flexion	Hamstrings	Sciatic
	L4/L5	Ankle Dorsiflexion	Tibialis Anterior	Deep Peroneal
	S1/S2	Ankle Plantarflexion	Gastrocnemius	Tibial
	L5	Hallux Extension	Extensor Hallucis Longus (EHL)	Deep Peroneal
	L5/S1	Ankle Eversion	Peronei	Superficial Peroneal

UK MRC POWER GRADING:

0: No Movement

1: Contraction Flicker

2: Movement Without Gravity

3: Movement Against Gravity

4: Movement Against Resistance

5: Full Power

Remember to test both sides for coordination.

COORDINATION	Interpretation
UPPER LIMB	• **Finger–Nose Test:** Place your finger tip within reach of the patient. Ask the patient to touch their nose then your finger tip, each time moving your finger to another position. Then test the contralateral arm. • **Dysdiadochokinesia:** Ask the patient to hold out 1 hand, palmar side up, keeping it still. Instruct the patient to clap this hand with their other hand, rapidly alternating between using the palmar & dorsal surfaces. Then test the contralateral arm. This may have already been tested in the cerebellum screen.
LOWER LIMB	• **Heel–Shin Test:** Ask the patient to use their heel to touch the anterior ankle joint of the contralateral leg. Instruct them to 'sweep' this heel proximally to touch the anterior knee joint, then distally again, **without lifting their heel** off their leg at any time. Then test the contralateral leg.

Remember to test all dermatomes for sensation (Fig 13.2).

SENSATION	Ascending Tract	Interpretation
ANTEROLATERAL SPINOTHALAMIC TRACT	Pain	Use a sharp pin & instruct the patient to close their eyes. Test a 'normal' dermatome for 'sharpness'. Instruct the patient to compare this intensity of sharpness quality to the remaining areas being tested. Ask the patient to say 'yes' each time they feel the pin with the same intensity. If they do not respond, ascertain if this intensity is more or less than 'normal'.
	Temperature	Use cold & warm metal tubes, incubated in a beaker of ice & hot water, to test each dermatome. Do this in a similar manner to pain.

SENSATION	Ascending Tract	Interpretation	
DORSAL COLUMNS	Light Touch	Use a strand of cotton wool to touch each dermatome gently. Do this in a similar manner to pain & do not sweep the strand across the skin.	
	Proprioception	Test the position of the DIPJs using gentle extension & flexion. It is important to move the joints by holding the digits on their lateral surfaces, otherwise pressure will guide the patient's interpretation of proprioception. Do this in a similar manner to pain, however the patient should say 'up' or 'down' instead of 'yes'. If proprioception is absent, work proximally until a joint is found where proprioception is preserved. Record this joint.	
	2 Point Discrimination	Use a pair of compasses to touch each dermatome. Do this in a similar manner to pain, however the patient should say '1' or '2' points felt instead of 'yes'. Discrimination of 3mm on the pads of the fingers, 1cm on the palm of the hand & 3cm on the sole of the foot is normal.	
	Vibration	Use a 128Hz tuning fork to test the dorsal aspects of DIPJs (hand) or IPJ (hallux). Do this in a similar manner to pain. If vibration sensation is absent, move proximally from joint to joint until it is detected.	

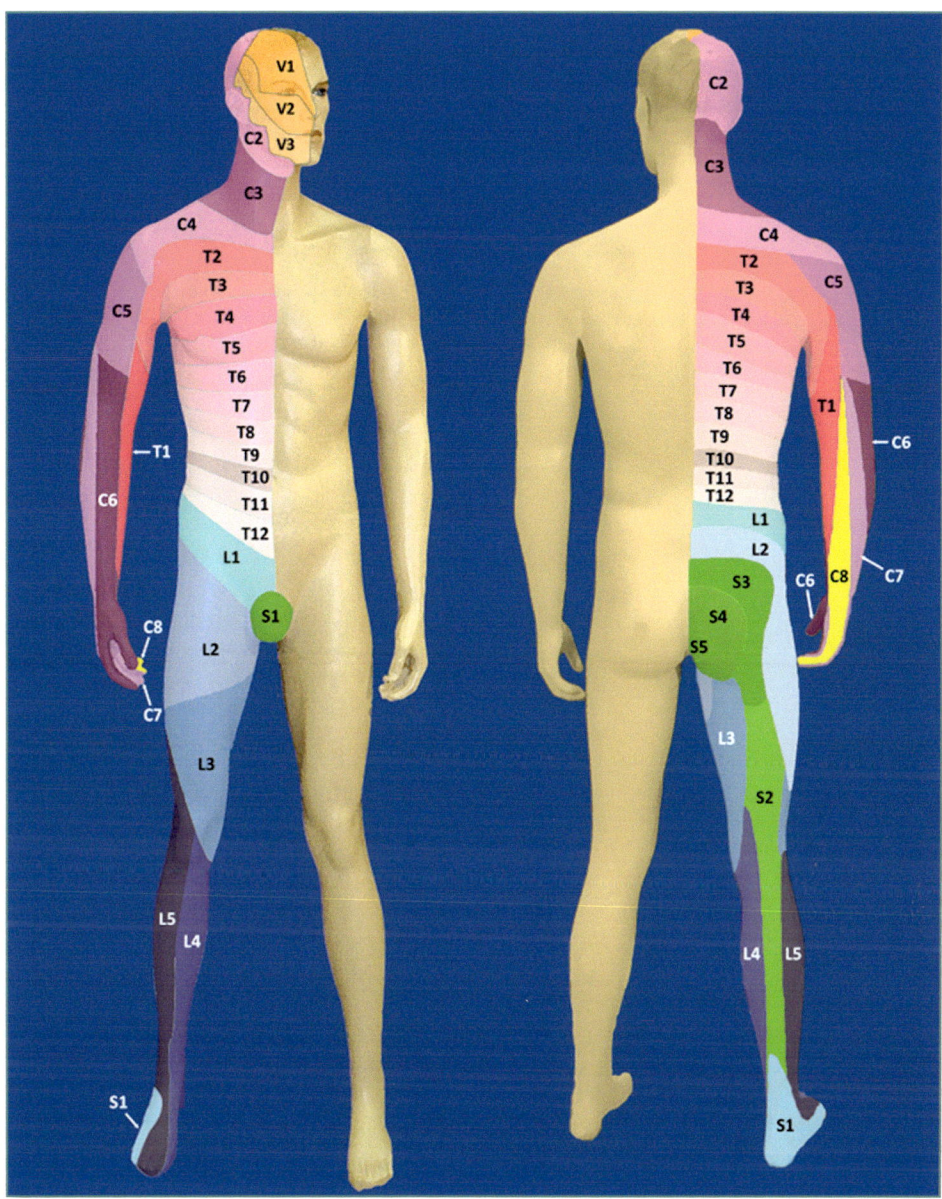

Fig 13.2: Dermatomes of the body. Left = anterior view. Right = posterior view.

Remember to test both sides for reflexes on both sides & compare each side.

Grade the reflex response where possible *(see box below)*.

REFLEXES	Arc	Interpretation
Ankle	S1/S2	Abduct & externally rotate the patient's hip & flex their knee. Use your hand to slightly plantarflex the foot at the ankle. Using the tendon hammer, strike the patient's Achilles tendon swiftly & accurately. The foot should be seen to plantarflex in response.
Knee	L3/L4	Support the patient's leg by 'hooking' your arm underneath, just proximal to the knee. Position the leg, flexed at the hip, so that the knee is flexed to approximately 60°. Using the tendon hammer, strike the patient's infrapatellar tendon swiftly & accurately. The knee should be seen to extend in response.
Biceps	C5/C6	Position the patient's arm, adducted at the shoulder & slightly flexed at the elbow, resting across their body. Place the pulp of your thumb on the biceps tendon. Using the tendon hammer, strike your thumb swiftly & accurately using a pendular motion. The biceps tendon should contract in response. This will be felt under the pulp of the thumb.
Supinator	C5/C6	Position the patient's arm as for the biceps reflex, ensuring the arm is slightly pronated. Place your index & middle fingers on the radial border of the patient's radius, approximately 5cm proximal to the wrist. Using the tendon hammer, strike your fingers swiftly & accurately. The elbow should be seen to flex, accompanied by finger flexion. If finger flexion only is observed, a spinal cord lesion involving C5 or C6 may be present. This response is termed an inverted reflex & may be associated with an absent biceps jerk. Causes of an inverted reflex include trauma, syringomyelia & prolapsed intervertebral disc.
Triceps	C7/C8	Position the patient's arm as for the biceps reflex & lean on the patient's resting hand. Using the tendon hammer, strike the patient's triceps tendon swiftly & accurately. The triceps muscle should be seen to contract in response.
Babinski	L4–S2	Immobilise the patient's leg by placing a firm hand just proximal to the ankle joint. Using the tendon hammer tip, purposefully swipe the lateral aspect of the foot in a proximal-distal motion. Whilst you are doing this, look at the toes for a flicker of motion that usually occurs as the tip reaches the level of the ball of the foot. The moment this flicker is detected, swipe the tip across the ball of the foot in a lateral-medial motion. The toes should be seen to flex. If an UMN lesion is present, the toes will abduct & extend.
Abdominal	T7–T12	Ensure the patient is lying completely relaxed. Use the tendon hammer tip to gently stroke the periumbilical skin, anticlockwise in a continuous motion. Each quadrant of the abdomen should be seen to contract as the tip enters the region.
Cremasteric	L1/L2	Gently stroke the proximal-medial aspect of the thigh. The ipsilateral testicle should be seen to retract.

REFLEXES	Arc	Interpretation
Anal	S2–S4	Prick the skin at the anal margin. The anal sphincter should be seen to contract. This is important in suspected cauda equina syndrome as it may often be absent. **Memory: S2/S3/S4 keeps the faeces off the floor!**
Bulbocavernosus	S2–S4	Squeeze the glans penis, clitoris or tug on an indwelling urinary catheter. The anal sphincter should be felt to contract. After spinal trauma, presence of this reflex with no motor / sensory function implies complete injury & suggests poor prognosis.

GRADING REFLEXES:

     0   Absent

     ±   Present With Reinforcement

     +   Hyporeflexia

     ++   Normal

     +++   Hyperreflexia

     ++++   Hyperreflexia & Clonus

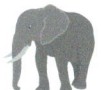

FINISH:

DrEXAM'S TIPS FOR REMEMBERING MYOTOMES & NERVE ROOTS

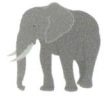

Myotomes & dermatomes are often feared by OSCE candidates, however there is no need to be afraid! A number of recognisable patterns exist & this knowledge may be 'layered' as follows:

1. Learn the arcs for the main limb reflexes first:

Memory:	1,2,3,4,5,6,7,8
Ankle:	S1/S2
Knee:	L3/L4
Biceps:	C5/C6
Triceps:	C7/C8

2. Note that the **myotomes correspond to the reflex arcs** i.e. ankle plantarflexion = S1/S2, knee extension = L3/L4, elbow flexion = C5/C6 & elbow extension = C7/C8. You now know 2 major myotomes for both the upper & lower limbs, so it should now be easier to work out the remaining myotomes!

3. Note some **important patterns in the lower limb** as follows:

Anterior movements of the lower limb begin with the last nerve root from the proximal joint, hence hip flexion = L2/L3, knee extension = L3/L4, ankle dorsiflexion = L4/L5.

Posterior movements of the lower limb begin with the last nerve root from the proximal joint, hence hip extension = L4/L5, knee flexion = L5/S1, ankle plantarflexion = S1/S2.

Anterior & posterior movements of the same joint follow directly on from each other, hence hip flexion & extension = L2/L3 & L4/L5, knee extension & flexion = L3/L4 & L5/S1, ankle dorsiflexion & plantarflexion = L4/L5 & S1/S2.

4. **Practise these movements** on your own limbs. This also applies for the dermatomes.

OSCE QUESTIONS

Low Back Pain & Prolapsed Intervertebral Disc

Q: What is the epidemiology of low back pain?

- Lifetime incidence >85%.
- It is the most common reason for disability in patients aged <45 years.
- No significant sex / race differences.
- Prevalence increases with age & pregnancy.

Q: What are the causes of low back pain?

Classification	Examples
Congenital	Kyphosis, Scoliosis, Spina Bifida, Spondylolisthesis.
Degenerative	OA, Spondylosis, Facet Joint Hypertrophy.
Gynaecological	Endometriosis, Pelvic Inflammatory Disease, Tumours.
Infective	Osteomyelitis , TB, Discitis.
Inflammatory	Ankylosing Spondylitis.
Metabolic	Osteoporosis.
Musculoskeletal	Posture Related Muscle Spasm (commonly in the lumbar region).
Neurological	Spinal Canal Stenosis, Prolapsed Intervertebral Disc, Spinal Haematoma.
Neoplastic	Primary (uncommon), Secondary Metastases (more common).
Psychiatric	Functional Overlay.
Renal	Calculi, Renal Cell Carcinoma.
Traumatic	Vertebral Fractures, Muscle Tears, Ligamentous Injuries.
Vascular	AAA.

Q: What is the mechanism of a prolapsed intervertebral disc?

- Posterior herniation of the central nucleus pulposus, through the annulus fibrosis, into the spinal canal.
- 50% are at the level L4/5 & 40% at L5/S1.
- Caused by a degenerative cascade, described in stages as follows:

Stage	Mechanism	Clinical Features
Dysfunction	'Acute' injury. Tear of the annulus fibrosis & prolapse of the inner nucleus pulposus with cartilage destruction. An inflammatory facet joint reaction occurs.	Back pain (worse on movement), localised tenderness on palpation, muscle spasm.
		Significant prolapse may impinge nerve root(s) causing radiculopathy or cauda equina syndrome.
Instability	Disc resorption & loss of height. Facet joints may become lax, predisposing to subluxation.	Intermittent back pain. Possible detectable instability on movement. Neurological deficit may persist or worsen.
Restabilisation	Osteophyte formation & progressive stenosis.	Chronic back pain but with reduced severity. Neurological deficits stabilise.

Q: What investigations would help your diagnosis of a prolapsed intervertebral disc?

After taking a full history & performing a thorough clinical examination, I would consider the following diagnostic investigations:

Investigation	Notes
MRI (gold standard)	Urgent if cauda equina syndrome is suspected *(see below)* (Fig 13.3).
CT (myelogram)	In absence of MRI / MRI contraindicated.

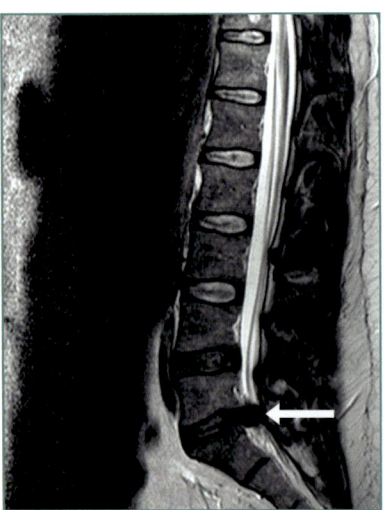

Fig 13.3: Sagittal T2 weighted lumbar spine MRI demonstrating a large disc prolapsed at the L5 / S1 level.

Q: What are the clinical features of lumbar radiculopathy secondary to a prolapsed intervertebral disc?

These are dependent on the level of involvement as follows:

L4 / L5 (compression of ipsilateral L5 nerve root)	L5 / S1 (compression of ipsilateral S1 nerve root)
L5 dermatome pain & sensory impairment	S1 dermatome pain & sensory impairment
Weak foot dorsiflexion	Weak foot plantarflexion
Weak extensor hallucis longus	Depressed / absent ankle jerk

Q: What are the treatment options for lumbar radiculopathy, secondary to a prolapsed intervertebral disc?

Conservative	Medical	Surgical
Lifestyle Modification & Patient Education	Analgesic Ladder	Lumbar Discectomy (>90% improvement, 5% recurrence rate)
OT / PT	Epidural & Nerve Root Injections	Lumbar Discectomy & Laminectomy (for canal stenosis)
Heat / Hydrotherapy		Lumbar Arthrodesis (for spondylosis)
TENS Machine		

Note: <20% of patients will require surgical intervention. Indications for surgery include cauda equina syndrome, intractable pain & progressive motor deficit (MRC Grade ≤3).

Cauda Equina Syndrome

Q: What is cauda equina syndrome & what are the characteristic features?

Cauda equina syndrome results from compression of the cauda equina nerve roots, secondary to a prolapsed intervertebral disc (most commonly) & constitutes a surgical emergency. Other causes include haematoma, infection, inflammatory conditions, malignancy & trauma.

Q: What are the clinical features of cauda equina syndrome?

Clinical features are characterised by the following 'red flags':

- Severe Low Back Pain
- Bilateral Sciatica
- Saddle Anaesthesia & Genital Sensory Deficit
- Bowel & Bladder Sphincter Dysfunction
- Sexual Dysfunction

3 typical presentations are well recognised:

1. **Sudden Onset** (in previously 'well' patient)
2. **Acute Bladder / Bowel Dysfunction** (in patient with low back pain & sciatica)
3. **Gradual Progression** (no acute / rapid deterioration)

Q: How would you classify cauda equina syndrome?

This may be classified as incomplete or complete as follows:

Incomplete	Complete
Difficulty urinating	Painless urinary retention ± overflow
Altered sensation on defecating	Altered / no sensation on defecating
Unilateral / partial perianal & genital sensory deficit	Bilateral perianal & genital sensory deficit
Some residual anal tone	Absent anal tone

Q: What questions are important to ask in the history & what examination features are essential to document in cauda equina syndrome?

When taking a full history & performing a thorough examination, I would ensure that the following are addressed:

History	Examination
Do you have pain in both legs? Is it worse than the back pain?	Assess & document genital sensation.
When did you last pass urine / open your bowels?	Assess & document perianal sensation & anal sphincter tone (per rectum examination).
Do you have difficulty urinating? Is there dribbling / leakage?	On catheterisation, document residual urine & catheter tug sensation.
Can you feel the paper when you wipe your bottom?	Document lower limb tone, power, coordination, sensation & reflexes.
Do you have numbness in your bottom & genitals?	

CHAPTER 13

DrExam™

334

Q: What are the treatment options for cauda equina syndrome caused by disc prolapse?

This is a neurosurgical emergency as irreversible nerve ischaemia begins to occur at 6 hours. Surgical decompression is via discectomy & decompressive laminectomy of 1–2 vertebrae typically. Incomplete cauda equina syndrome has a good prognosis if surgery is performed <12 hours of onset. Complete cauda equina syndrome has a limited prognosis, however reasonable recovery may still occur if surgery is performed <24 hours of onset.

Head Injury

Q What is the epidemiology of head injuries?

- Estimated 1,000,000 A&E attendances per year.
- Approximately 200,000 hospital admissions.
- Approximately 4,000 patients undergo neurosurgery for head injury per year.

Q: What important specific points would you consider in the history of a patient with a suspected head injury?

History	Notes	
Mechanism	Was there a history of assault, falls or RTA? If there is a history of falls, ascertain any precipitating syncopal events.	
Loss of Consciousness	What was the duration? Was it witnessed? Obtain 3rd-party history if possible.	
Amnesia	**Retrograde:**	Unable to recall events prior to the injury.
	Anterograde:	Unable to recall events after the injury.
Raised ICP Symptoms	Headache, nausea & vomiting, visual disturbances, focal neurological deficit.	
General	Medical & surgical co-morbidities, medications e.g. anticoagulants / antiplatelets, allergies, last meal.	

Q: What signs would you look for to confirm a head injury?

Specific points to consider include:

Examination	Notes
External Trauma	Ecchymoses, lacerations, haemorrhage.
Base of Skull Fracture	Periorbital bruising (**panda / raccoon eyes**), retroauricular bruising (**Battle's Sign**), CSF otorrhoea / rhinorrhoea, bleeding from ear / behind tympanic membrane.
GCS	Compare at scene & post-resuscitation. GCS ≤8 is associated with a need for intubation.
Pupils	Asymmetry, reaction to light.
Focal Neurological Deficit	Cranial nerve palsy, limb motor weakness, sensory deficit.
Associated Spinal Trauma	Bruising, vertebral fractures, poor anal sphincter tone (PR).

Q: When would you request a CT brain (& cervical spine) after a head injury?

These are based on NICE guidelines & include:

CT Modality	Notes
Immediate CT Brain	**Absolute Indications:** • GCS <13 on initial assessment in A&E • GCS <15 more than 2 hours after injury • Suspected open, depressed or base of skull fracture • Post traumatic seizure • Focal neurological deficit • ≥2 or episodes of vomiting (≥3 in children) • Amnesia of events >30 minutes before impact **Consider High Risk Criteria:** • Age >65 years • Coagulopathy • Dangerous mechanism of injury e.g. ejection from vehicle, pedestrian vs vehicle
CT Cervical Spine (in addition to brain)	• GCS <13 on initial assessment in A&E • Intubated patient • Suspected abnormality on plain film or technically inadequate • Patient being scanned for multi-region trauma

Q: How would you classify the severity of a head injury?

According to whether it is **open** (stabbing, gunshot, compound fracture) or **closed** (blunt trauma) & according to GCS as follows:

Minor (80%)	Moderate (10%)	Severe (10%)
GCS 14–15	GCS 9–13	GCS ≤8

Q: When would you refer a patient with a head injury to a neurosurgeon?

All moderate & severe head injuries should be discussed with a neurosurgeon. In addition, the following criteria necessitate discussion:

- New 'surgically significant' abnormality on CT
- GCS ≤8 persisting after resuscitation
- Unexplained confusion >4 hours
- Deterioration in GCS (by ≥2 points)
- Progressive focal neurological deficit
- Seizure without full recovery
- Open or suspected open injury
- CSF leak

Q: What are the principles of management of a minor head injury in a non-neuroscience centre?

- Manage according to **ATLS** resuscitation principles
- For patients admitted with GCS = 15, observations should include RR, pulse, BP, saturations, GCS, pupils & focal neurological deficit & should be:
   - ½ hourly for first 2 hours
   - Hourly for next 4 hours
   - 2 hourly thereafter.
- Ensure adequate analgesia (caution with opiates).
- Ensure adequate hydration & check electrolytes (especially Na⁺).
- Consider antiepileptics (discuss with neurosurgeon).
- Consider rescan & rediscussion with neurosurgeon if GCS deteriorates, worsening headache, nausea or vomiting.
- Consider referral to neurorehabilitation for post concussional syndrome.

Q: What are the indications for emergency neurosurgery following head injury?

Depends on individual circumstances (age, neurological status, co-morbidities, other injuries) but the following are a guide:

- Extradural or subdural haematoma with >5mm midline shift.
- Intracerebral haematoma >40cm^3 in surgically accessible area.
- Depressed skull fracture with depression > skull thickness.
- Potentially all open injuries for wound exploration *(no role for prophylactic antibiotics in base of skull fractures).*

Q: What are the management principles for severe head injuries that *do not* require immediate neurosurgery?

Primary Goals:

Prevention of secondary brain injury, cerebral ischaemia & herniation. A rise in ICP generally results in a fall in CPP, with a reduction in O_2 supply (resulting in ischaemia) & CO_2 clearance (resulting in vasodilation). This precipitates a vicious cycle that worsens brain injury & increases ICP further.

General Management Principles:

- Follow **ATLS** principles for patients with multi-system trauma.
- Intubation & ventilation in ICU.
- Insertion of ICP monitor (see ICP section).

*Aim is to optimise potential for recovery using medical & surgical strategies to maintain:

- CPP > 65 mmHg
- ICP < 25 mmHg

Specific Management Principles:

The following specific measures are considered in a stepwise 'tiered' fashion depending on response:

Tier	Medical	Surgical
1	• **Elevate Head (30–45°).** • *Avoid Hypoxia & Hypercapnoea.* • **Sedation & Paralysis:** Decreases O_2 demand & cerebral blood flow, therefore decreasing ICP. • **Control P_aCO_2 (4-4.5kPa):** Moderate hyperventilation 'blows off' CO_2 to help prevent cerebral vasodilation. • **Maintain MAP:** This helps maintain CPP. • **Ensure Normothermia.**	• **External Ventricular Drainage**: Therapeutic CSF withdrawal to control ICP.
2	*Tier 1 +* • **Increase Sedation**: Use boluses if required. • **Induce Hypothermia (33-35°C):** Reduces metabolic demand. • **Mannitol** (osmotic diuretic) / **Hypertonic Saline** (target Na^{2+} 145-155mmol/l)**:** Reduces cerebral oedema. There is a risk of renal impairment when serum osmolality >320mOsm/kg water.	• **External Ventricular Drainage**: Therapeutic CSF withdrawal to control ICP.
3	*Tiers 1 & 2 +* • **Barbiturate Coma** (e.g. thiopentone)**:** Induces 'total cerebral narcosis' & reduces brain metabolic demand to minimum requirement. Risks include myocardial depression, hepatic & renal impairment.	*Tiers 1 & 2 +* • **Consider Decompressive Craniectomy:** Remove skull section(s) to allow cerebral herniation into defect.

Q: What are the possible neurological sequelae for survivors of severe head injury?

Sequela	Notes
Vegetative State	No Physical Recovery
Cognitive Impairment	Concentration & Memory Impairment
Epilepsy	Partial / General Seizures
Location Specific	**Brainstem:** 'Locked In' Syndrome
	Frontal: Disinhibition, Emotional Disturbance, Personality Disorder
	Temporal: Aphasia
	Motor Cortex: Mono-, Hemi- or Tetraparesis
Psychiatric	Delirium, Depression, Psychosis

Traumatic Intracranial Haemorrhage

Q: What are the most common causes of intracranial haemorrhage?

1. Trauma (most common)
2. Spontaneous Intracerebral Haemorrhage (haemorrhagic stroke)
3. Subarchnoid Haemorrhage

Q: What are the underlying mechanisms & features of traumatic intracranial haemorrhages?

Classification & Location		Mechanism & Features
EXTRA-AXIAL	**Extradural Haematoma (EDH) (Fig 13.4)**	• High pressure arterial origin (middle meningeal artery most commonly). • >85% associated with skull fracture. • Decreased GCS & contralateral hemiparesis is common. • <30% have classic presentation of LOC → lucid interval → rapid deterioration ('talk & die'). • Variable underlying brain injury is present. • High density bi-convex lesion on non-contrast CT scan.
	Subdural Haematoma (SDH) (Fig 13.5)	• Generally venous origin. • Cortical laceration in young (often with significant underlying brain injury). • Bridging veins between inner table of skull & brain in elderly. • Decreased GCS & contralateral hemiparesis is common. • High density, concave lesion on non contrast CT scan.
INTRA-AXIAL	**Intracerebral Haematoma / Contusion (ICH) (Fig 13.6)**	• Due to direct brain injury. • Most commonly in inferior frontal lobe & temporal lobe due to anatomy of skull base (85%). • Decreased GCS & focal neurological deficit is characteristic. • Symptoms may worsen after 24–48 hours. • High density lesion in affected area on CT scan, with surrounding low density (cytotoxic) oedema. • **Coup** = direct injury. • **Contrecoup** = injury on opposite side of direct injury.

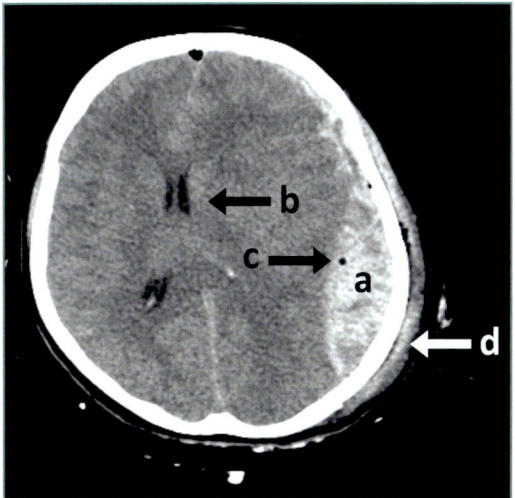

Fig 13.4: Axial CT brain (non contrast) demonstrating large left parietal / frontal extradural haematoma (EDH) (a) with midline shift (b). There are locules of air (c) within the EDH that may suggest an actively enlarging haematoma or possible open injury. There is also an extracranial scalp haematoma (d).

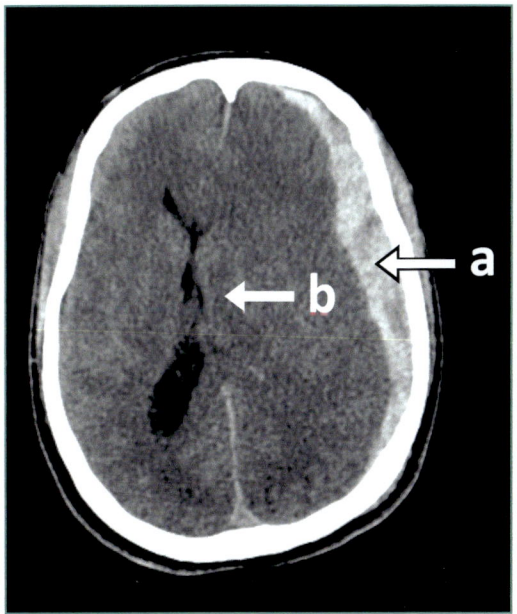

Fig 13.5: Axial CT brain (non contrast) demonstrating large left acute subdural haematoma (SDH) (a) & midline shift (b).

Q: What are the management options for traumatic intracranial haemorrhages?

Management is according to **ATLS** resuscitation & head injury principles *(see head injuries).* Specific options include:

Extradural	Subdural	Intracerebral
Conservative (if small)	**Conservative** (if small / chronic)	**Conservative** (mostly)
Endovascular Embolisation (if small & stable)	**Consider Trial of Steroids** (if chronic)	**Craniotomy & Evacuation** (if >40cm³ or with inferior temporal lobe / cerebellum involvement due to risk of brainstem compression)
Craniotomy & Evacuation (if increasing in size / >0.5cm thick with >5mm midline shift / deteriorating GCS)	**Burr Hole Drainage** (if chronic with mass effect)	**Bifrontal Decompressive Craniectomy** (consider for small, diffuse bifrontal contusions with mass effect)
	Craniotomy & Evacuation (if >1cm thick with midline shift / focal neurological deficit / deteriorating GCS)	**Note: Delayed deterioration is common due to 'maturation' of contusions, peaking at days 3–6.**

Spontaneous Intracranial Haemorrhage

Q: What is the difference between intracerebral & subarachnoid haemorrhage?

Haemorrhage	Notes
Intracerebral	Haemorrhage into brain parenchyma (Intra-axial)
Subarachnoid	Haemorrhage into subarachnoid space (Extra-axial)

Q: What are the risk factors for spontaneous intracerebral haemorrhage?

Spontaneous intracerebral haemorrhage has an annual incidence of approximately 10–15 / 100,000. >80% are secondary to hypertension & amyloidosis. Risk factors include:

Classification	Examples
Unavoidable	• **Age** (>55 years)
	• Race (Afro-Caribbean > Caucasian)
Iatrogenic	• Post Operative (especially malignant tumours)
Medical	• Coagulopathy (hepatic failure / antigcoagulation)
	• **Hypertension (affects basal ganglia & brainstem)**
	• **Amyloidosis (amyloid angiopathy weakens blood vessel walls)**
Vascular	• Aneurysm
	• AVM
Social	Illicit Drugs The most common cause in patients <30 years (amphetamines, cocaine)

Q: What are the treatment principles of spontaneous intracerebral haemorrhage?

Conservative	Medical	Surgical
Modify Risk Factors	Resuscitation	Craniotomy & Evacuation
	Control Hypertension	
	Reverse Anticoagulation	

Note: Current evidence base overall does not support surgical intervention. In general, right hemisphere peripheral parietal haematomas are most favourable for surgery. Basal ganglia & brainstem haematomas are least favourable for surgery.

Q: What is the epidemiology of subarachnoid haemorrhage?

- Annual incidence 10–15 per 100,000   (not changed in last 40 years)
- Increased prevalence in patients aged 50–65 years
- Sex difference   (female : male = 1.5 : 1)
- Race difference   (Afro-Caribbean : Caucasian = 2 : 1)

Note: Estimated prevalence of intracranial aneurysms is 4-7%. This implies that that most aneurysms *do not* rupture & remain asymptomatic.

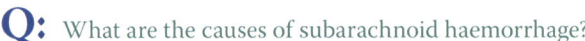

Q: What are the causes of subarachnoid haemorrhage?

Approximately 80% are due to rupture of an aneurysm. 15% of patients have multiple aneurysms. Causes may therefore be classified as follows:

Cause	Notes
Idiopathic	No cause found
Aneurysm	Berry Aneurysm (saccular) Rupture >75%
	Infective e.g. Endocarditis
	Inflammatory
Arteriovenous Malformation	AVM Dural Arteriovenous Fistula (these are mostly acquired)
Trauma	Uncommon & usually with a different radiological distribution of blood vs. spontaneous bleeds.

Q: What features on history & examination suggest subarachnoid haemorrhage?

Consider in any patient presenting with a sudden onset, severe headache. 5–10% die immediately & 15% are comatose on arrival to A&E. Also consider the following headache history & examination findings:

Headache History	Examination
Very Sudden Onset (reaching maximum intensity <1min)	**May Be Entirely Normal**
Persisting	**Meningism**
Usually Worst Ever Experienced	**Focal Neurological Deficit** (hemiparesis / monoparesis) (cranial nerve (III) palsy = posterior communicating artery aneurysm)
Variable Location (classically occipital)	**Visual Defect** (ophthalmic artery aneurysm)
Dull / Boring Character	**Papilloedema** (uncommon acutely as develops >6 hours from onset)
Associated Nausea & Vomiting	**Drowsiness**
Associated LOC	**Coma**
Associated Seizure	

Q: What investigations would you order / perform to confirm subarachnoid haemorrhage?

Investigation	Examples
CT Brain (Fig 13.6) **(non-contrast)**	• Sensitivity >96% in 1st 6 hours.
	• Sensitivity drops to 80% at 3 days.
	• CT is generally superior to MRI for detecting SAH.
Lumbar Puncture	• If CT is normal, perform at >12hours.
	• Sensitivity drops with time but is still worth doing up to 14 days.
	• CSF bilirubin indicates SAH.
	• A raised oxyhaemoglobin level may cause a false negative bilirubin reading.
	• Must obtain CSF WCC, RBC count, protein, oxyhaemoglobin & bilirubin absorbance ratios.

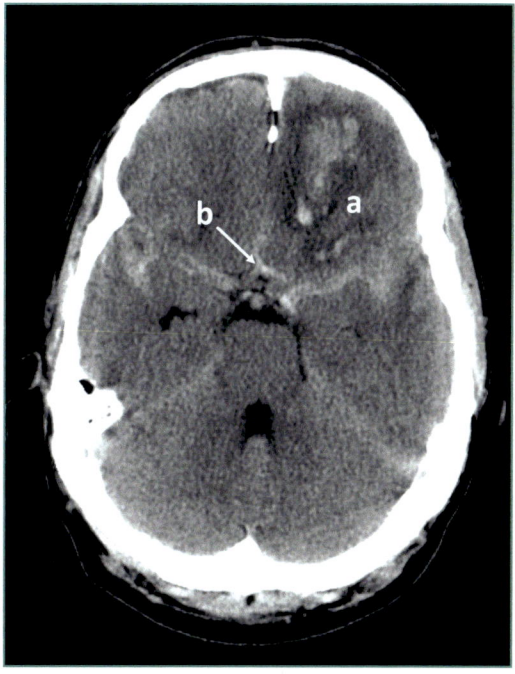

Fig 13.6: Axial CT brain (non contrast) at the level of the Circle of Willis.

There is patchy intracerebral haemorrhage in the left frontal lobe (a) & diffuse subarachnoid haemorrhage (SAH) in the basal cisterns (b).

Q: What radiological investigations would you order to detect an intracranial aneurysm?

- **CT- Angiogram**   (detects most aneurysms, except the smallest)
- **MR- Angiogram**   (better detection at skull base than CT)
- **Catheter Angiogram** ('gold standard' but invasive & carries 1/1000 risk of stroke)

Q: What are the treatment options for a proven aneurysmal subarachnoid haemorrhage?

Treatment is aimed at securing the aneurysm & reducing the risk of re-bleeding:

Treatment	Notes
Conservative	Supportive treatment should be considered in patients with a poor recovery from an initial SAH, elderly patients & patients with major co-morbidities.
Interventional	Endovascular embolisation with coils (for >80% of patients with aneurysms in the UK, but only 50% in USA). Procedure involves femoral catheterisation, passage of microcatheters to the cerebral vasculature & deployment of coils into the aneurysm sac. This is most suitable for aneurysms with a large dome & narrow neck. Some require stent assistance to assist access.
Surgical	Craniotomy & titanium clipping of the aneurysm neck (prevents aneurysm filling). Performed when coiling has failed, is technically unfeasible or when there is an existing requirement for craniotomy e.g. evacuation of large haematoma due to SAH.

Stroke (CVA)

Q: What is a stroke?

Clinical syndrome, with an underlying vascular cause, of rapidly developing clinical features of focal or global disturbance in cerebral function lasting >24h or leading to death.

*Note: Transient ischaemic attacks (TIAs) are similar, however clinical features last <24h.

Q: What is the epidemiology?

- 3rd most common cause of death in developed countries.
- Affects 200 per 100000 people per year.
- Commonly in 65-75 year age group.
- Significant cause of morbidity in aging populations

Q: What is the pathophysiology of stroke?

- Cerebrovascular accidents (CVAs / strokes) may be **haemorrhagic** *(see spontaneous Intracranial haemorrhage section)*, **thrombotic** or **embolic**.
- Thrombotic CVAs are due to atherosclerosis resulting in atheroma formation within the affected blood vessel & subsequent acute occlusion.
- Embolic CVAs most commonly originate from a site of thrombus e.g. at the carotid artery bifurcation / from the cardiac atria in AF. Other emboli include fat, air & foreign bodies.
- The result of the above CVA mechanisms is brain parenchyma damage (Fig 13.7).

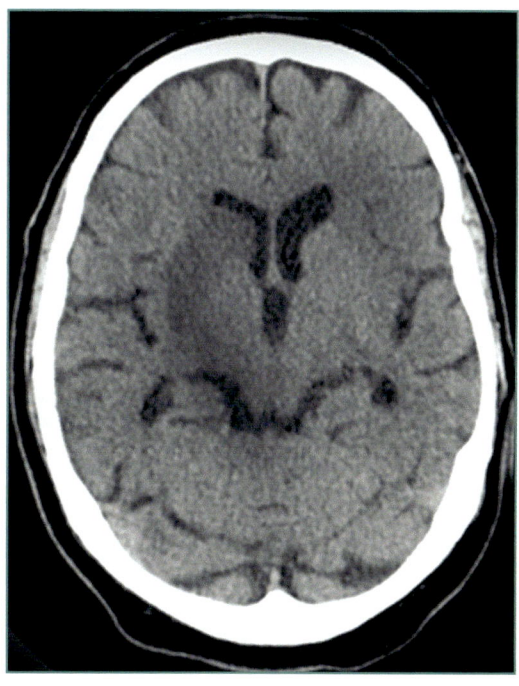

Fig 13.7: Embolic CVA CT.

CT scan illustrating right middle cerebral artery infarction.

Q: What are the risk factors for stroke?

These may be classified as non-modifiable & modifiable as follows:

Non-Modifiable	Modifiable
Age	Hypertension
Gender (more common in males)	Hypercholesterolaemia
Diabetes	Obesity
Genetic Predisposition	Poor Diet
Essential Medications e.g. Warfarin (haemorrhagic stroke)	Smoking
	Alcohol
	Sedentary Lifestyle
	Stress

Q: What are the management strategies for stroke?

- Hospital admission for thorough investigation & diagnosis (CT / Angiogram).
- Treatment:

Preventative measures are most important, medical & surgical treatment options depend on the underlying pathology e.g. anticoagulants & thrombolysis are contraindicated in haemorrhagic strokes. Treatment options include:

Prevention	Medical	Surgical
Reduce Risk Factors	Anticoagulants	Carotid Endarterectomy
Treat Predisposing Conditions	Thrombolysis	Superficial Temporal to Middle Cerebral Artery Anastomosis
	Calcium Antagonists e.g. Nimodipine	
	Aspirin	
	Good INR Control (if on warfarin)	

- Risk factor identification & reduction e.g. on a stroke unit.
- Rehabilitation e.g. physiotherapy & occupational therapy.
- Care plan implementation e.g. district nurse / care home.
- Psychological support.

Hydrocephalus

Q: What is hydrocephalus?

- Hydrocephalus is an imbalance between CSF production & absorption usually due to increased CSF volume & pressure.
- May cause increased ICP, progressive head enlargement, convulsions, mental disability, coma & death.

Q: What do you know about CSF production?

- Average adult ventricular system contains 150mls CSF.
- CSF is produced by the **choroid plexus** & **ependyma** at 20mls/hour (480mls/day).
- CSF is reabsorbed by the **arachnoid villi**.

Q: How would you classify hydrocephalus?

Classification	Sub-Classification	Examples
INCREASED CSF PRODUCTION	(rare)	• Choroid Plexus Papilloma. • Choroid Plexus Carcinoma.
IMPAIRED CSF CIRCULATION	**Obstructive:** Impairment within ventricular system. Ventricles DO NOT communicate with subarachnoid space.	• Congenital Aqueduct Stenosis (obstructs aqueduct of Sylvius). • Congenital Arnold-Chiari Malformation (obstruction at foramen magnum). • Thalamic Tumour (obstructs 3rd ventricle). • Cerebellar Tumour (obstructs 4th ventricle).
	Communicating: Impairment within subarachnoid space. Ventricles DO communicate with subarachnoid space.	• Head Injury. • Infection e.g. brain abscess / meningitis. • Subarachnoid Haemorrhage.
IMPAIRED CSF ABSORPTION	–	• Sinus Thrombosis. • Subarachnoid Haemorrhage. • Superior Vena Cava Syndrome.
Other	–	• Benign Intracranial Hypertension. • Normal Pressure Hydrocephalus.

Q: How does hydrocephalus present?

This depends on several factors including patient age, speed & duration of onset & cause. Clinical features may generally be classified according to onset as follows:

Classification	Examples
Acute (hours – days)	• **Infants:** Poor feeding, drowsiness / irritability, bulging anterior fontanelle, 'sunsetting' eyes (downward gaze & lid retraction = Parinaud's Syndrome), distended scalp veins, increasing head circumference. • **Adults:** Severe headache, nausea & vomiting, visual disturbance, gait disturbance, focal neurological deficit, papilloedema, drowsiness, coma.
Subacute (days – weeks)	More insidious onset with morning headaches, nausea & vomiting, upward gaze failure, delayed deterioration after an initial recovery.
Chronic (months)	Cognitive impairment, gait disturbance, bowel incontinence, neck pain.

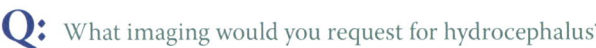

Q: What imaging would you request for hydrocephalus?

After taking a **full history** & performing a **thorough clinical examination**, I would consider the following:

Imaging	Notes
USS	Useful for infants & may be done on ward (via anterior fontanelle).
CT	Reveals ventricular size & configuration.
MRI	Reveals small space occupying lesions missed on CT & other associated brain abnormalities.

Q: What are the treatment options & prognoses for diagnosed hydrocephalus?

Treatment	Examples	Notes
MEDICAL	**Acetazolamide & Furosemide**	Reduce CSF secretion. *Ineffective in long term.*
	Isosorbide	Increases CSF absorption. *Ineffective in long term.*
INTERVENTIONAL	**Serial Anterior Fontanelle CSF Taps (infants).**	Useful in patients with 'transient' communicating hydrocephalus e.g. post SAH. Avoids risks of surgery. *Not practical in long term.*
	Serial Lumbar Puncture (adults – up to twice daily).	
SURGICAL	**Ventriculoperitoneal (VP) Shunt**	Most common procedure. Usually extends from right lateral ventricle (in the right parietal region), to the peritoneum. Prone to blockage (50% <2 years), tubing fracture & infection. *Very effective.*
	Ventriculoatrial (VA) Shunt	Usually extends from right lateral ventricle to jugular vein. Used when abdomen not suitable e.g. peritonitis / multiple abdominal surgery. Rare association with glomerulonephritis. *Very effective.*
	Endoscopic 3rd Ventriculostomy (ETV)	Endoscopic fenestration of 3rd ventricle floor 'creating' new CSF flow channels. Most efficacious in adults with obstructive hydrocephalus (70%). *Less effective than shunts.*
	Ventriculopleural shunt	'Last resort' shunt when Abdomen / cardiac shunt not suitable. Pleural effusion common complication. *Very effective.*
	Lumbar-Peritoneal Shunt	Can be used for benign intracranial hypertension & some types of communicating hydrocephalus. *Very effective in select cases.*

CNS Infections

Q: What are the most common CNS infections?

Remember to consider involved micro-organisms as viral, bacterial, fungal & parasitic. The most common & most significant micro-organisms are bacteria. CNS infections may be broadly classified as cranial vs. spinal:

CRANIAL	Common Bacteria	Notes
Brain Abscess	**Often multiple including:** • *Staphylococcus aureus.* • *Streptococcus milleri.* • *Bacteroides spp.* • *Pseudomonas aeruginosa.*	*(see below)*
Subdural Empyema	• *Streptococcus milleri* >60%. • *Haemophilus spp.* • Anaerobes.	Pus rapidly spreads along the subdural space, but does not cross boundaries e.g. falx cerebri & tentorium cerebellum. **Cause:** Iatrogenic e.g. post-operative. Spread of pus from sinusitis, otitis media & mastoiditis. **Features:** Fever, lethargy, reduced consciousness, focal neurological deficit, seizures in 70% of cases. **Investigations:** Diagnosis may be difficult, even with CT. **Treatment:** As for brain abscess *(see below)*.
Meningitis	**Neonates:** • Group B / D *Streptococcus.* • *Escherichia coli.* • *Staphylococcus aureus.* **Infant / Young Child:** • *Neisseria meningitidis.* • *Streptococcus pneumoniae.* • *Haemophilus influenzae.* **Teenager / Adult:** • *Neisseria meningitidis.* • *Streptococcus pneumoniae.* **Trauma / Post-Operative:** • *Staphylococcus aureus.* • *Pseudomonas spp.* • *Enterobacter spp.* • *Mycobacterium tuberculosis.*	Inflammation of the meninges of the brain & spinal cord. **Cause:** • Infection. • Iatrogenic e.g. post-operative. • Chemicals e.g. intrathecal drugs. • Tumour e.g. brain tumour / lymphoma. • Inflammatory sarcoidosis. • Traumatic e.g. penetrating head injury, base of skull fracture. **Features:** Meningism, decreased GCS, focal neurological deficit, sepsis (petechial rash in meningococcal sepsis). **Investigations:** Blood tests e.g. FBC, U&E, CRP. Blood Cultures. CT Brain (excludes mass lesion). LP (*microbiology* - gram stain, MC+S / *biochemistry* - protein, glucose, WCC / *virology & immunology* as required). **Treatment:** Resuscitation, broad spectrum antibiotics immediately (gram -ve cover essential), analgesia, possibly corticosteroids, definitive management depends on cause.

CRANIAL	Common Bacteria	Notes
Ventriculitis	• Coagulase -ve *Staphylococcus*. • *Escherichia coli*.	Inflammation of the ventricular cavity & ependymal lining. **Cause:** V/P Shunt, intrathecal chemotherapy, post-meningitis (rarely aseptic). **Features:** Markedly decreased GCS, sepsis, enhancing ventricles on imaging **Investigations:** LP (CSF sample establishes diagnosis). **Treatment:** Intrathecal & intravenous antibiotics until CSF clear. Remove shunt / re-site EVD if present.

SPINAL	Common Bacteria	Notes
Primary Discitis	• *Staphylococcus epidermidis* (most common post-op). • *Staphylococcus aureus*. • *Escherichia coli*. • *Proteus spp.* • *Pseudomonas spp.* (common with IVDU).	Infection of nucleus pulposus, then vertebral body. **Cause:** Iatrogenic e.g. post-operative (0.2–4% incidence after lumbar discectomy). Immunocompromise e.g. HIV, IVDU, DM. Obesity, multiple surgeries & sepsis at time of surgery are risk factors. **Features:** Severe localised pain that is worse on spinal movement, radicular symptoms, tenderness, muscle spasm. Investigations: **Investigations:** Blood tests e.g. FBC, U&E, CRP. Blood Cultures. MRI. Spine X-ray usually normal in 1st week. **Treatment:** Brace, bed rest, analgesia, antibiotics 4–8 weeks, surgery (for associated abscess / unstable spine).

Q: What factors predispose to brain abscess development?

Factors	Notes
Contiguous Spread (most common)	From ENT infection into adjacent brain: • Sinusitis (spreads to inferior frontal lobe). • Mastoiditis (spreads to inferior temporal lobe).
Head Injury	Penetrating Head Injury.
Immunocompromise	HIV, Steroids, DM.
Systemic	Bacterial Endocarditis, Congenital Cyanotic Heart Disease.

Q: What are the common clinical features of brain abscesses?

Most patients present with a history of symptoms <2 weeks:

Features	Frequency	Features	Frequency
Headache	70%	Nausea & Vomiting	40%
Mental State Changes	65%	Seizures	30%
Focal Neurological Deficit	65%	Nuchal Rigidity	25%
Fever	50%	Papilloedema	25%

Q: What are the treatment options for brain abscesses?

Medical	Surgical	Follow-Up
Empirical Antibiotics (initially)	Image Guided Burr Hole & Abscess Aspiration (repeat if necessary)	Clinical Progression
Anticonvulsants (>6months)	Craniotomy & Surgical Excision	Serial Imaging
Specific Antibiotics (after MC+S)	Ventricular Drainage (for intraventricular extension)	Serial Inflammatory Markers
Intrathecal Antibiotics (for intraventricular extension)		

Brain Tumours

Q: What are the causes of an intracranial mass lesion?

Classification	Examples
Congenital	Arachnoid Cyst, Hamartoma, Dermoid Cyst.
Infective	Abscess, Toxoplasmosis, Subdural Empyema, Hydatid Cyst.
Inflammatory	Multiple Sclerosis, Reaction Around Foreign Body.
Neoplastic	Primary (Fig 13.8) & Secondary Tumours *(see below)*.
Trauma	Extradural Haematoma, Subdural Haematoma, Intracerebral Haematoma.
Vascular	Aneurysm, AVM, Cavernoma.

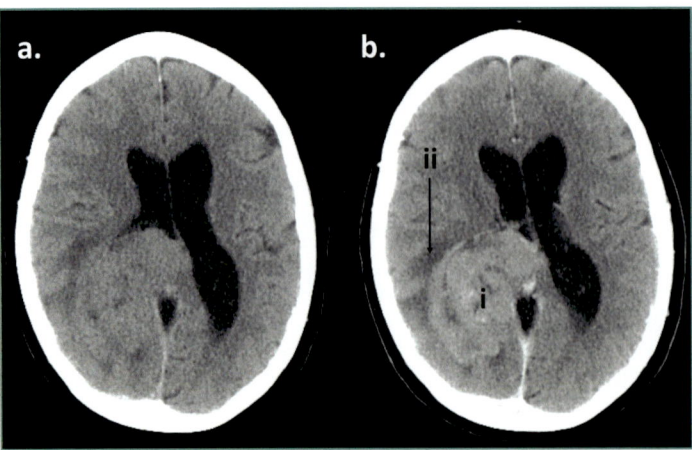

Fig 13.8: Non-contrast (a) & contrast enhanced (b) axial CT brain demonstrating large right parietal enhancing space occupying lesion (i), with extension into the ventricular system. There is surrounding low density that represents oedema (ii). These features are consistent with a malignant primary tumour.

Q: What is the epidemiology of brain tumours?

- Primary brain tumours have an annual incidence of 7.5/100,000 & result in >3,500 deaths/year.
- It is the 15th most common cancer in adults & 2nd most common in children (after leukaemia).
- Metastases account for 50% of brain tumours & prevalence increases with age.
- Metastases are found in 25% of post mortems (with brain examinations).
- Despite modern treatments, primary malignant brain tumours have a poor outcome.
- Outcome for metastatic brain tumours depends on the primary pathology & extent of metastatic spread.

Q: What risk factors are associated with development of a brain tumour?

- Most arise in patients without an obvious predisposing factor.
- <5% are associated with genetic conditions including Von Recklinghausen's Disease (NF1 gene), tuberous sclerosis (TSC1 & TSC2 genes), Li-Fraumeni syndrome (P53 gene).
- Radiation exposure e.g. previous whole brain radiotherapy.
- Immunocompromise e.g. HIV & primary CNS lymphoma.
- Possible increased risk from certain chemical exposures.
- No proven link with mobile phone use or previous head injury.

Q: How would you classify brain tumours?

These may be **benign or malignant, primary or secondary** & may be classified **according to location** as follows:

Tumour	Classification		Notes
PRIMARY (45%)	*Intra-Axial (within brain parenchyma)*		
	Glioma (69%)	Astrocytoma (61.5%)	Arise from astrocytes in any part of the brain. Diffusely infiltrative, with ill-defined capsule around tumour.
			WHO grading 1–4 (increasingly malignant)
			• Grade 1 (2%): Pilocytic – median age 13
			• Grade 2 (23%): Diffuse – median age 40
			• Grade 3 (30%): Anaplastic – median age 45
			• Grade 4 (45%): Glioblastoma Multiforme – median age 55+
		Oligodendroglioma (5%)	Arise from oligodendroglial cells. 1p19q co-deletion is 'genetic signature'. Frontal lobe involvement common.
		Ependymoma (2.5%)	Arise from ependymal cells e.g. 4th ventricle. 2 peaks of incidence at ages 5 & 35 years.
	Lymphatic (3%)	Lymphoma	Often intraventricular. Increased risk with immunocompromise. May regress with steroids.
	Extra-Axial (outside brain parenchyma)		
	Meningioma (20%)		Arise from arachnoid cap cells. More common in females. Mostly parasagittal (attached to midline) & convex (over hemisphere surface). Slow growing & usually benign.
	Pituitary (5%)		Usually benign adenomas. May present with endocrine hyper- / hypofunction. Bitemporal hemianopia is due to upward compression of the optic chiasm.
	Cerebellopontine (3%)		Acoustic neuroma often presents with sensorineural hearing loss & facial nerve palsy. Usually benign & surgery / radiosurgery is curative.

Tumour	Classification	Notes
SECONDARY	*Intra-Axial / Extra-Axial*	
(50%)	**Metastases**	Small, often multiple, lesions with disproportionately excessive oedema. More common in patients aged >60 years. Most are intra-axial but some are extra-axial (attached to dural surface). Common primary lesions include: • **Lung** (60%): Especially small cell carcinoma. • **Breast** (20%): Oestrogen receptor positivity predicts favourable response to chemotherapy. • **Others** (20%): Colon, melanoma, prostate, renal, testicular.
OTHER	**Vascular**	Haemangioma (Von Hippel-Lindau Syndrome).
(5%)	**Midline**	Dermoid cyst, epidermoid cyst.
	Pineal	Pinealblastoma / pinealcytoma, germ cell tumours.

Q: What are the clinical features of brain tumours?

These depend on the mechanism of involvement e.g. direct infiltration & destruction of neurones, local pressure on neighbouring structures or generalised increase in ICP. Clinical features therefore include:

- Headaches (morning), nausea & vomiting, papilloedema (all due to raised ICP).
- Drowsiness.
- Seizures.
- Focal neurological deficits (depending on location) including:
    - Hemiparesis (contralateral frontal involvement)
    - Dysphasia (Broca / Wernicke involvement)
    - Cranial nerve palsy, cardiorespiratory disturbance (brainstem involvement)
    - Ataxia, incoordination, hydrocephalus (cerebellum involvement)

Q: What are the radiological features of common brain tumours?

These are dependent on the imaging modality & tumour. CT requires pre- & post-contrast scan comparison. MRI demonstrates if metastases are solitary or multiple. Magnetic resonance spectroscopy (MRS) can generate useful information about tumour activity. Common imaging findings are as follow:

Diagnosis	Findings
Glioma (high grade)	Large lesion (often) with central low density (necrosis).
	Ring enhancement.
	Rapid progression.
Metastases	Small & multiple (often).
	Less ring enhancement than glioma.
	Disproportionately excessive peri-tumour oedema.
Meningioma	Extra-axial.
	High density on non-contrast CT.
	Slow progression.

Q: What are the surgical treatment options & prognoses of common brain tumours?

Tumour	Treatment	Prognosis
Glioma	**Grade 1:** Gross total surgical resection ± radiotherapy.	Likely to be curative with total excision, especially in children.
	Grade 2: Surgical debulking depending on location. Chemotherapy has proven benefit.	30% survival at 5 years. 85% transform to a higher grade.
	Grade 3: Surgical debulking depending on location & adjuvant radiotherapy. Chemotherapy has proven benefit.	Median survival 2 years (with treatment).
	Grade 4: Surgical debulking depending on location & adjuvant radiotherapy. Chemotherapy has proven benefit.	Median survival 10 months (with treatment).
Metastases	**Non Small Cell Lung:** Surgical debulking / biopsy & radiotherapy.	Poor prognosis. Depends on resection of primary tumour & other extracranial metastases.
	Breast: Surgery, chemotherapy & radiotherapy.	Can be >5 years with full resection of a solitary brain metastasis & chemosensitive tumour.
Meningioma	Curative surgery is usually feasible even with bone involvement. Radiotherapy indicated for all malignant meningiomas.	>90% cure. 5–10% recurrence if benign. 5% are malignant & have a poor outcome.

CHAPTER 14
UPPER LIMB NERVES

BH Miranda
K Asaad
M Nicolaou
SK Al-Ghazal

CHAPTER CONTENTS

RADIAL NERVE EXAMINATION

START: Patient sitting opposite you, with hands resting on a table / supported by a pillow.

Expose patient to at least above the elbows. However, some nerve injuries may originate more proximally, so exposing the entire upper limb & cervical spine is ideal.

Look for any aids e.g. splints.

LOOK	Interpretation
Scars	Check for scars indicating penetrating trauma of the upper limb: • Upper arm (fractured humerus) • Radial side of elbow (fractured radial head)
Swelling	Soft tissue / bony mass.
Symmetry	Symmetrical disease is associated with RA.
Deformity	Wrist drop (ask the patient to hold their hands & arms out straight).
Erythema	Inflammation.
Sinus	Post-operative, infective.
Muscle Wasting	Wrist extensors, triceps.

Ask about pain.

Feel for temperature changes (dorsal & ventral) with the back of your hand.

SENSATION	Interpretation
1st Dorsal Web Space	Innervated by the superficial radial nerve.
Dorsal Forearm	High lesion.

Remember to test like-for-like

MOTOR	Interpretation
Triceps	Triceps extension affected with high lesions (nerve branch is proximal to spiral groove).
Brachioradialis	Elbow flexion affected with lesions above the elbow (nerve branch is distal to spiral groove).
Supinator	Supplied by the posterior interosseous branch of the radial nerve (PIN). The PIN branches off at the level of the elbow, passing deep between the 2 heads of supinator.
MCPJ Extension	The radial nerve supplies all long digital extensors.
Extensor Pollicis Longus (EPL)	Patient keeps palmar surface of hand flat on a table & lifts thumb. EPL is usually visible & palpable.

SPECIAL TESTS	Interpretation
Functional Assessment	Assess global & fine function (*see hand examination*).

COMPLETION	Interpretation
Upper Limb Neurovascular Status	Full examinations required *(see relevant sections)*.
	Particularly focus on pulses, dermatomes & myotomes.
Neck Examination	Exclude cervical spine pathology.
QoL Impingement & Sleep	Asking patient about these helps to assess impact on life & therefore necessity for intervention.
Help Patient Dress	Good practice if patient has functional limitation.
Radiology	Humerus fracture (radiograph). Cervical spine (MRI).
Nerve Conduction Studies	Assist in further diagnosis of underlying pathology e.g. degeneration, demyelination, conduction block.

FINISH:

MEDIAN NERVE EXAMINATION

START: Patient sitting opposite you, with hands resting on a table / supported by a pillow.

Expose patient to at least above the elbows. However, some nerve injuries may originate more proximally, so exposing the entire upper limb & cervical spine is ideal.

Look for any aids e.g. splints.

LOOK	Interpretation
Scars	Carpal tunnel decompression / previous trauma.
Swelling	Soft tissue / bony mass.
Symmetry	Symmetrical disease is associated with RA.
Deformity	Benediction sign (when the patient makes a fist), ape hand, simian thumb.
Erythema	Inflammation.
Sinus	Post-operative, infective.
Muscle Wasting	Thenar eminence, forearm flexors.

Ask about pain.

Feel for temperature changes (dorsal & ventral) with the back of your hand.

Feel for reduced sweating.

SENSATION	Interpretation
Thenar Eminence	Innervated by the palmar cutaneous branch, this passes over the flexor retinaculum. It branches from the median nerve proximal to the carpal tunnel.
Digital Nerves	Test all ulnar & radial digital nerves. The median nerve classically supplies sensation to the radial 3½ digits after it has passed through the carpal tunnel.

Remember to test like-for-like.

MOTOR	Interpretation
Pronator Teres	Pronation is affected with high lesions.
Opponens Pollicis	Ask the patient to touch each finger, in succession, with their ipsilateral thumb.
Abductor Pollicis Brevis (APB)	Ask the patient to place their hand on the table (palm up) & point their thumb to the ceiling. Tell the patient to stop you from pushing their thumb down & simultaneously palpate the bulk of APB.
Flexor Pollicis Longus (FPL)	**Pincer Grip:** The patient makes an 'OK' sign with each hand, by pinching their thumb & index finger together. A piece of paper is slipped between the pinched grips of both hands (thumbs facing up). Using your own pincer grips, gently pull the paper away from the patient, asking them to prevent you from doing this. If FPL is affected, the patient's thumb will flatten to prevent the paper from being pulled away. This occurs as the patient switches to using adductor pollicis (ulnar nerve). FPL is supplied by the anterior interosseous nerve (Fig 14.1).

SPECIAL TESTS	Interpretation
Tinel's Test	Carpal tunnel syndrome *(see hand examination)*.
Phalen's Test	Carpal tunnel syndrome *(see hand examination)*.
Functional Assessment	Assess global & fine function *(see hand examination)*.

COMPLETION	Interpretation
Upper Limb Neurovascular Status	Full examinations required *(see relevant sections)*. Particularly focus on pulses, dermatomes & myotomes.
Neck Examination	Exclude cervical spine pathology.
QoL Impingement & Sleep	Asking patient about these helps to assess impact on life & therefore necessity for intervention.
Help Patient Dress	Good practice if the patient has functional limitation.
Radiology	Cervical spine (MRI).
Nerve Conduction Studies	Assist in further diagnosis of underlying pathology e.g. degeneration, demyelination, conduction block.

FINISH:

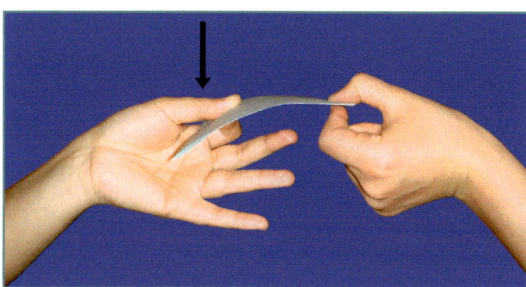

Fig 14.1: Pincer grip test. Flexion at the thumb IPJ is maintained in the normal hand. This is due to the innervation of FPL by the anterior interosseous nerve. On the abnormal hand, adductor pollicis takes over, innervated by the ulnar nerve, such that there is flattening of the thumb (arrowed). Compare with Froment's Test (Fig 14.3).

ULNAR NERVE EXAMINATION

START: Patient sitting opposite you, with hands resting on a hand table.

Expose to at least above the elbows. However, some nerve injuries may originate more proximally, so exposing the entire upper limb & cervical spine is ideal.

Look for any aids e.g. splints.

LOOK	Interpretation
Scars	Cubital tunnel decompression scar posterior to the medial epicondyle / previous trauma.
Swelling	Soft tissue / bony mass.
Symmetry	Symmetrical disease is associated with RA.
Deformity	Claw hand (when the patient extends their fingers).
Erythema	Inflammation.
Sinus	Post-operative, infective.
Muscle Wasting	Hypothenar eminence, interosseous muscles (intermetacarpal wasting).

Ask about pain.

Feel for temperature changes (dorsal & ventral) with the back of your hand.

Feel for reduced sweating.

Palpate the ulnar nerve behind the medial epicondyle.

SENSATION	Interpretation
All Digital Nerves	Test all ulnar & radial digital nerves.
	The superficial cutaneous branch of the ulnar nerve classically supplies sensation to the ulnar 1½ digits, via the digital nerves, after it has passed through Guyon's Canal.
Little Finger Metacarpal (dorsal aspect)	Innervated by the dorsal sensory branch. It branches from the ulnar nerve, approximately 1 hand's breadth proximal to the wrist.

Remember to test like-for-like.

MOTOR	Interpretation
Flexor Digitorum Profundus (ulnar)	Test the ulnar ½ of FDP (ring & little fingers), by testing distal interphalangeal joint (DIPJ) flexion.
Palmar Interossei	Get the patient to adduct their fingers, placing a sheet of paper between adjacent fingers. Place the opposite end of the paper between your adducted fingers, tell the patient to prevent you from pulling the paper away, & pull. Palmar interossei weakness will result in the paper slipping from the patient's fingers. **Memory:**　　　　　　**'PAD'** The **p**almar interossei **ad**duct the fingers relative to middle finger:
Dorsal Interossei	Test abduction of the fingers against resistance (Fig 14.2). **Memory:**　　　　　　**'DAB'** The **d**orsal interossei **ab**duct the fingers relative to middle finger.
Froment's Test	Ask the patient to put their fists together, making a 'thumbs up' sign with both hands. Put a piece of paper between their thumbs & closed fists & ask them to hold it in place with their thumbs. Adopting the same position, place the opposite end of the paper between your thumbs & closed fists. Tell the patient to prevent you from pulling the paper away & pull. Weakness of adductor pollicis will result in the patient flexing their thumb to prevent the paper being pulled away. This occurs as the patient switches to using flexor pollicis longus (median nerve).

SPECIAL TESTS	Interpretation
Guyon's Canal Percussion	May reproduce ulnar nerve symptoms, if compression is within Guyon's Canal.
Cubital Tunnel Syndrome	Ask the patient to fully flex their elbows & tuck them closely into the sides of their abdomen. Reproduction of ulnar symptoms suggests cubital tunnel syndrome. Percussion over the cubital tunnel may also reproduce symptoms.

COMPLETION	Interpretation
Upper Limb Neurovascular Status	Full examinations required *(see relevant sections)*. Particularly focus on pulses, dermatomes & myotomes.
Neck Examination	Exclude cervical spine pathology.
QoL Impingement & Sleep	Asking patient about these helps to assess impact on life & therefore necessity for intervention.
Help Patient Dress	Good practice if patient has functional limitation.
Radiology	Cervical spine (MRI).
Nerve Conduction Studies	Assist in further diagnosis of underlying pathology e.g. degeneration, demyelination, conduction block.

FINISH:

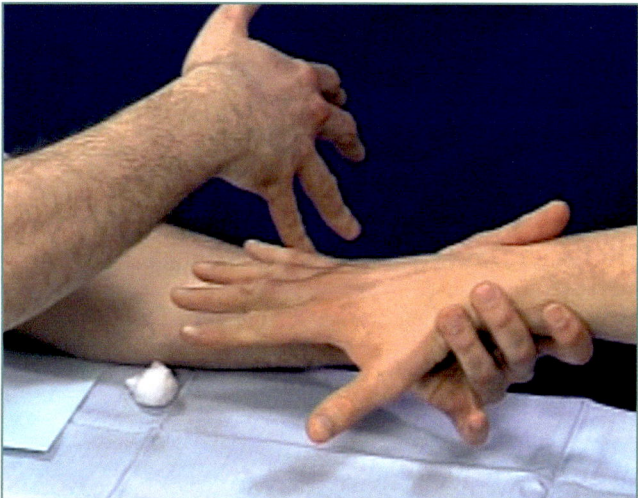

Fig 14.2: Abduction of the little finger, tested like-for-like.

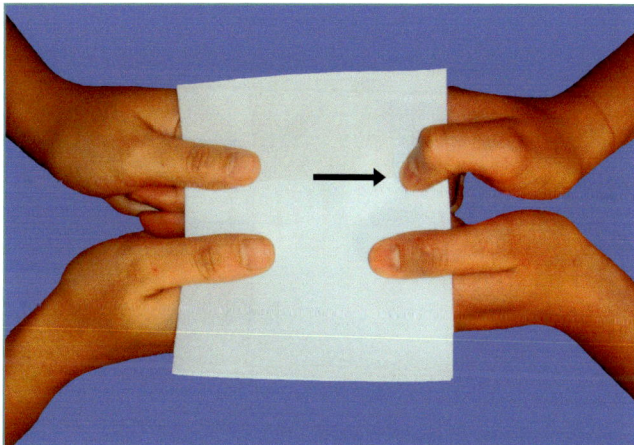

Fig 14.3: A positive Froment's Test. The thumb IPJ flexes to grip the paper. This is due to FPL action (innervated by the anterior interosseous branch of the nerve) taking over from adductor pollicis (innervated by the ulnar nerve). Compare with the pincer grip test (Fig 14.1).

OSCE QUESTIONS

Radial Nerve

Q: What is the course of the radial nerve?

- Roots C5–T1.
- Arises from the posterior cord of the brachial plexus.
- Passes through the triangular space.
- Descends the posterior humerus in the spiral groove between the medial & lateral heads of triceps.
- Gives a nerve branch to **triceps** & **anconeus**.
- Above the elbow it gives a nerve branch to **brachioradialis** & **ECRL**.
- At the level of the lateral epicondyle it divides into 2 branches:

Superficial Radial Nerve (superficial branch)	Posterior Interosseous Nerve (PIN) (deep branch)
Descends the dorsal-radial aspect of the forearm, beneath brachioradialis.	Winds around the neck of the radius & passes between the superficial & deep heads of supinator (Arcade of Frohse).
Emerges to a subcutaneous position at the junction of its middle & distal third.	Supplies **wrist extensors & supinators, hand extensors** & **APL**.
Supplies **sensation on the dorsal 1st web space**.	Supplies **ECRB**.

Q: What is the typical appearance of the hand in radial nerve palsy?

This will depend on the level of injury:

- A high radial nerve palsy results in complete wrist drop due to loss of all extensors.
- A palsy affecting the PIN alone will result in loss of extension of all digits, with preservation of wrist extension (as ECRL is still functioning via innervation from the main radial nerve more proximal to the PIN). A small patch of sensory loss on the dorsal 1st web space may also be identified.

Median Nerve

Q: What is the course of the median nerve?

- Roots C5–T1.
- Arises from the medial & lateral cords of the brachial plexus.
- Passes with the brachial artery.
- Passes through or under pronator teres & continues beneath FDS.
- Supplies **pronator teres, palmaris longus, FCR & FDS.**

- Gives off the **anterior interosseous nerve.** This supplies **FPL, radial ½ FDP, pronator quadratus.**
- Gives off the **palmar cutaneous branch** 5cm proximal to wrist. This supplies **sensation to the palm of the hand (in line with the radial 3½ digits)**.
- Enters the carpal tunnel & gives off:
  - **Recurrent motor branch** to the **LOAF muscles** (**l**umbricals (radial 2), **o**pponens pollicis, **a**bductor pollicis brevis & **f**lexor pollicis brevis)
  - **Digital branches** which supply **sensation to the volar-radial 3½ digits.**

Q: What is the appearance of the hand in a high median nerve palsy?

Appearance	Notes
Thenar Eminence Wasting	Lose innervation to **abductor pollicis brevis, flexor pollicis brevis** & **opponens pollicis.**
Benediction Sign	The index & middle fingers remain extended when the patient tries to make a fist.
Ape Hand Deformity	Wasting of the thenar muscles, results in the thumb coming to lie in line with the remaining digits. Thumb movement is limited to flexion & extension, with loss of abduction & opposition.

Ulnar Nerve

Q: What is the course of the ulnar nerve?

- Roots C8, T1.
- Arises from the medial cord of the brachial plexus.
- Descends the posterior-medial aspect of the humerus.
- Pierces the medial intermuscular septum.
- Passes posterior to the medial epicondyle in the cubital tunnel.
- Passes between the 2 heads of FCU to enter the anterior compartment of the forearm.
- Gives branches to **FCU & FDP (ulnar ½).**
- Gives off the **dorsal sensory branch** at the distal ⅓ of the forearm. This perforates deep fascia & runs on the ulnar side of the dorsum of the wrist & hand, supplying **sensation to the dorsal-ulnar aspect of the hand**.
- The ulnar nerve continues through Guyon's Canal (medial to the ulnar artery) & divides into:

Deep Motor Branch	Superficial Sensory Branch
Supplies **all intrinsic hand muscles except LOAF (median nerve).**	Supplies **sensation to the volar-ulnar 1½ digits via digital nerve branches.**

Q: What is the typical appearance of the hand in ulnar nerve palsy?

- Ulnar clawing of the ring & little fingers.
- This is characterised by MCPJ hyperextension (lumbrical paralysis) & flexion at the PIPJ & DIPJ.
- The clawing becomes more obvious when the patient is asked to straighten their fingers.
- The middle & index fingers are not affected as those 2 lumbricals are supplied by the median nerve (LOAF).

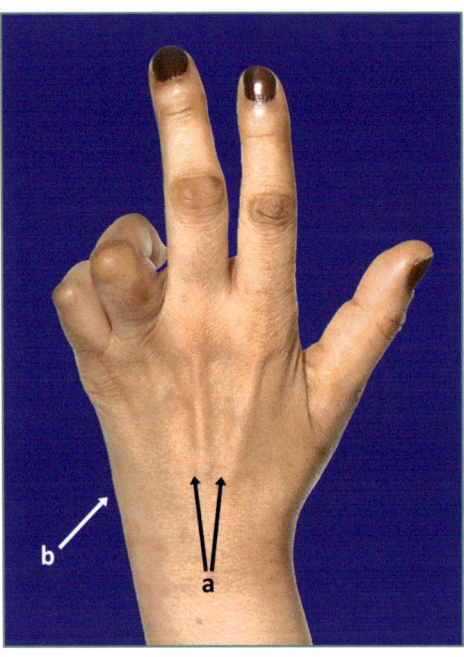

Fig 14.4: A clawed left hand due to ulnar nerve injury. Note the intermetacarpal (a) & hypothenar (b) wasting. There is sparing of the thenar eminence as these muscles are supplied by the median nerve. Compare this with fig 8.2 which shows Dupuytren's Contracture. A thorough systematic examination is necessary to reach the correct diagnosis.

Q: What is the ulnar paradox?

The claw appears worse in a lower (less severe) ulnar nerve injury.

- Clawing is caused because the ulnar 2 lumbricals are paralysed.
  - Lumbricals flex the MCPJ & extend the DIPJ & PIPJ.
- FDP & FDS flex the DIPJ & PIPJ in the fingers.
  - FDP to the ring & little fingers is supplied by the ulnar nerve (flexes DIPJ).
  - FDS is supplied by the median nerve (flexes PIPJ).
- In a high ulnar nerve injury (e.g. at the elbow) there is loss of FDP function to the ring & little fingers, so there is no flexion at the DIPJ & a less-severe looking claw.
- In a low ulnar nerve lesion (e.g. at the wrist) the FDP branch is spared, so flexion occurs at the DIPJ of the ring & little fingers, & the claw appears worse.

Q: What is a tardy ulnar nerve palsy?

- Valgus deformity in the area of the medial epicondyle.
    - E.g. caused by malunion / non-union of a condylar fracture.
    - E.g. caused by epiphyseal injury to the lateral side of the elbow.
- Chronic stretching of the ulnar nerve occurs.
- This leads to a late (tardy) ulnar nerve palsy.

Nerve Injuries & Palsies

Q: What are the common sites of radial, median & ulnar nerve compression in the upper limb?

Radial Nerve	Median Nerve	Ulnar Nerve
Thoracic Outlet	Medial Intermuscular Septum	Medial Intermuscular Septum
Axilla	Ligament of Struthers	Cubital Tunnel
Radial Tunnel Syndrome	Pronator Teres	Guyon's Canal
Arcade of Frohse	Anterior Interosseous Syndrome	
ECRB	Carpal Tunnel	
Supinator		

Q: What fractures may be associated with radial, median & ulnar nerve injuries?

- Humeral shaft fractures are associated with radial nerve injuries.
- Median nerve injuries may be associated with wrist fractures.
- Ulnar nerve injuries are associated with supracondylar humeral fractures.
- Phalangeal or metacarpal fractures may be associated with digital nerve injuries.

Q: Can you summarise the effects of nerve injuries in the upper limb?

Nerve	Injury	Muscles Affected	Sensory Loss	Appearance
R A D I A L	Axilla	• Triceps • Brachioradialis • Supinator • ECRL & ECRB • Extensors	1st Dorsal Webspace	• Reduced / Absent Elbow Flexion • Reduced / Absent Supination • Wrist Drop • Absent Digital Extension
	Spiral Groove	• Brachioradialis • Supinator • ECRL & ECRB • Extensors	1st Dorsal Webspace	• Reduced / Absent Supination • Wrist Drop • Absent Digital Extension
	Proximal Forearm	• Extensors	1st Dorsal Webspace	• Milder Wrist Drop • Absent Digital Extension
M E D I A N	Elbow	• FDS • FDP (to index & middle fingers) • FPL • FCR • Pronator Teres • Palmaris Longus • LOAF Muscles	Radial 3 ½ Digits & Palm	• Benediction Sign • Ape Thumb
	Wrist	• LOAF Muscles	Radial 3½ Digits	• Ape Thumb
U L N A R	Elbow	• FDP (to ring & little fingers) • FCU • Interossei • Ulnar 2 Lumbricals • Adductor Pollicis • Hypothenar Muscles	Ulnar 1½ Digits	• Less Severe Clawing (of little & ring fingers) • Interosseous Wasting • Hypothenar Wasting
	Wrist	• Interossei • Ulnar 2 Lumbricals • Adductor Pollicis • Hypothenar Muscles	Ulnar 1½ Digits	• More Severe Clawing (of little & ring fingers) • Interosseous Wasting • Hypothenar Wasting

SECTION B: COMMUNICATION SKILLS & ETHICS

CHAPTER 15
COMMUNICATION SKILLS & ETHICS

M Epstein
LK McMurray
BH Miranda

CHAPTER CONTENTS

INTRODUCTION

The OSCE may include dedicated ethics & communication skills stations. However these domains are assessed throughout the OSCE stations, so it is important for an appropriate ethical & communicative framework to be used throughout the examination process.

The stations which specifically test ethics & communication skills can be presented in a variety of formats. The candidate may be expected to role play a scenario with an actor whist being observed by the examiner. Other stations are unmanned e.g. writing a patient transfer letter or filling out an investigation request form. Some example themes & stations include:

Theme	Example Stations
Information Gathering	• Taking a history from a patient.
	• A consultation with a relative of a patient.
Information Giving	• Writing a patient transfer letter.
	• Conducting a telephone conversation.
	• Taking a patient history & presenting it to a consultant.
	• Completing investigation request forms.
Appropriate & Factual Communication	• Obtaining informed consent.
	• Breaking bad news.
	• Discussing investigations.
	• Discussing a diagnosis.
	• Discussing treatment options, including complications & relevant prognoses.
	• Discussing a management plan with a colleague.

POINT SCORING

In order to maximise points, consider the following patient & surgeon factors. These are based on General Medical Council & Intercollegiate Surgical Curriculum Project guidelines.

Patient Factors	Surgeon Factors
Consider age, culture, ethnicity, religion & disability.	Address patients or relatives from a variety of cultural, religious & ethnic backgrounds.
Establish rapport through empathy & honest communication.	Treat all patients, relatives & colleagues with courtesy & respect.
Allow time to listen to the patient's account.	Address a spectrum of pre-existing emotional states of patients or relatives.

Patient Factors	Surgeon Factors
Identify & respond to the patient's or relative's verbal & non-verbal cues.	Address a spectrum of emotional responses from patients or relatives.
Be non-judgemental, non-paternalistic & non-patronising towards the patient or relatives.	Address complaints & questions appropriately, including those beyond the candidate's level of competence.
Respect patients' views about their health, responding to their ideas, concerns & expectations.	Ensure patients are well informed about their care & how their information will be shared within involved medical & surgical teams.
Use a holistic approach to patients & relatives.	Address time constraints.

KEY COMPETENCIES

There are numerous potential scenarios that assess communication skills. The candidate should be prepared to interact with a patient, relative, carer or allied healthcare professional. Although it is impractical to approach the station with a rigid framework, a few competencies will have to be demonstrated:

Competency	Explanation
Interpersonal Skills	• The ability to form a good rapport.
Information Gathering	• Effectively eliciting important information, including ideas, concerns & expectations.
	• Summarising the patient's agenda to confirm understanding.
Information Giving	• Explaining the issues fully, to a level that is clearly understood.
	• Avoiding the use of jargon.
	• Providing an appropriate management plan within the framework of the patient's ideas, concerns & expectations.
	• Ensuring that summaries are clear & concise if writing a patient referral letter.
Ethical & Legal Principles *(see later)*	• Ensuring the consultation respects the basic ethical principles.
	• Ensuring the consultation is within the correct legal framework.

Interpersonal Skills

Interpersonal skills are required to build up the doctor–subject relationship. These encompass a number of verbal & non-verbal attributes throughout the consultation:

Interpersonal Skill	Examples
Body Language	• Open body language, avoiding crossed legs or arms. • Maintaining an appropriate distance. • Appropriate, non-threatening eye contact.
Active Listening (verbal & non-verbal)	• Using verbal phrases such as *"Okay..." "Yes..." "I see..."*. • Head nodding. • Echoing the patient.
Empathy	• Using phrases such as *"That must be difficult for you..."* & *"I can see why that must be a problem..."*. • Using silence during the consultation. • Offering a tissue if the subject cries.
Cues Identification & Response	• Responding to verbal & non-verbal cues, which inform you of the patient's needs, desires & feelings. • Using phrases such as *"You mentioned that things were difficult at home, can you tell me more about this?"*.

Information Gathering

The first part of the consultation should be used to elicit the salient points from the subject:

Consultation Step	Explanation	Examples
Introduce	• Use a well-practised phrase. • Give your name to the patient. • Explain your role.	• *"Hello, my name is Dr ... "* • *"I am the surgical doctor on the ward..."*
Check Patient Identity	• Check the name of the patient. • If speaking to a 3rd party, establish their relationship to the patient & ascertain whether the patient is aware of the consultation.	• *"Is it Mr/Mrs ... ?"* • *"Can I ask what your relationship is with Mrs X?"* • *"Does Mrs X know that we are speaking today?"*

Consultation Step	Explanation	Examples
Elicit Reason for Consultation	• Use a well-rehearsed open question. • Do not interrupt the patient as they give their answer. • Listen carefully for cues which you will have to address.	• *"What can I do for you today?"* • *"What is the problem which has bought you here today?"* • *"I'm told you would like to speak to me about Mrs X?"*
Encourage Patient to Provide Information	• Use open questions & active listening techniques to encourage the patient to reveal more information.	• *"Can you tell me a bit more about that…"*

Memory: 'ICE'

It is important to elicit the patient's ideas, concerns & expectations (ICE). This will ensure the consultation is tailored towards the patient's agenda. Marks will be scored if these are identified early in the consultation, reflected upon & applied appropriately.

Consultation Step	Explanation	Examples
Ideas	• What the patient thinks is happening.	• *"What do you know about what has been going on so far?"* • *"What do you think is going on?"*
Concerns	• What worries the patient has that need to be addressed.	• *"Is there anything particular that you are concerned about"* • *"What concerns you most about the current situation?"*
Expectations	• What the patient wants from the consultation.	• *"What do you feel we can do for you today?"* • *"What would you like to achieve from today's consultation?"* • *"How would you like to take this forward?"* • *"What is your understanding of what we are going to do next?"*

Memory: Summarise!

Before you formulate the management plan, briefly summarise the key points. Summarising demonstrates to the patient that you have listened & understood what they have said. It also demonstrates to the examiner that you have elicited the salient issues & addressed the patient's agenda. You may want to ask:

- *"Can I just summarise what you have told me so far?"*
- *"From what I understand you have told me..."*

After summarising, give the patient the opportunity to divulge any information not picked up during the information gathering process. You may want to ask:

- *"Is there anything else you want to tell me about?"*

Information Giving & Referral Letters

Many communication skills scenarios test the candidate's ability to effectively communicate an explanation & management plan to the patient:

Consultation Step	Explanation	Examples
Explain Issue	• Use simple language. • Avoid medical jargon. • Avoid abbreviations.	• *"Blocked blood vessels"* rather than *"arteriosclerosis"* • *"Do not resuscitate"* rather than *"DNR"*
Ensure Understanding	• Deliver the information in small chunks. • Regularly check that the patient understands your explanation.	• *"Does this all make sense to you so far?"* • *"Do you have any questions about this so far?"*
Formulate Management Plan	• The management plan must be shared. • Avoid being prescriptive, ensure you provide management options to the patient. • Formulate the plan within the patient's ICE.	• *"The options available to us are..."* • *"Are you happy for us to proceed this way?"* • *"We should be able to address your concerns with this test."*
Follow Up	• Arrange a follow up appointment. • Alternatively arrange a contact point for the patient.	• *"I would like to see you in 2 weeks once you have had more time to think about it."* • *"I am on call next week, my bleep number is ..."*
Finish Consultation	• Ask the patient whether they have any further questions. • Always thank the patient.	• *"Do you have any questions before we finish?"*

Candidates may also be expected to read a set of medical or surgical patient notes & then write a referral or transfer letter to a colleague. Due to time constraints, it is important to gather relevant information from the notes as quickly as possible. Remember that some details may be written down prior to reading through the notes e.g. referring doctor or surgeon details, date, patient details etc. The following information should be included in any transfer letter:

Information	Explanation
Referring Doctor or Surgeon Details	• Name of referring doctor or surgeon. • Details of referring department & hospital. • Contact details.
Referral Date	• Date letter.
Address Referral	• Direct referral with title where possible *"Mr X, Consultant Cardiothoracic Surgeon..."* • An alternative is a speciality referral *"Dear Consultant Cardiothoracic Surgeon..."*
Patient Details	• 1st name, surname, date of birth, age, sex & NHS number
Patient Contact Details	• House number, street name, city & postcode • Include telephone number if possible.
Referral Reason	• Introduce the problem that precipitated the referral. • Ask for an opinion.
Surgical History of Presenting Complaint	• Include onset, duration, course, severity, precipitating factors, relieving factors, associated features & previous episodes.
Other Relevant Medical Details	• Additional current & past medical & surgical problems. • Medications. • Investigation results e.g. blood tests & imaging.
Interpreter	• Mention if required or not.

Here is an example layout for a referral letter:

Mr J Tomkins (A&E SpR)
County Hospital
1 County Street
London L1 1NE
020 7xxx xxxx ext. 1000

Mr H Ali (Consultant Orthopaedic Surgeon)
District Hospital
1 District Street
London L1 1NE
London L1 1NE
020 7xxx xxxx ext. 3000

Referral Date: 21st Jan 2010

Dear Mr Ali,

Re: Jenny Smith, DoB 19/12/1990, Female, Hospital #123456.

Thank you for your kind referral acceptance of the above patient whom I discussed with your trainee doctor, Mr C Jenkins. Ms Smith presented to A&E on the 21st Jan 2010, after sustaining a comminuted fracture of the shaft of the left humerus with shortening & rotation. She sustained this after a mechanical fall onto the edge of a stone step whilst gardening. This was witnessed by her friend who was helping her. There were no other injuries sustained, neither was there loss of consciousness. The patient has no other medical or surgical history & does not take any medication. The AP & lateral view radiographs that were taken are included with the patient notes. No blood test results are currently available for this patient. Ms Smith will not require an interpreter.

Yours sincerely,

Mr J Tomkins

ETHICAL & LEGAL PRINCIPLES

The scenario may be written to test the candidate's ability to identify & appropriately manage an ethical or legal issue.

The four basic ethical principles are:

Ethical principle	Explanation	Example
Autonomy	• Respecting the patient's attitude & wishes with regard to their own health & future.	• Advanced directives. • Do not resuscitate decisions. • Informed consent.
Justice	• Being fair to the wider community in terms of the consequence of a decision.	• Driving after a surgical procedure.
Beneficence	• Ensuring all decisions are **in the patient's best interest.**	• Not undertaking an unnecessary investigation. • Weighing up the benefits & side effects of a medication.
Nonmaleficence	• Ensuring actions **do not harm** the patient.	• Resuscitation resulting in a vegetative state. • Dealing with an unfit colleague.

Capacity

The Mental Capacity Act (2005) provides a framework to assess whether a patient is able to make a decision about their management. This became law in 2007 & applies to anyone over the age of 16. In order to decide if a patient is competent, a number of principles must be followed:

Principles of Capacity	Explanation
Assume the patient is competent unless proven otherwise.	• Do not make assumptions based on appearance, behaviour or current medical condition.
The patient should be in an optimal position to process information & make a decision, prior to assessing capacity.	• Ensure they have adequate time to process the information. • Use appropriate communication aids e.g. interpreters & diagrams.
If competent, the patient has the right to make a decision, even though the decision may be deemed 'unwise'.	• A competent patient may refuse treatment even if it is life saving.
Decisions made on behalf of a non-competent patient must always be **in the patient's best interest**.	• No adult can make a decision for another adult, unless they have lasting power of attorney *(see later)*. • This is regardless of 3rd-party wishes such as family & friends. • Management decisions for non-competent patients must be made by medical or surgical teams & be **in the patient's best interest.**

Assessment of capacity is both decision & time specific. It is only valid for the action being proposed & only for the moment it was taken. A patient's capacity can change over the course of time & from one situation to another.

To prove capacity, the patient needs to demonstrate:

Assessing Capacity	Explanation
Understanding	The patient must understand their: • Condition. • Prognosis. • Proposed management options, including purpose of intervention, risks, benefits & alternatives.
Information Retention	• The patient must be able to retain the information for long enough to make a decision.
Information Evaluation	• The patient must be able to weigh up the risks & benefits of their actions.
Decision Communication	• Communication may include talking, signing or use of any other communication aid.

If a patient lacks capacity, the Mental Capacity Act states:

- Any decisions made must be in **the patient's best interest**.
- The decision should be the least restrictive on the patient's human rights.
- Family & friends can represent the patient's wishes, feelings, beliefs & values, but cannot make a decision on behalf of the patient unless they have lasting power of attorney (see below).
- If the patient has no family or friends to represent them, an independent mental capacity advocate can be appointed.

If a patient lacks capacity, there are 2 situations where a decision can be made on behalf of the patient:

- **Lasting Power of Attorney:** Empowers the patient to appoint an attorney to make health decision for them, if they lack capacity in the future.
- **Court Appointed Deputies:** A deputy is appointed to make decisions, as authorised by the Court of Protection.

Gillick Competence

Patients under the age of 16 are considered to lack capacity unless proven otherwise. When capacity is lacking, parents have the right to make medical decisions on behalf of their child. A patient under the age of 16 who demonstrates capacity, is said to be Gillick competent. There are a number of principles relating to Gillick Competence:

Principles of Gillick Competence	Explanation
Sufficient Intelligence & Understanding	• The child must have a sufficient level of intelligence & understanding in order to process information relating to their management & formulate an informed decision about their treatment. • There must be understanding of the nature, purpose & possible consequences of proposed investigations & treatments. • There must be understanding of the consequences of not having treatment.
Situation Dependent	• Different treatments have varying levels of complexity & life impact, hence they require different levels of intelligence & maturity in order to understand them fully. • If a child is competent to consent for a treatment, their competence should be specifically reassessed prior to a decision about another treatment.
Case-by-Case Decisions	• Each case must be evaluated on its own merit.
Gillick Competent Children's Decisions Can't be Overridden	• Gillick competent children have the right to make an uncoerced decision about their management.

Note: It is important not to confuse Gillick Competence & Fraser guidelines. The latter relates specifically to decisions regarding contraception in minors.

Consent

The candidate should be prepared to fill out a consent form accurately, as part of an unmanned station, or to obtain consent from a patient in a consultation scenario.

Under usual circumstances, consent for a procedure is obtained from a **competent patient with the capacity to make a decision** (discussed earlier). In order for consent to be valid, it must be obtained **without coercion, from a patient who has been well informed** about the treatment options available, including complications & relevant prognoses.

There are 4 consent forms, available from the Department of Health, that apply to various circumstances:

Consent Form	Application
1	Patients able to consent for themselves.
2	Those with parental responsibility, consenting on behalf of a child or young person.
3	Patients able to consent for themselves & those with parental responsibility consenting on behalf of a child, where the procedure does not involve consciousness impairment.
4	Adults unable to consent for themselves.

There are various points in the consent forms that need to be considered by the candidate:

Consent Form Point	Explanation
Patient Details	• These include 1st name, surname, date of birth, age, sex & NHS number.
	• There is also a space to enter the name of the responsible healthcare professional.
Name of Procedure	• This must be filled in as specifically as possible, avoiding the use of abbreviations.
Benefits of Procedure	• These must be specified.
	• Examples include diagnosis, symptom improvement & removal of cancer.
Procedure Complications	• These must be specified according to each procedure.
	• Include the most common & most severe complications only.
Anaesthetic	• GA or Regional Anaesthetic.
	• LA.
	• Sedation.
Requirement for Additional Procedures	• Each possible additional procedure must be specified & consented for.
	• This includes blood transfusion.
Interpreter	• If there is an interpreter present, they must also sign the form.
Patient / Responsible Adult's Signature	• The patient must sign & date the form.
	• With children, the adult with parental responsibility must sign, though there is a space for the child to sign too, if they so wish.
	• When adults are unable to give consent for themselves there are spaces for 2 doctors to sign for a procedure that is **in the patient's best interests**.
Capacity	• When adults are unable to give consent for themselves, a capacity assessment must be made that indicates this.
	• The patient must either be unable to comprehend & retain information, unable to evaluate this information in the decision making process or be unconscious.
Best Interests	• When adults are unable to give consent for themselves, a statement must be made that indicates why the procedure is in the patient's best interests e.g. to save life.
Family Involvement	• When adults are unable to give consent for themselves, it is good practice to involve the family in the management process. They may sign the consent form indicating their approval for treatment. Despite this, they may not override the medical or surgical team's management, unless they have lasting power of attorney.
Medical Signature	• The surgeon undertaking the operation should consent the patient prior to surgery.
	• In the case of invasive or diagnostic procedures, the doctor undertaking the procedure should consent the patient prior to it.

Advanced Directives

Advanced directives allow competent patients to decide on withdrawal of life-saving treatments should they lose capacity. It can apply to anyone over the age of 18.

The basic principles underlying advanced directives include:

- The patient must have capacity at the time it is created.
- They must not be made under duress.
- They must be signed, dated & witnessed.
- They must specify the circumstances to which they apply.
- Patients can specify treatments to be refused, but cannot demand treatment which are deemed inappropriate.
- Once signed, they cannot be modified verbally or in writing.
- Assuming capacity is present, they can be revoked at any time.

Organ Donation

Organ donation is currently an 'opt out' policy in the UK. Absolute contraindications to organ donation include HIV & CJD. Organs can be obtained from either living or deceased donors:

Living Donors

Altruistic donors require mental capacity to be assessed to ensure they are competent to make a decision.

Full informed consent must be obtained prior to donation including success rate, risks to donor & recipient & the requirement for virology assessment.

The Human Tissue Authority must approve all donations from living donors to ensure the decisions were free of coercion or reward.

Living donors can donate their kidney, segment of liver or small bowel.

Deceased Donors

This includes both brainstem death & non-heart-beating donors.

Efforts should be made to ascertain whether the potential donor had expressed a wish to donate.

Evidence includes a written will, donor card, being on the NHS organ donor register or wishes communicated to relatives.

Even if there is evidence of an expression of interest, in practice if the relatives strongly object their views are normally respected.

Relatives of deceased donors are not able to express a preference for the recipient.

Organs which can be donated from deceased donors include heart, lungs, kidney, liver, pancreas, bowel, bone, skin, cornea, face (skin & muscle).

Confidentiality

GMC guidelines state *"Patients have a right to expect that you will not disclose any personal information which you learn during the course of your professional duties, unless they give permission. Without assurances about confidentiality patients may be reluctant to give doctors the information they need in order to provide good care."*

The basic principles of confidentiality include:

- Confidential information should be protected against improper disclosure when stored, transmitted or disposed.
- When a patient has given consent to disclose information, they must be aware of what will be disclosed & the likely consequences.
- Patients must be informed whenever information about them is likely to be disclosed.
- Requests by patients not to submit information to 3rd parties must be respected, unless withholding the information may result in risk to others.
- If confidential information is discussed, only as much information as is necessary to address the issue should be disclosed.
- Health workers should be made aware that the information has been given in confidence.

When confidentiality cannot be breached:

- Casual breaches in & out of the work environment.
- To prevent minor crime or help conviction in minor crime.
- To prevent minor harm to another individual.
- Disclosing information to a 3rd party e.g. insurance company without the patients' consent.

Some situations where confidentiality can be breached:

- Notifiable diseases.
- Drug addiction.
- Births & deaths.
- Court orders.
- When patients who are not medically fit to drive, continue to do so.
- When there is a 3rd party at significant risk of harm. For example, the partner of an individual who has expressed a desire to kill them.

COMMUNICATION SKILLS OSCE SCENARIOS

It is important to practise communication skills scenarios before the OSCE. This allows the candidate to become familiar with the process & timings of the station. The following section provides some example communication skills scenarios. Each case has separate briefings for the doctor & actor. The actor could be anything from a patient to an angry relative.

Practise with a colleague, taking turns between playing the role of doctor & actor. Playing the actor provides valuable insight into how the actor will perceive & respond to the candidate in the exam. If the resources are available, it is useful to have an impartial observer to make notes & give feedback after the consultation.

SCENARIO 1: *"The angry patient"*

DOCTOR BRIEFING

You are the surgical CT2 on the ward & have been managing Mr Bukley, a 65-year-old admitted last night with a critically ischaemic leg. On admission he was found to have:

- Right ABPI - 0.3
- Left ABPI - 0.5
- Absent pedal pulses bilaterally
- No evidence of gangrene or ulcers
- The rest of the cardiovascular assessment was normal
- BP - 138/80
- Blood sugar - 7.8

He was due for an angiogram this afternoon but the procedure has been postponed due to an emergency. It has been rescheduled as the 1st case on the list tomorrow morning. Your consultant has asked you to tell the patient.

ACTOR BRIEFING

You are John Bukley, a 65-year-old retired baker.

Appearance & Behaviour: Anxious, concerned about your condition & upset about the news of the postponement.

Background:

- For the past few years you have had intermittent pains in both legs.
- You saw your GP a few months ago who thought it may be arthritis or a muscle sprain.
- Initially the pain only started after walking about 100 yards but it has been progressively worsening.
- Over the past few weeks you have been getting pain on mobilising a few yards.
- In addition you have been experiencing pain during the night which is helped when hanging the leg out of the bed.
- The pain feels like cramp in the back of your thigh & calf.
- You called an ambulance yesterday evening after the pain became severe & your right foot looked pale & felt cold.
- You were admitted into hospital as an emergency last night.
- After a few tests in A&E you were referred to the surgical doctors who were concerned your leg may not be getting enough blood.
- You were informed of a special test which was urgently required to assess circulation.
- They explained the risks of not getting enough blood to the leg including gangrene & amputation.
- You are currently on the ward.
- You are still in some pain but occasional morphine is helping.

ICE:

- When told of the delay you get angry & are particularly concerned as the doctors in A&E had seemed very concerned about the leg. Why would have they admitted you if the procedure wasn't an emergency?
- You are still in pain & your foot is pale, you feel it may go gangrenous at any time.
- You cannot contemplate living as an amputee; you have seen pictures of amputees from various wars on television.
- Your wife & children are on route to be with you for the procedure, but now you have to tell them that the procedure has been postponed.

Past Medical History:

- You have high BP & are a diet-controlled diabetic.
- You are well otherwise.

Drug History:

- You take a BP tablet called ramipril.
- You have no drug allergies.

Social History:

- You live with your wife in a house.
- You drive & are dependent on your car.
- You started smoking at the age of 22. You stopped about 10 years ago but restarted 5 years ago after retirement.
- You have 2 children who both live nearby.

Family History:

- There is no family history of medical illness as far as you are aware.

First words to the doctor: *"Are you here to prepare me for the procedure?"*

Key Principles:

- The station tests the candidate's ability to deal with an angry / upset patient.

- The candidate should aim to diffuse the situation & reassure the patient.

- It is important to be truthful, direct & to apologise sincerely for the current situation.

Introduce Yourself	• *"Hello, my name is Dr ... I am the surgical CT2."*
Check Patient Identity	• Confirm the patient's name.
	• Check the patient's wristband.
Break News	• Inform the patient that the investigation has been delayed until tomorrow.
	• Explain the reason for the delay.
Apologise	• The patient may be too angry to acknowledge an apology so be sure to repeat it later in the consultation.
Diffuse Situation	• Let the patient talk & don't interrupt them.
	• Remain polite & avoid confrontation.
Empathise	• Empathise that you understand why he is anxious about getting treatment as soon as possible.
Identify ICE	• Listen carefully to pick up cues & elicit fears & concerns from the patient.
Address Ideas & Concerns	• Address his fear regarding the immediacy of the investigation.
	• Reassure him that he is still considered to be high priority by the vascular team.
	• Ensure he is aware that he is the first case on the list tomorrow morning.
	• Advise that you are happy to speak to him again with his family when they arrive.
	• Ensure his pain is controlled as he may need more analgesia overnight.
	• Suggest that he can speak to the consultant if he wishes.
Summarise & Check Patient Questions	• Summarise the plan.
	• Offer to answer any further questions.
Close Consultation	• Ask the patient whether they have any questions.
	• Explain that he can contact the ward doctor at any time.
	• Thank the patient for their understanding.

SCENARIO 2: "Breaking bad news"

You are the surgical ST4 in out-patient clinic. Your next patient is Mrs Susan Arnold, a 70-year-old referred with a 2 month history of dysphagia & weight loss. She has undergone a barium swallow which shows an irregular narrowing, highly suspicious of malignancy.

Explain the suspicion to her & the need for a staging CT.

You are Susan Arnold, a 70-year-old retired GP receptionist.

Appearance & Behaviour: You are highly anxious about coming for the results of your test.

Background:

- For the past 2 months, you have been experiencing a sensation of food getting stuck when swallowing & upper abdominal pain.
- You have lost weight (about 1 stone in 6 weeks).
- You went to the GP who was very efficient & sorted out a quick consultation with the hospital doctor.
- You have undergone a test called a barium swallow where you swallowed dye to look at your 'food pipe'.
- You have come for the results of the test.
- Your husband is ill with seasonal flu so unfortunately couldn't attend.

ICE:

- You are worried about cancer but your GP said there were a few possible reasons to explain your symptoms.
- You were a receptionist in a GP surgery & remember a few patients with oesophageal cancer who passed away quickly after diagnosis.
- You wish your husband was with you in the consultation but he is at home with the seasonal flu.
- Your main physical problem at the moment is not being able to eat proper meals because food keeps getting stuck.
- When you are told it looks like cancer, you want to know whether you should call your son back from Australia.

Past Medical History:

- You had your appendix removed at the age of 22.
- You have suffered from irritable bowel syndrome for many years.

Drug History:

- You take occasional mebeverine for your irritable bowel syndrome.
- You have no drug allergies.

Social History:

- You live with your husband who is your "rock" of support.
- You smoked many years ago.
- You drink the occasional glass of wine (about twice a week).
- You have 3 children, 1 in Australia, the other 2 live locally.

Family History:

- There is no family history of medical illness as far as you are aware.

First words to the doctor: *"I've come for the results of my test."*

APPROACH TO STATION

Key Principles:

- This is a breaking bad news station.
- The patient may cry, regardless of your approach.
- Interpersonal skills are particularly important in this station.
- Ensure the patient doesn't sense you are pressured for time.
- Ensure there is adequate support available for the patient.

Introduce Yourself	• *"Hello, my name is Mr ... I am the surgical ST4."*
Check Patient Identity	• Confirm the patient's name.
Initiate Consultation	• Establish whether the patient would like someone to be in the consultation with them.
Elicit ICE	• Establish what the patient knows already about their condition & the test performed. • This will help gauge whether the patient has any insight into the diagnosis.
Break News	• It is always difficult to break bad news. • Ensure you are honest, sincere & give the patient adequate time during the process. • Break the news in small chunks. • Fire a warning shot before mentioning cancer, for example *"I'm afraid the results are worrying"*. • Avoid jargon, mention cancer rather than "growth", "neoplasm" or "malignancy". • Despite the need for confirmatory tests, avoid giving false hope to the patient about an alternate diagnosis. • Advise that there is a strong possibility of cancer but further tests need to be carried out.

APPROACH TO STATION	
Empathic Response	• If there is silence, avoid the temptation to fill it, give the patient a few moments to respond & ensure the consultation pace isn't rushed. • If the patient cries offer them a tissue & allow them to express their emotions. • Be empathetic *"I can see & understand that you are distressed by the news."* • Ask if cancer had been considered by the patient, this will help establish whether the patient had mentally prepared for the news.
Patient Questions or Concerns	• Ask the patient if they have any questions or concerns. • This will help steer the consultation to address the patient' agenda. • The patient may volunteer that she was a medical receptionist & knew a few patients who died of oesophageal cancer.
Explain Plan	• It is important to give a clear plan but avoid giving too much technical information. • Advise the patient of the need for a CT scan & biopsy. • Despite the news, it is important to give hope to the patient about management options. • Mention that there are treatment options including radiotherapy, surgery & symptom-relieving palliation e.g. stents.
Ask About Support	• Ask about family & friends. • Advise of other support networks including the nurse specialist & GP.
Summarise & Check Further Patient Questions	• If the patient is too overwhelmed to think of questions, suggest she can write a list of questions & speak to one of the team or their GP later. • If the patient asks how long they have to live, never give a precise answer. • Ask why they would like to know, there may be a specific reason e.g. wanting to know whether she should call her daughter back from Australia urgently.
Arrange Follow Up	• Arrange a follow up appointment as appropriate. • Leave contact details e.g. bleep number as appropriate.
Close Consultation	• It is important to finish the consultation with a definite plan. • Ensure the patient is safe to travel home. • Thank the patient.

SCENARIO 3: *"Don't tell dad about the diagnosis"*

DOCTOR BRIEFING

You are the surgical doctor, looking after Mr Levent Ali, an 80-year-old man admitted with bowel obstruction. He currently has a naso-gastric tube in situ & is undergoing fluid rehydration. His clinical condition is stable. An abdominal CT scan has revealed a suspicious bowel mass & the appearance of metastatic lesions in the liver. The patient has not been told the news.

The son of Mr Ali would like to have a discussion with you.

ACTOR BRIEFING

You are Mr Imran Ali, the son of Mr Levent Ali. You are 44 years old.

Appearance & Behaviour: You are concerned about your father & feel you know what is in his best interests.

Background:

- Your father has been unwell recently, he has been losing weight & had vomited a number of times before admission to the hospital.
- Since admission the vomiting has stopped & he feels better.
- Currently he is not allowed any food & has had a tube placed into his stomach.
- Your father told you that there may be a blockage in the bowel & a CT scan had been arranged.
- He had the CT scan today but you haven't heard the results yet.

ICE:

- You are suspicious that he may have cancer.
- He has been low in mood for a number of years since your mother died 5 years ago.
- You are concerned that if he finds out about the cancer, he would not cope with the news & sink further into depression.
- He has been in a residential home for the past year & gets carers twice daily who help with meals & bathing.
- He is occasionally forgetful, but you are not concerned about his memory.
- You speak to him every 2–3 days & visit him every weekend.
- Ideally you would like him to go back to the residential home & you will liaise with the GP about managing his further care in the residential home.
- You want to speak to the doctor & get the results of the CT scan before she speaks to your father.
- If it is cancer, you would like the doctor to withhold this information from your father.
- Your father has never mentioned whether he would or wouldn't like to know about a potential serious diagnosis, neither has he mentioned an advanced directive.

First words to the doctor: *"Can I have a quick chat with you about dad?"*

APPROACH TO STATION

Key Principles:

- This station tests the candidate's ability to communicate & negotiate with a relative that has an agenda that differs from yours.
- It is important to discuss the issues within an appropriate ethical framework.
- The discussion must be balanced & care should be taken to avoid having to deal with an angry relative!

Introduce Yourself	• *"Hello, my name is Dr ... I am the surgical doctor."*
Check Relationship to Patient	• *"I have been asked to come & talk to you, how are you related to the patient?"*
Initiate the consultation	• Ask an open question such as *"I believe you wanted to have a chat about your father?"* • Actively listen to the son & avoid interrupting him.
Elicit ICE	• Establish what he already knows about his father's condition. • His main concern will be regarding the potential diagnosis of cancer & withholding this information from his father. • Don't be judgemental & try to establish why he has these concerns.
Explain the Difficulty of the Situation	• Be empathic & acknowledge his concerns. • Explain that the CT has been performed, but because of patient confidentiality you should speak to his father first. • Establish whether his father has ever expressed a wish for potentially serious news to be withheld from him. • Explain that if his father were to ask the result of the CT scan, it would not be ethical to lie to him.
Address Concerns & Negotiate	• Try to address the son's concerns & explain why it is important for the father to know the results of the scan. • You cannot consent for any treatment if the patient doesn't know their diagnosis. • If he deteriorates & is unsure of a diagnosis, this may cause him psychological distress. • He may have issues to sort out before he deteriorates further e.g. a will or advanced directive. • Advise that he could ask his father whether he wants to know all the details of his illness & if he chooses not to, you will respect his wishes. • You are happy if the son wants to ask this question of his father. • Reassure him that in your experience, patients like to know their diagnosis & with the right support, cope well with bad news.
Summarise & Check Patient Questions	• Summarise the plan. • Confirm the son understands the issues. • Offer to answer any questions.
Arrange Follow Up	• Arrange a follow up appointment as appropriate. • Leave contact details e.g. bleep number as appropriate.
Close Consultation	• Thank the son.

SCENARIO 4: *"Refusal of treatment"*

You are seeing Mr Trevor Rogers in urology out-patient clinic.

Mr Rogers is a 54-year-old gentleman with TCC (with carcinoma in situ). He has undergone a course of chemotherapy & radiotherapy but a recent biopsy has shown persistence. He has undergone a CT & bone scan which has shown organ-confined disease.

A recent MDT meeting has concluded that whilst BCG treatment is an option, the approach that would be in the patient's best interests, would be cystectomy with neobladder formation.

The patient is aware of the recent histology results but not the CT & bone scan. Discuss the results of the scan & management plan.

You are Mr Trevor Rogers, a 54-year-old postman.

Appearance & behaviour: Anxious about your diagnosis, but firm about which treatment plan you want.

Background:

- You were diagnosed with bladder cancer 8 months ago after developing blood in your urine.
- You have undergone a course of chemotherapy & radiotherapy but unfortunately the bladder cancer has persisted.
- You had a CT & bone scan & understand that this was to see whether the cancer has spread elsewhere.
- You don't know the results but have come today to get them.
- Your only urinary symptom at present is frequency. You have been told that this is likely due to the chemotherapy & radiotherapy, rather than infection & this may be chronic.

ICE:

- You are concerned the cancer has spread elsewhere & are pleased to hear the results of the scans.
- You are aware that a previously discussed treatment option was removal of the bladder & formation of an artificial bladder.
- You do not want a surgical procedure & are keen to explore all other options before undergoing an operation.
- You have heard of a *"BCG treatment"* & want to know more about it.
- You have a strong belief that even if there is just a small chance of success, you want to try this before losing your bladder.
- You are aware there is a risk the cancer may spread if you choose the BCG treatment, but are firm that this is your preferred choice.
- Currently the cancer doesn't trouble you too much. You work as a postman & occasionally have to find a toilet due to urinary frequency. You are able to carry out all duties.

Past Medical History:

- You are a well-controlled asthmatic, requiring occasional use of the *"blue inhaler"*.

Drug History:

- You are only taking a *"blue inhaler"*, which you don't use often.
- You have no allergies.

Social History:

- You work full time as a postman.
- You have a wife & 2 sons aged 16 & 13 years.
- You do not smoke.
- You do not drink any alcohol.

Family History:

- There is no family history of medical illness as far as you are aware.

First words to the doctor: *"I've come for the results of my test."*

Key Principles:

- This station tests the candidate's ability to effectively communicate treatment options within an appropriate ethical framework.
- The candidate should demonstrate to the examiner that capacity is being gauged during the consultation.
- Avoid being judgemental & respect the patient's right to autonomy.

Introduce Yourself	• *"Hello, my name is Dr ... I am the urology doctor."*
Check Patient Identity	• Confirm the patient's name.
Establish Baseline Knowledge	• Ask what treatments he has already undergone. • Confirm he understands why the CT & bone scans were performed.
Explain Scan Results	• Explain the good news that the scans did not show metastases.
Explain MDT Decision	• Explain the MDT's view that cystectomy with neobladder formation is in his best interest. • This decision is based on the previous ineffective chemotherapy & radiotherapy. • Briefly explain the surgical procedure to the patient, avoiding jargon & emphasising that patients cope very well with neobladders.
Elicit ICE	• Listen to the patient's concerns about surgery & preferences for BCG treatment. • Empathise that making the decision about surgery must be difficult for him.
Explain Risks	• Advise that surgery would be curative, whilst a conservative approach would not eliminate the risk of metastasis. • Ensure he fully understands this.
Respect Autonomy	• Mr Rogers is not keen on surgery & is competent to make a decision. • Advise he does not have to make a decision today & can discuss the options with his family or the nurse practitioner. • If his decision is final, ensure you fully support it & avoid being judgemental.
Explain BCG Treatment	• Establish what he knows about BCG treatment. • Explain that the treatment involves catheterisation & introduction of BCG into the bladder through a catheter. • This can stimulate the immune response to attack the tumour. • A number of courses will be required.
Summarise & Check Patient Questions	• Summarise the plan. • Offer to answer any questions.
Arrange Follow Up	• Arrange a follow up appointment as appropriate. • Leave contact details e.g. bleep number as appropriate.
Close Consultation	• Inform Mr Rogers that you will report his decision back to the MDT & they will contact him shortly. • Thank the patient.

SCENARIO 5: *"Explaining a diagnosis"*

You are seeing Mr Trevor Gregory in vascular out-patient clinic.

Mr Gregory is a 58-year-old gentleman who presented to his GP with abdominal pain. Blood tests were normal apart from a raised ALP of 140. USS revealed a fatty liver & an incidental 4.1cm AAA. The rest of the ultrasound was normal. He has been referred by his GP to the vascular clinic for further assessment of the AAA.

Physical examination is normal.

Explain the findings & the need for surveillance.

ACTOR BRIEFING

You are Mr Gregory, a 58-year-old estate agent.

Appearance & Behaviour: Anxious about the need for referral to the vascular clinic.

Background:

- You went to your GP a few months ago with some intermittent abdominal pains.
- You had some blood tests & were told that a liver test called the "ALP" had come back slightly raised at 140.
- In view of this, your GP sent you for an ultrasound to assess the liver.
- You saw the GP afterwards for the results & were informed that the liver looked a bit "fatty", which might explain the abnormal liver test. However, you were concerned to hear that one of the big blood vessels in your abdomen was enlarged.
- The GP reassured you but advised that you should be assessed by one of the hospital doctors.
- The abdominal pains have resolved & you suspect it may have been due to some stress at work.
- You do not suffer from any back pain.
- You do not have any problems with circulation in your feet.

ICE:

- You have looked up abdominal aortic aneurysms on the internet & are particularly worried that it can burst at any time!

Past Medical History:

- You have high BP. The last reading by the nurse was 160/90. You were told to come back in a few weeks for a recheck but haven't had time due to your job.
- You have high cholesterol & are on tablets.

Drug History:

- You take a drug called ramipril 2.5mg for your BP & simvastatin 20mg for your cholesterol.
- You do occasionally forget to take your tablets.

Social History:

- You work as an estate agent.
- The job has been very stressful recently.
- You live with your wife who doesn't work.
- You have a daughter who is at university.
- You smoke 15 cigarettes a day & have smoked for about 26 years.
- Your wife also smokes.
- You do occasionally think about giving up but due to stress at work, you have not attempted to stop.
- You would consider speaking to the NHS smoking services if suggested.

Family History:

- There is no family history of medical illness as far as you are aware.

First words to the doctor: *"My GP sent me here for assessment of my aneurysm!"*

APPROACH TO STATION	
Key Principles:	
• The station tests the candidate's ability to communicate a diagnosis & management plan to the patient.	
• It is important to assess risk factors & provide appropriate health education to the patient.	
Introduce Yourself	• *"Hello, my name is Dr … I am one of the vascular doctors."*
Check Patient Identity	• Confirm the patient's name.
Establish Baseline Knowledge	• Find out what he knows so far about the USS. • Establish his ideas about the condition.
Explain Investigation Results	• Explain what an AAA is without using any medical jargon. • Give the explanation in small chunks, checking understanding throughout the process. • It may be appropriate to draw a small diagram for the patient.
Elicit ICE	• Establish his concerns, in this case his fear of sudden death. • Make reference to his concerns when explaining the diagnosis & management plan. • Empathise & reassure him that at its current size, the aneurysm only requires monitoring. • Reassure him that there are no other worrying features on examination.
Explain Management Plan	• Advise that he will be closely followed up with 6-monthly USS. • Explain that surgery is considered if the aneurysm increases to over 5.5cm in size, grows >1cm a year or if he becomes symptomatic. • Reassure him that the rupture risk for an aneurysm this size is very low.

APPROACH TO STATION	
Address Risk Factors	• Assess modifiable risk factors including BP, cholesterol & smoking cessation.
	• Emphasise that addressing these will slow progression of the aneurysm.
	• Check his compliance with medications & ensure his BP is being monitored.
	• If he admits to forgetting his tablets, suggest that he builds it into his daily routine e.g. leaving tablets by his toothbrush in morning.
	• Empathise that it is difficult to quit smoking. Explain that there are services & support groups available.
	• Explain it is often easier if all smokers in the household give up together.
	• Advise that he can contact the NHS smoking cessation services.
Summarise & Check Questions	• Summarise the plan.
	• Confirm he understands the issues.
	• Offer to answer any questions.
Arrange Follow Up	• Arrange USS in 6 months.
	• Arrange outpatient appointment.
Close Consultation	• Thank the patient.

SCENARIO 6: *"Organ donation"*

DOCTOR BRIEFING

You have been looking after Mrs Jenny Thomas, a 22-year-old who was admitted with sudden loss of consciousness secondary to a subarachnoid haemorrhage. She has been on a ventilator in the intensive care unit but has recently been pronounced brain dead by 2 attending consultants. You have been asked to speak to her father, Robert Thomas, to inform him of the loss & ask about organ transplantation.

ACTOR BRIEFING

You are Mr Robert Thomas, a 53-year-old accountant.

Appearance & Behaviour: Emotionally upset about the news of your daughter, but prepared for this outcome.

Background:

- You called an ambulance for your daughter yesterday after you found her unconscious in her bedroom.
- Your wife is currently at home but will be coming to the hospital in a few hours.
- The incident was sudden & there was no warning this was going to happen.
- You have been told that she has had a bleed into the brain.
- You are aware that she is not conscious & is on a machine to help her breathing.
- You were told yesterday that the outlook was poor & she may not survive.
- When told she has died you are shocked but had been prepared for the news.
- Jenny has never mentioned her wishes for organ donation in the past.
- She has never carried a donor card.

ICE:

- When the doctor explains the possibility of organ donation, you feel it is a difficult decision to make right now.
- However you do feel Jenny would have wanted to donate organs.
- You would like to know:
    - If you can wait to discuss with your wife?
    - Which organs they may take?
    - You are concerned about face transplant & wouldn't want this to be done.
    - Would organ donation delay the funeral arrangement?

First words to the doctor: *"I believe you wanted to have a chat about my daughter?"*

APPROACH TO STATION

Key Principles:

- The station tests 2 key skills, breaking bad news & discussing organ donation.
- It is important to remain empathic throughout the discussion & avoid applying any pressure for a decision on donation.

Introduce Yourself	• *"Hello, my name is Dr..."*
Check Relationship to Patient	• Confirm this is the father.
Establish Baseline Knowledge	• Find out what the father knows already about his daughter's condition & prognosis.
Break News	• Ask if there is anyone else he would like present. • Explain that unfortunately his daughter has passed away. • Explain that she has been pronounced brain dead & explain what this means. • It is important to emphasise that whilst she is still on a respirator, she has died. • You can explain that if the respirator was to be turned off she would not be able to breathe for herself.
Empathic Response	• Ensure you give time for the father to reflect on the news. • Use silence if appropriate. • Be empathic.
Discuss Organ Donation	• This issue must be approached slowly & tactfully. • Ask the father if he has any knowledge about organ donation. • Explain that organ transplant gives the opportunity to improve the quality of life for other sick people awaiting organ donations. • Empathise that this must be a difficult decision given the current situation. • Explain organs for donation can include heart, lungs, kidneys, pancreas & cornea.
Check if Daughter was in Favour of Organ Donation	• Did they ever have a discussion about organ donation? • Did she carry a donor card? • Did she put herself on the organ donation register? • If donation had never been discussed, what does he think his daughter's views would have been?
Elicit ICE	• Explain he doesn't need to make a decision immediately & has time to talk to his wife about the decision. • Explain that organs are removed in a way to minimise any visible signs on the body. • Advise that the body will be available for the funeral shortly after the organs are removed. • Reassure him that face transplantation has to be specifically agreed upon.

APPROACH TO STATION		
Explain Next Step	•	Do not pressurise the father & ensure he knows that his decision will be respected.
	•	If he agrees, explain that you will inform the transplant co-ordinator & the family will be kept up to date throughout the process.
	•	If he decides to wait for his wife, respect this decision.
Summarise & Check Questions	•	Confirm he understands the issues.
	•	Offer to answer any questions.
Close Consultation	•	Thank the father for his patience & understanding.

SCENARIO 7: *"Apologise for a mistake"*

DOCTOR BRIEFING

You are the ST5 looking after Mr Albert Knox who has had a routine hernia repair. He is recovering but is in pain. He is a type 1 diabetic & normally self administers insulin, however as he is in some discomfort, the nurses are giving his evening dose. Your F1 doctor wrote the insulin dose, but unfortunately due to illegible handwriting on the drug chart, 40 Units of insulin were given to the patient instead of 20 Units. He subsequently had a hypoglycaemic attack which required emergency intravenous dextrose administration by the ward team. Mr Knox has recovered fully & is now alert & well.

Mr Knox would like to speak to you about the hypoglycaemic episode. He is unaware of the drug chart error.

You are Mr Albert Knox, a 48-year-old artist.

Appearance & Behaviour: Worried about the recent hypoglycaemic episode & concerned about why it occurred.

Background:

- You have been admitted for a routine hernia repair, which occurred yesterday.
- You are recovering but are in some pain from the operation.
- You are a type 1 diabetic & this evening suffered a hypoglycaemic attack.
- This is strange as your diabetic control is normally very good & you haven't had a hypoglycaemic event for many years.
- At the time you felt sweaty & drowsy.
- You remember a bit of commotion around the ward but had no real insight into what was happening.
- You now feel fine.

ICE:

- You are concerned about why you had the hypoglycaemic event & are keen to discuss this with the doctor.
- When the error on the drug chart is explained, you cannot believe what has happened.
- You are concerned about how the team has cared for you & have lost trust in them.
- You want to know what will happen to the doctor concerned.
- You want to make sure this will not happen again.
- You wish to personally administer your own insulin again.

Past Medical History:

- You are a well-controlled type 1 diabetic, diagnosed at the age of 8 years.
- You have not had a hypoglycaemic attack for many years & are followed up by your GP & the hospital endocrinology department.
- You have not had any previous hospital admissions.

Drug History:

- Apart from insulin you take no other medication.
- You do not have any allergies.

Social History:

- You are an artist.
- You live alone.
- You do not smoke.
- You drink 2–3 glasses of wine a week.

Family History:

- There is no family history of medical illness as far as you are aware.

First words to the doctor: *"I wanted to have a chat with you about my diabetes…"*

APPROACH TO STATION

Key principles:

- The station tests the candidate's ability to be honest with the patient & sincere in apology.

- Never lie & do not apportion blame to any particular individual.

Introduce Yourself	• "Hello, my name is Mr ... I am the ST5 surgeon."
Check Patient Identity	• Confirm the patient's name.
	• Check the patient's wristband.
Establish Baseline Knowledge	• Ask if he knows what happened to him.
Explain Mistake & Apologise	• Explain that he had a hypoglycaemic attack earlier which required emergency intravenous glucose administration.
	• Explain that it seems he was given too much insulin by the ward staff.
	• Advise that this was because an error had been made when interpreting the dosage on the drug chart.
	• Ensure you apologise sincerely to the patient, accept that there was an error.
Elicit ICE	• Allow the patient to express his concerns & respond to them appropriately.
	• Advise that medical errors are rare & are taken very seriously.
	• Do not divert blame onto the nurse or the F1 doctor.
	• If he expresses concerns about the team, empathise but reinforce that such mistakes are very rare.
	• Reassure him that the episode will not affect his recovery.
Explain Next Step	• Explain that there is a formal system to ensure the risks of such an error recurring are minimised.
	• Advise that the consultant will be involved.
	• Advise that if he is upset he can discuss the issue with the consultant.
	• If the patient wants to formally complain, explain there is a PALS system which can facilitate this.
Summarise & Check Questions	• Confirm that he understands the complaints procedure.
	• Offer to answer any questions.
Close Consultation	• Apologise again & thank the patient.

SCENARIO 8: *"Resuscitation decision"*

You are looking after Mrs Ruby Rose, an 88-year-old lady who has been admitted with a fractured neck of femur (complete fracture with full displacement). She is known to have dementia & has been admitted from a residential home. She is on the operating list for surgery tomorrow. She is currently confused & you have been asked to speak to the son regarding a resuscitation decision.

You are Phillip Rose, the son of Ruby Rose. You are 56 & work in information technology.

Appearance & Behaviour: Concerned about your mother & keen she gets optimal treatment regardless of her age.

Background:

- Your mother has been in a residential home for the past 3 years.
- You were called by the home today & told that she had a fall & was in hospital.
- You have been told that she has a fractured hip.
- At present she is confused & does not seem to understand what is happening.
- She was put into the home a year after your father died because she was suffering from worsening dementia & could not cope alone.
- You had some guilt about putting her in a home, but she has settled & seems content there.
- At the home she can wash & dress herself, but needs supervision.
- She can feed herself & the meals are prepared by the home.
- She walks with a Zimmer frame & has had 2–3 falls over the past 12 months.
- She has been fairly well & active & you feel she has an adequate quality of life.
- She still participates in activities around the home & has friends who she sits with.
- You are unsure on her exact past medical history but you know she has high BP & an irregular heartbeat.
- If asked, you are not sure what tablets she is on but know she is definitely not on warfarin.

ICE:

- When asked about the resuscitation decision you are not happy as you feel she still has a good quality of life.
- You are concerned the team may give her suboptimal care once this decision is made.
- Some of your concerns will be addressed if the doctor explains that the "do not resuscitate" decision does not mean she will receive inferior treatment & that it will only apply if her heart was to stop.
- If she were able to express her wish, you are sure she wouldn't want any prolongation of her life if she were gravely ill.

First words to the doctor: *"How is my mother getting on?"*

APPROACH TO STATION

Key Principles:

- The station requires effective communication of the current situation & prognosis.
- Listen carefully to the son's concerns regarding resuscitation & try to address them.
- Avoid being prescriptive & try to reach a shared decision.

Introduce Yourself	• "Hello, my name is Dr ... I am one of the orthopaedic doctors..."
Check Relationship to Patient	• Confirm he is the son.
Establish Baseline Knowledge	• Find out what he knows about the current situation & plan.
Empathic Response	• Acknowledge that this is a difficult time for the family.
Explain Plan & Prognosis	• Explain that his mother needs surgery. • Convey the risks associated with surgery.
Elicit ICE	• Ask if his mother had ever conveyed an opinion about resuscitation. • Establish what his current ideas are about resuscitation. • Advise that it is often better to have a clear resuscitation plan to avoid unnecessary distress.
Emphasise that Resuscitation is Unlikely to be Successful	• Mention the poor success rate & outcome. • Advise that resuscitation may cause more harm & distress to her. • Explain it can involve prolonged cardiac massage & even if her heart restarts, she would be unlikely to regain consciousness.
Reassure About the Meaning of "Not For Resuscitation"	• Reassure him that this does not mean his mother will receive suboptimal treatment. • Reassure him that any active medical or surgical problems will be managed regardless of the "do not resuscitate" decision.
Empathic Response	• Be empathic about the situation. • Allow time for a response. • Use silence if appropriate. • Reassure him that he can talk to other family members if he wishes. • Offer the hospital religious or spiritual support services if appropriate. • If he questions the decision, always respect his view & try & establish why he feels this way. • Advise that if his mother's confusion settles, the decision will also be discussed with her.
Summarise & Check Questions	• Summarise the plan. • Confirm he understands the issues. • Offer to answer any questions.
Arrange Follow Up	• Leave contact details e.g. bleep number as appropriate.
Close Consultation	• Thank the son.

SCENARIO 9: *"Self discharge"*

You are looking after Mr Robert Curren, a 44-year-old gentleman who was admitted yesterday with upper abdominal pain & vomiting. He was diagnosed with acute pancreatitis. This is his first presentation. He drinks half a bottle of vodka a day & this is thought to be the cause.

Blood Tests on Admission: Amylase – 2000U/l

LFT & Albumin – Normal

WCC – 14×10^9/l

U&E - Normal

CRP – 18mg/l

MCV – 104fl

Current Observations: Temperature - 37.8°C

HR- 98bpm

BP - 136/72

His is nil by mouth & is having intravenous rehydration. His pain is controlled by pethidine.

He has asked to speak to you on the ward.

ACTOR BRIEFING

You are Mr Robert Curren. You are 44 years old & unemployed. You live alone in a flat.

Appearance & Behaviour: Agitated & keen to leave hospital.

Background:

- You have been feeling generally unwell for the past week & developed severe abdominal pain & vomiting yesterday.
- You called an ambulance & were taken into hospital.
- You had some blood tests & were told you had "acute pancreatitis".
- You had never heard of this condition until it was explained by the doctor. You don't understand how severe acute pancreatitis can be.
- You were told this was likely due to alcohol consumption.
- Since admission, you have been told not to eat & are currently on a fluid drip.
- You were given an injection for the pain & sickness.
- You last received an injection for the pain about 4 hours ago.
- You feel much better now but still have some slight nausea.

ICE:

- You were under the impression that once the pain had settled you could be discharged.
- You don't like hospitals & have decided you don't want to stay in hospital any more.
- You are feeling anxious about not having any alcohol.
- You will be happy to stay in hospital once the risks of self discharge are explained & you are reassured about alcohol withdrawal.

ACTOR BRIEFING

Social History:

- You are unemployed.
- You have smoked 10 cigarettes a day for 20 years.
- You have been drinking alcohol excessively for about 6–7 years.
- You drink about half a bottle of vodka a day.
- You normally start drinking at about midday.
- If you don't drink you do get shakes.
- You know you are drinking too much & have been to the GP to discuss this.
- You realise it is harmful & do have feelings of guilt after a drinking session.
- You were given the number for an alcohol cessation service but did not attend.
- If offered, you will be willing to accept some help.
- You have been depressed since losing your job & the GP has signed you off sick.
- You do not take illicit drugs.
- You have not travelled recently.

Past Medical History:

- You have had occasional episodes of abdominal pain & vomiting in the past but nothing as severe as this.
- You have been to your GP with depression & alcohol dependence.

Drug History:

- You are not on regular medications, but take occasional paracetamol for headaches.
- You have no allergies.

First words to the doctor: *"Doctor, I have to get out of here..."*

APPROACH TO STATION

Key Principles:

This is a difficult station which tests the candidate's ability to:

- Explain a diagnosis.
- Assess competency.
- Explain the risks of self-discharge.
- Address concerns.
- Offer lifestyle advice.

Introduce Yourself	*"Hello, my name is Dr ... I am one of the surgical doctors."*
Check Patient Identity	Confirm the patient's name.
Elicit ICE	The key to this scenario is establishing his concerns about staying in hospital & addressing them efficiently.
	Find out what he understands about pancreatitis, including the cause.

APPROACH TO STATION	
Empathic Response	• Convey that you understand how difficult & frustrating it is, being in hospital. • Advise that people are only kept in hospital when absolutely necessary.
Explain Necessity to Remain in Hospital	• Explain his condition has improved because of the fluids & painkillers. • Ensure he understands that unless this continues, the pain & vomiting may recur. • Be clear about the complications & risks of pancreatitis, including death.
Address Concerns About Alcohol	• Empathise that you understand the difficulties in stopping alcohol. • Stress the importance of cessation to prevent pancreatitis & other alcohol related illnesses. • Establish whether he is motivated to stop drinking. • Reassure him that there are some medications which can be prescribed to help with the withdrawal process. • Advise that there are alcoholic support services available.
Explain Self Discharge Procedure	• Advise him that if he does self discharge, he will have to take responsibility for the decision, by signing a legal document.
Assess Competency	• Ensure he has understood all of the information & risks of self discharge. • Ask him to summarise the key points back to you.
On Self Discharge	• Ensure you still "safety net" with advice of what to do if symptoms return. • Encourage the patient to see their GP & advise that a letter will be urgently sent to the GP in advance.
Summarise & Check Questions	• Summarise important points. • Ask the patient if they have any further questions.
Close Consultation	• Thank the patient. • Document in the notes. • Discuss with your consultant.

SCENARIO 10: *"Consent to a trial"*

You are seeing Mr Gary Stevens in outpatient clinic. He is 61 years old & is being managed for intermittent claudication with lipid lowering therapy, aspirin & exercise. You feel he is suitable for entry into a double-blind randomised controlled trial looking at the effect of a new peripheral vasodilator (treatment X) against placebo. The trial is being carried out in the hospital you are working at. The new drug is to be given for 1 year, with 3-monthly follow up via symptom questionnaires & clinical assessment including ABPIs.

In addition there is a hotline which the patient can call if they have any side effects or questions.

Phase I & II trials have only revealed rare side effects such as rash, ankle swelling & headache. At present the patient is taking simvastatin, aspirin & an ACE inhibitor which he will remain on throughout.

You are Mr Gary Stevens, a 61-year-old working in a paper mill. You live with your wife in a house.

Appearance & Behaviour: Relaxed, interested in your condition & keen for further management.

Background:

• You have come for a routine review of your intermittent claudication.

• You understand that the condition is fairly stable & you have made necessary lifestyle changes including starting medication, weight loss & exercise.

• You do not feel the symptoms are worsening, but still get claudication after about 150 yards when walking uphill.

• It does not significantly affect your activities of daily living but you do find it a nuisance.

• If asked, you do not get leg pain at night.

ICE:

• You are being asked whether you would like to be entered into a clinical trial.

• You have heard of clinical trials in the press & remember a recent case in the papers where participants were severely hurt by side effects from a trial drug.

• You are concerned that you would be used as a guinea pig.

• If explained properly by the doctor, you will be happy to be enrolled, especially because you will be followed up regularly.

Past Medical History:

• You have peripheral vascular disease as described above.

• You have high BP.

Drug History:

• You currently take aspirin, simvastatin & ramipril.

• You have no allergies.

Social History:

• You gave up smoking 2 years ago.

• You do not drink any alcohol.

• You work in a paper mill.

• You live with your wife & are totally independent.

First words to the doctor: *"Hello doctor..."*

APPROACH TO STATION

Key Principles:

- This station tests the candidate's ability to discuss the principles of a clinical trial.
- The patient must be fully informed of the risks & benefits of participating.
- Ensure the consultation is a discussion & avoid pressurising the patient to participate.

Introduce Yourself	• "Hello, my name is Dr ... I am one of the vascular doctors."
Check Patient Identity	• Confirm the patient's name.
Explain Agenda	• Tell him you would like to invite him to participate in a research trial.
	• Explain the aims of the study.
Elicit ICE	• Find out what he knows about clinical trials.
	• Find out what his concerns are about clinical trials if he indicates that he is worried.
Explain Trial	• He will be given either the trial drug or a placebo for 12 months.
	• Explain the placebo is to eliminate bias from the study
	• Which tablet he is given will be selected at random.
	• Neither he nor the people running the trial will know which tablet he is taking.
	• He will be followed up regularly to assess his progress.
	• If he has any problems such as side effects, this will be acted upon immediately.
	• His identity will be kept confidential during the trial & if the results are published; however registration authorities or the hospital ethics committee may need to see his identity.
Explain Trial Benefits	• He will be monitored more closely than usual.
	• There is a possibility that his condition will improve, although there is no guarantee.
	• The trial will be helpful to develop future treatments.
Explain Possible Side Effects	• Explain there may be side effects, as shown in the phase I & II trials.
	• Reassure him that these have been rare & minor.
	• Advise that there is a telephone hotline he can call or leave a message on 24 hours a day.
Emphasise Choice	• Explain that participation is voluntary & he can think about the decision.
	• Advise he can withdraw at anytime during the trial if he wishes.
	• If he agrees, reiterate that his contribution will be valuable to people with his condition.
Summarise & Check Questions	• Summarise important points.
	• Ask the patient if they have any further questions.
Close Consultation	• Thank the patient.

SECTION C: HISTORY TAKING

CHAPTER 16
STRUCTURED HISTORY

AD Ebinesan
BH Miranda

CHAPTER CONTENTS

STRUCTURED HISTORY

It is important to have a systematic approach to history taking stations during the OSCE. This ensures that the candidate gathers all of the relevant information, in a slick & efficient manner. It is important to stay focused throughout & avoid diverting from the topic. Here follows a suggested framework & tips:

- Presenting Complaint
- History of Presenting Complaint
- Past Medical & Surgical History
- Drug History
- Family History
- Social History
- Activities of Daily Living
- Systems Review.

PRESENTING COMPLAINT

- Must be in the patient's own words.
- Get the most 'recent' symptoms 1ˢᵗ & number them.*

*If a patient has multiple presenting complaints, or a complicated history extending back many years, it may be better to begin by focusing on the most recent complaint. Continue by numbering other complaints in reverse chronological order & complete the remainder of the history-taking process for each complaint. Numbering in reverse chronological order will assist the candidate in separating which complaints are still part of the current problem, part of a separate problem, or part of the past medical history.

HISTORY OF PRESENTING COMPLAINT

- Start with events leading up to most recent symptoms.
- If the above events are complicated or unrelated, then subcategorise by number & address in reverse chronological order.
- Obtain a concise history, using a protocol such as the one presented below.
- Present your history, in the same order as your protocol.

Memory: 'Only Do Clinical Stations, Properly Relaxed & Prepared'

History of Presenting Complaint	Interpretation
Onset	• Did this start suddenly or gradually?
Duration	• When did it start?
	• How long have you had this for?
Course	• Does it come & go?
	• Does it get progressively worse?
	• Is it worse in the morning or at night?
Severity	• How bad is it?
	• How much would you rate the pain out of 10? *(see box below)*
	• Does it wake you up at night?
	• Does it stop you from doing your daily routine?
	• Does it stop you from working?
Precipitating Factors	• Is there anything that makes it worse?
Relieving Factors	• Is there anything that makes it better?
Associated Features	Ask specifically about the clinical features associated with each system being addressed in the history of the presenting complaint. These are listed in the systems review.
Previous Episodes	• Have you ever had this before?

 Memory: 'SOCRATES' for pain

If the history of the presenting complaint involves pain, then ask the following:

Site: Where is the pain?

Onset: When did the pain start & was this sudden or gradual?

Character: What is the pain like? An ache? Sharp or stabbing?

Radiation: Does the pain radiate anywhere?

Associations: Any other signs or symptoms associated with the pain?

Time Course: Does the pain follow any pattern?

Exacerbating/Relieving Factors: Does anything make the pain better / worse?

Severity: Ask patient to score between 1 (mild) – 10 (severe).

PAST MEDICAL & SURGICAL HISTORY

- Classify this as **medical** or **surgical**.
- It is useful to quickly screen the patient for the following:

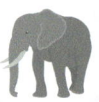

Memory: 'MI THREADS JCAT'

MI

TB

Hypertension

Rheumatic Fever

Epilepsy

Angina

Diabetes

Stroke

Jaundice

Cholesterol

Atopy (asthma / eczema / hayfever)

Thyroid

DRUG HISTORY

- Don't forget to ask about allergies.

FAMILY HISTORY

- Take a relevant family history only.

SOCIAL HISTORY

- **Accommodation:**   Do you live in a house or a flat?
- **Profession:**   Are you working? What job do you do?
- **Alcohol:**   How many units per week? (limits: ♂ = 21 units & ♀ = 14 units).
- **Smoking:**   How many pack years? (20 cigarettes/day for 1 year = 1 pack year).

ACTIVITIES OF DAILY LIVING

- Should be asked in all patients with conditions that may affect function.
- Should be asked in all elderly or frail patients.

 Memory: Remember these according to what your morning routine might be after waking up!

Routine	Activities of Daily Living
Wash	Are you able to wash / bath / shower yourself? Do you need assistance? Do you need hoisting into the bath?
Dress	Are you able to dress yourself? Do you need assistance?
Go Downstairs	Are you able to use stairs? Do you need assistance? How many people assist you?
Cook Breakfast	Are you able to cook? Do you use have deliveries e.g. meals on wheels?
Clean Up	Are you able to clean? Do you need a cleaner?
Use Toilet	Are you able to use toilet facilities independently? Do you need assistance?
Walk Outside	Are you able to walk independently? Do you use a stick or a walker? Do you need assistance? How many people assist you? Do you require use of a wheelchair?
Shopping	Are you able to go to the shops & do your shopping independently? Do you use shopping delivery services? Do you need assistance?
Care Package	Finish by asking if the patient either has a care package already, or requires one. Establish what level of care the patient may already have & assess if the patient is coping with this. If a higher care package is required, communication with a district nurse, the patient's family & relevant support groups is required.

SYSTEMS REVIEW

At the end of the history, the candidate must ensure that a systems review is conducted. This will assist in uncovering any additional problems that may have been overlooked or forgotten during the history taking process.

When addressing associated features during the history of the presenting complaint, the candidate should ensure that all clinical features are enquired about from the relevant system below.

GASTROINTESTINAL	CARDIOVASCULAR
Abdominal Pain	Angina / Chest Pain
Constipation / Diarrhoea	Ankle Swelling
Flatus	Orthopnoea
Haematemesis	Paroxysmal Nocturnal Dyspnoea
Jaundice	Shortness of Breath on Exertion
Nausea / Vomiting	**RESPIRATORY**
Oedema	Chest Pain
Pruritis	Cough & Sputum
Stool Description	Haemoptysis
MUSCULOSKELETAL	Shortness of Breath
Joint Pain / Swelling	**UROLOGICAL**
Loss of Function	Dysuria
Morning Stiffness	Frequency
Power Decrease	Haematuria
Swelling	Incontinence (stress / urge)
Muskuloskeletal Chest Pain	Polyuria / Polydipsia
Associated Urethritis	Poor Stream
NEUROLOGICAL	Terminal Dribbling
Bladder / Bowel Dysfunction	Urgency
Diploplia	Associated Arthritis
Epilepsy / Fits	**GENITAL**
Focal Neurological Defecit	Amenorrhoea
Headaches	Impotence
Hearing Loss	Menorrhagia
Memory Problems	Penile Discharge
Paraesthesia	Period Cycle Abnormalities
Power Decrease	Vaginal Discharge

ABBREVIATIONS

αFP	Alpha Fetoprotein
βhCG	Beta Human Chorionic Gonadotropin
AAA	Abdominal Aortic Aneurysm
ABG	Arterial Blood Gas
ABPI	Ankle Brachial Pressure Index
ACE	Angiotensin Converting Enzyme
ACJ	Acromioclavicular Joint
ACL	Anterior Cruciate Ligament
ACS	Acute Coronary Syndrome
ACTH	Adrenocorticotropic Hormone
ADH	Antidiuretic Hormone
AF	Atrial Fibrillation
AIDS	Auto-Immune Deficiency Syndrome
AJCC	American Joint Committee on Cancer
AMTS	Abbreviated Mental Test Score
ANA	Anti-Nuclear Antibody
ANDI	Aberrations of Normal Development & Involution
AP Resection	Abdominoperineal Resection
APB	Abductor Pollicis Brevis
APL	Abductor Pollicis Longus
ARDS	Acute Respiratory Distress Syndrome
AS	Ankylosing Spondylitis
ASIS	Anterior Superior Iliac Spine
AVF	Arterio-Venous Fistula
AVM	Arteriovenous Malformation
AXR	Abdominal X-Ray / Radiograph
BAL	Bronchoalveolar Lavage
BCC	Basal Cell Carcinoma
BCG	Bacillus Calmette-Guérin

BP	Blood pressure
Ca	Calcium
CAP	Community Acquired Pneumonia
CBD	Common Bile Duct
CCF	Congestive Cardiac Failure
CD	Crohn's Disease
CEA	Carcinoembryonic Antigen
CF	Cystic Fibrosis
CMCJ	Carpometacarpal Joint
CML	Chronic Myeloid Leukaemia
CMV	Cytomegalovirus
CNS	Central Nervous System
CO_2	Carbon Dioxide
COPD	Chronic Obstructive Pulmonary Disease
CPP	Cerebral Perfusion Pressure
CRP	C-Reactive Protein
CRPS	Complex Regional Pain Syndrome
CRT	Capillary Refill Time
CSF	Cerebrospinal Fluid
CTA	Computed Tomography Angiogram
CTPA	Computed Tomography Pulmonary Angiogram
CVA	Cerebrovascular Accident
CWP	Coal Workers' Pneumoconiosis
CXR	Chest X-Ray / Radiograph
DDH	Developmental Dysplasia of the Hip
DFSP	Dermatofibrosarcoma Protuberans
DIC	Disseminated Intravascular Coagulation
DIPJ	Distal Interphalangeal Joint
DM	Diabetes Mellitus
DNA	Deoxyribonucleic Acid
DP	Dorsalis Pedis
DPLD	Diffuse Parenchymal Lung Disease
DVT	Deep Vein Thrombosis
DXT	Radiotherapy
EBV	Epstein Barr Virus

ECG	Electrocardiogram
Echo	Echocardiogram
ECRB	Extensor Carpi Radialis Brevis
ECRL	Extensor Carpi Radialis Longus
EDC	Extensor Digitorum Communis
EDH	Extradural Haemorrhage
EHL	Extensor Hallucis Longus
ENT	Ears, Nose & Throat
EPL	Extensor Pollicis Longus
ERCP	Endoscopic Retrograde Cholangiopancreatography
ETOH	Alcohol / Ethanol
EVAR	Endovascular Aneurysm Repair
EVLT	Endovenous Laser Therapy
FAP	Familial Adenomatous Polyposis
FBC	Full Blood Count
FCR	Flexor Carpi Radialis
FCU	Flexor Carpi Ulnaris
FDP	Flexor Digitorum Profundus
FDS	Flexor Digitorum Superficialis
Fe	Iron
FNE	Flexible Nasendoscopy
FPB	Flexor Pollicis Brevis
FPL	Flexor Pollicis Longus
GA	General Anaesthetic / General Anaesthesia
GCS	Glasgow Coma Scale
GI	Gastro-Intestinal
GN	Glomerulonephritis
GnRH	Gonadotrophin Releasing Hormone
GORD	Gastro-Oesophageal Reflux Disease
HAP	Hospital Acquired Pneumonia
HAV	Hepatitis A Virus
HBV	Hepatitis B Virus
HCC	Hepatocellular Carcinoma
hCG	Human Chorionic Gonadotropin
HCV	Hepatitis C Virus

HDU	High Dependency Unit
HIV	Human Immunodeficiency Virus
HNPCC	Hereditary Non-Polyposis Colorectal Carcinoma
HR	Heart Rate
HSV	Herpes Simplex Virus
IADSA	Intra-Arterial Digital Subtraction Angiography
IBD	Inflammatory Bowel Disease
ICE	Ideas, Concerns & Expectations
ICH	Intracerebral Haematoma
ICP	Intracranial Pressure
IFN	Interferon
IJV	Internal Jugular Vein
IL	Interleukin
ILD	Interstitial Lung Disease
IPJ	Interphalangeal Joint
ITU	Intensive Therapy (Care) Unit
IVC	Inferior Vena Cava
IVD	Intervertebral Disc
IVDU	Intravenous Drug Use
IVU	Intravenous Urogram
JVP	Jugular Venous Pressure
KUB	Kidneys Ureters Bladder X-Ray / Radiograph
LDH	Lactate Dehydrogenase
LFT	Liver Function Tests
LMN	Lower Motor Neuron
LOAF	Lateral (Radial) 2 Lumbricals
LSV	Long Saphenous Vein
MC+S	Microscopy Culture & Sensitivity
MCPJ	Metacarpophalangeal Joint
MDT	Multidisciplinary Team
MEN	Multiple Endocrine Neoplasia
MMS	Mini Mental State Examination
MRA	Magnetic Resonance Angiography
MRI	Magnetic Resonance Imaging
MRV	Magnetic Resonance Venography

MTPJ	Metatarsophalangeal Joint
Na⁺	Sodium
NGT	Nasogastric Tube
OA	Osteoarthritis
OP	Opponens Pollicis
OT	Occupational Therapy
P$_a$Co$_2$	Partial Pressure of Arterial Oxygen
PCKD	Polycystic Kidney Disease
PCL	Posterior Cruciate Ligament
PCR	Polymerase Chain Reaction
PDGF	Platelet-Derived Growth Factor
PE	Pulmonary Embolism
PEFR	Peak Expiratory Flow Rate
PEG	Percutaneous Endoscopic Gastrostomy
PEJ	Percutaneous Endoscopic Jejunostomy
PET	Positron Emission Tomography
PFL	Patellofemoral Ligament
PIN	Posterior Interosseous Nerve
PIPJ	Proximal Interphalangeal Joint
PR	Per Rectum
PT	Physiotherapy
PTHrP	Parathyroid Hormone Related Protein
QoL	Quality of Life
RA	Rheumatoid Arthritis
RAD	Right Axis Deviation
RBBB	Right Bundle Branch Block
RCC	Renal Cell Carcinoma
ROM	Range of Motion
RR	Respiratory Rate
RSV	Respiratory Syncytial Virus
RTA	Road Traffic Accident
SAH	Subarachnoid Haemorrhage
SCC	Squamous Cell Carcinoma
SCFE	Slipped Capital Femoral Epiphysis
SCJ	Sternoclavicular Joint

SCM	Sternocleidomastoid
SDH	Subdural Haematoma
SFJ	Sapheno-Femoral Junction
SIADH	Syndrome of Inappropriate Antidiuretic Hormone Secretion
SLE	Systemic Lupus Erythematosus
SOB	Shortness of Breath
SPJ	Sapheno-Popliteal Junction
SSV	Short Saphenous Vein
STD	Sexually Transmitted Disease
SUFE	Slipped Upper Femoral Epiphysis
SVC	Superior Vena Cava
TA	Tibialis Anterior
TB	Tuberculosis
TCC	Transitional Cell Carcinoma
TFT	Thyroid Function Tests
THC	Tetrahydrocannibinol
TIA	Transient Ischaemic Attack
TMJ	Temporomandibular Joint
TNM	Tumour, Lymph Nodes (local/regional), Metastasis Staging System
TOE	Trans-Oesophageal Echocardiogram
TP	Tibialis Posterior
TPN	Total Parenteral Nutrition
U&E	Urea & Electrolytes
UC	Ulcerative Colitis
UMN	Upper Motor Neuron
USS	Ultrasound
UTI	Urinary Tract Infection
V/P Shunt	Ventriculoperitoneal Shunt
VEGF	Vascular Endothelial Growth Factor
VF	Ventricular Fibrillation
VL	Vastus Lateralis
VMO	Vastus Medialis Obliquus
VT	Ventricular Tachycardia
VV	Varicose Veins
X-Ray	Radiograph
ZN	Ziehl-Neelsen

INDEX